Polymer Materials in Biomedical Application

Polymer Materials in Biomedical Application

Editors

Faisal Raza
Bramasta Nugraha

MDPI • Basel • Beijing • Wuhan • Barcelona • Belgrade • Manchester • Tokyo • Cluj • Tianjin

Editors

Faisal Raza	Bramasta Nugraha
School of Pharmacy	Biopharmaceuticals RD
Shanghai Jiao Tong University	Cardiovascular
Shanghai	Renal and Metabolism
China	AstraZeneca
	Gothenburg
	Sweden

Editorial Office
MDPI
St. Alban-Anlage 66
4052 Basel, Switzerland

This is a reprint of articles from the Special Issue published online in the open access journal *Polymers* (ISSN 2073-4360) (available at: www.mdpi.com/journal/polymers/special_issues/Polymer_Materials_in_Biomedical_Application).

For citation purposes, cite each article independently as indicated on the article page online and as indicated below:

LastName, A.A.; LastName, B.B.; LastName, C.C. Article Title. *Journal Name* **Year**, *Volume Number*, Page Range.

ISBN 978-3-0365-3336-0 (Hbk)
ISBN 978-3-0365-3335-3 (PDF)

Contents

About the Editors . . . . **vii**

Ali Alqahtani, Bhavana Raut, Shagufta Khan, Jamal Moideen Muthu Mohamed, Adel Al Fatease and Taha Alqahtani et al.
The Unique Carboxymethyl Fenugreek Gum Gel Loaded Itraconazole Self-Emulsifying Nanovesicles for Topical Onychomycosis Treatment
Reprinted from: *Polymers* **2022**, *14*, 325, doi:10.3390/polym14020325 . . . . **1**

María Z. Saavedra-Leos, Manuel Román-Aguirre, Alberto Toxqui-Terán, Vicente Espinosa-Solís, Avelina Franco-Vega and César Leyva-Porras
Blends of Carbohydrate Polymers for the Co-Microencapsulation of *Bacillus clausii* and Quercetin as Active Ingredients of a Functional Food
Reprinted from: *Polymers* **2022**, *14*, 236, doi:10.3390/polym14020236 . . . . **15**

Payal Bhatnagar, Jia Xian Law and Shiow-Fern Ng
Chitosan Reinforced with Kenaf Nanocrystalline Cellulose as an Effective Carrier for the Delivery of Platelet Lysate in the Acceleration of Wound Healing
Reprinted from: *Polymers* **2021**, *13*, 4392, doi:10.3390/polym13244392 . . . . **31**

Chen-Ying Su, Lung-Kun Yeh, Yi-Fei Tsao, Wen-Pin Lin, Chiun-Ho Hou and Hsueh-Fang Huang et al.
The Effect of Different Cleaning Methods on Protein Deposition and Optical Characteristics of Orthokeratology Lenses
Reprinted from: *Polymers* **2021**, *13*, 4318, doi:10.3390/polym13244318 . . . . **53**

Zhepeng Liu, Jing Wang, Haini Chen, Guanyu Zhang, Zhuman Lv and Yijun Li et al.
Coaxial Electrospun PLLA Fibers Modified with Water-Soluble Materials for Oligodendrocyte Myelination
Reprinted from: *Polymers* **2021**, *13*, 3595, doi:10.3390/polym13203595 . . . . **63**

Felipe Orozco, Thomas Hoffmann, Mario E. Flores, Judit G. Lisoni, José Roberto Vega-Baudrit and Ignacio Moreno-Villoslada
Concentration Dependent Single Chain Properties of Poly(sodium 4-styrenesulfonate) Subjected to Aromatic Interactions with Chlorpheniramine Maleate Studied by Diafiltration and Synchrotron-SAXS
Reprinted from: *Polymers* **2021**, *13*, 3563, doi:10.3390/polym13203563 . . . . **75**

Maqusood Ahamed, Mohd Javed Akhtar, M. A. Majeed Khan and Hisham A. Alhadlaq
A Novel Green Preparation of Ag/RGO Nanocomposites with Highly Effective Anticancer Performance
Reprinted from: *Polymers* **2021**, *13*, 3350, doi:10.3390/polym13193350 . . . . **93**

Kamran Hidayat Ullah, Faisal Raza, Syed Mohsin Munawar, Muhammad Sohail, Hajra Zafar and Mazhar Iqbal Zafar et al.
Poloxamer 407 Based Gel Formulations for Transungual Delivery of Hydrophobic Drugs: Selection and Optimization of Potential Additives
Reprinted from: *Polymers* **2021**, *13*, 3376, doi:10.3390/polym13193376 . . . . **107**

Sindi P. Ndlovu, Kwanele Ngece, Sibusiso Alven and Blessing A. Aderibigbe
Gelatin-Based Hybrid Scaffolds: Promising Wound Dressings
Reprinted from: *Polymers* **2021**, *13*, 2959, doi:10.3390/polym13172959 . . . . **125**

Md Abdul Wahab, Li Luming, Md Abdul Matin, Mohammad Rezaul Karim, Mohammad Omer Aijaz and Hamad Fahad Alharbi et al.
Silver Micro-Nanoparticle-Based Nanoarchitectures: Synthesis Routes, Biomedical Applications, and Mechanisms of Action
Reprinted from: *Polymers* **2021**, *13*, 2870, doi:10.3390/polym13172870 . . . . **157**

Mohammad Mostakhdemin, Ashveen Nand and Maziar Ramezani
Articular and Artificial Cartilage, Characteristics, Properties and Testing Approaches—A Review
Reprinted from: *Polymers* **2021**, *13*, 2000, doi:10.3390/polym13122000 . . . . **179**

Heba A. Gad, Autumn Roberts, Samirah H. Hamzi, Haidy A. Gad, Ilham Touiss and Ahmed E. Altyar et al.
Jojoba Oil: An Updated Comprehensive Review on Chemistry, Pharmaceutical Uses, and Toxicity
Reprinted from: *Polymers* **2021**, *13*, 1711, doi:10.3390/polym13111711 . . . . **205**

Po-Sung Fu, Jen-Chyan Wang, Pei-Ling Lai, Shih-Ming Liu, Ya-Shun Chen and Wen-Cheng Chen et al.
Effects of Gamma Radiation on the Sterility Assurance, Antibacterial Ability, and Biocompatibility of Impregnated Hydrogel Macrosphere Protein and Drug Release
Reprinted from: *Polymers* **2021**, *13*, 938, doi:10.3390/polym13060938 . . . . **227**

About the Editors

Faisal Raza

Faisal Raza is from the School of Pharmacy at Shanghai Jiao Tong University (SJTU), China. He received his M.S. degree in Pharmaceutics from China Pharmaceutical University (CPU), Nanjing, China in 2019. His research focuses on the development of stimuli-responsive nanomedicine for the treatment of cancer. Such nanomedicine is based on novel biomimetic nanotechnologies derived from various cell sources and used for various biomedical applications with a particular focus on cancer drug delivery.

Bramasta Nugraha

A highly ambitious and passionate researcher in multidisciplinary and multicultural environments. A global citizen with experience studying and working in Indonesia, Singapore, Taiwan, Japan, USA, Switzerland, and Sweden. A quick learner and solid team player. My passion as an Associate Principal Scientist at AstraZeneca, Gothenburg, Sweden, is to lead research in complex cellular models and advanced in vitro imaging to evaluate cellular and molecular events in the early drug discovery within the research areas of cardiovascular, renal, and metabolic diseases.

polymers

MDPI

Article

The Unique Carboxymethyl Fenugreek Gum Gel Loaded Itraconazole Self-Emulsifying Nanovesicles for Topical Onychomycosis Treatment

Ali Alqahtani [1], Bhavana Raut [2], Shagufta Khan [2,*], Jamal Moideen Muthu Mohamed [3], Adel Al Fatease [4], Taha Alqahtani [1], Ali Alamri [4], Fazil Ahmad [5] and Venkatesan Krishnaraju [1]

[1] Department of Pharmacology, College of Pharmacy, King Khalid University, Guraiger, Abha 62529, Saudi Arabia; amsfr@kku.edu.sa (A.A.); ttaha@kku.edu.sa (T.A.); krishcology@gmail.com (V.K.)
[2] Institute of Pharmaceutical Education and Research, Borgaon (Meghe) Wardha, Wardha 442001, India; bhavanaraut23@gmail.com
[3] College of Pharmacy, Shri Indra Ganesan Institute of Medical Science, Tiruchirapalli 620012, India; jmuthumohamed@gmail.com
[4] Department of Pharmaceutics, College of Pharmacy, King Khalid University, Guraiger, Abha 62529, Saudi Arabia; afatease@kku.edu.sa (A.A.F.); aamri@kku.edu.sa (A.A.)
[5] Department of Anesthesia Technology, College of Applied Medical Sciences in Jubail, Imam Abdulrahman Bin Faisal University, Dammam 34212, Saudi Arabia; fmahmad@iau.edu.sa
* Correspondence: shaguftakhan17@rediffmail.com; Tel.: +91-75591-78862

Abstract: The novel itraconazole (ITZ) nail penetration enhancing self-emulsifying nanovesicles (ITZ-nPEVs) loaded in carboxymethyl fenugreek gum (CMFG) gel circumvent the systemic onychomycosis treatment. The ITZ-nPEVs were prepared by the thin film hydration technique, and the particle size (PS), zeta potential (ZP), drug content (DC), entrapment efficiency (% EE), deformity index (DI), viscosity, morphology, and physical stability of the ITZ-nPEVs were measured. In terms of nail hydration, transungual drug absorption, and antifungal efficacy against *Candida albicans*, the chosen ITZ-nPEVs, nPEV-loaded CMFG (CMFG-ITZ-nPEVs) gel, and the commercialized Itrostred gel were compared. The ITZ-nPEVs showed spherical structure with high DC, % EE, low PS and PDI and positive ZP of ITZ ranging from 95.36 to 93.89 mg/5 mL and 95.36–96.94%, 196.55–252.5 nm, 0.092–0.49, and +11.1 to +22.5 mV, respectively. Compared to the Itrostred gel, the novel ITZ-nPEVs exhibited hydration enhancement factor for 24 h (HE24) of 1.53 and 1.39 drug uptake enhancement factor into nail clippings. Moreover, zone of inhibitions for ITZ-nPEVs (27.0 ± 0.25 mm) and CMFG-ITZ-nPEVs (33.2 ± 0.09 mm) against *Candida albicans* were significantly greater than that of Itrostred gel (22.9 ± 0.44 mm). For clinical investigation on onychomycotic patients, a nail penetration enhancer containing ITZ-nPEV-loaded CMFG gel presents a highly promising approach.

Keywords: itraconazole; onychomycosis; self-emulsifying nanovesicles; transungual; anti-fungal

Citation: Alqahtani, A.; Raut, B.; Khan, S.; Mohamed, J.M.M.; Fatease, A.A.; Alqahtani, T.; Alamri, A.; Ahmad, F.; Krishnaraju, V. The Unique Carboxymethyl Fenugreek Gum Gel Loaded Itraconazole Self-Emulsifying Nanovesicles for Topical Onychomycosis Treatment. *Polymers* **2022**, *14*, 325. https://doi.org/10.3390/polym14020325

Academic Editors: Faisal Raza and Bramasta Nugraha

Received: 17 December 2021
Accepted: 11 January 2022
Published: 14 January 2022

1. Introduction

Onychomycosis is a fungal infection that affects both the fingernail and toenail. The documented negative effects of antifungal medication, as well as the restricted blood circulation to the afflicted nails, have impeded systemic therapy of onychomycosis. Approximately 19% of the global population is affected by the fungal infection of the human nail, which is known as onychomycosis or tinea unguium [1]. *Trichophyton rubrum*, followed by *Trichophyton mentagrophtes* var; interdigitale, are the anthropophilic dermatophytes that cause this illness. Non-dermatophytes molds, such as *Scopulariopsis brevicaulis* and *Aspergillus* spp., can be main and secondary pathogens in onychomycosis. Yeast, like *Candida albicans* and *Candida parapsilosis*, is the third cause of nail fungal infection [2].

Onychomycosis causes thickening and discoloration of nail. The nail becomes brittle and begins to break or completely come out of the toe or finger as the infection develops [3].

The toenail is determined to be the most impacted by the fungal infection of all the nails, whereas fingernails are the least affected [4]. Because of the low vascularity of the nail bed and barrier characteristic of the nail plate, penetration of drugs through the nail is very poor, the human nail is composed of 25 keratinized layers, which is 100-fold thicker than the stratum corneum. Current treatment strategies include both oral and topical delivery, but both suffer from poor diffusion of drugs through the nail [5]. Therefore, it is highly desirable to design formulations that can improve nail penetration of the antifungal drugs. To improve the therapeutic efficiency by the topical route, three key means include mechanical, physical and chemical. The mechanical therapy involves complete nail avulsion or filing the affected nail, the physical means include iontophoresis, phonophoresis, photodynamic therapy or laser therapy and chemical method uses chemical nail penetration enhancer [6]. Nanoparticles offer deep penetration of drug into the nail with prolonged retention in the nail and can avoid the painful surgical removal of the nail. Wang et al. (2018) demonstrated improved permeation of ketoconazole through the nail plate and longer its retention at the site when it was encapsulated in crosslinked fluorescent supramolecular nanoparticles [7]. Nail-penetrating nanovesicles have shown promise in improving diffusion of drugs through. Elsherif et al. (2018) formulated terbinafine hydrochloride-loaded spanlastic nanovesicular carrier for enhanced transungual drug delivery. The nanovesicles however have poor retention at the site. To improve both penetration and retention, nail penetration nanovesicles were dispersed in gel in the present investigation [8]. Itraconazole (ITZ) was used as a model drug and an attempt has been made to improve its solubility in the aqueous medium and improve its penetration.

The aim of research work is to develop an effective topical delivery system suitable for treatment of onychomycosis, to eliminate the need for systemic intervention. The nail penetration-enhancing vesicles open a new approach for topical treatment of nail-related fungal infection such as onychomycosis. In the present work for the formulation of nanovesicles, incorporation of the penetration enhancer labrasol, with the nail penetration enhancer N-acetyl-L-cysteine and the positive charge inducer stearylamine within aqueous deformable-natured nanovesicles (nPEVs) proved to be a promising combination for enhancing the transungual delivery of ITZ.

2. Results and Discussion

2.1. High-Performance Liquid Chromatography (HPLC)

Figure S1 shows the quantification and standard calibration curve for ITZ using the HPLC technique. With a correlation value of 0.9991, a linear response was seen in range of 5 to 50 μg/mL (Figure S1b and Table S1). The derivatized ITZ had a retention time of 7.8 min, a limit of identification of 110 μg/mL, and a limit of detection of 32 μg/mL (Figure S1a), respectively.

2.2. Preparation of ITZ-nPEVs

According to the earlier work [9], the ITZ-nPEVs were effectively produced by employing the thin film hydration approach. Briefly, amount of nail penetration enhancers was restricted to a maximum of 5% as greater concentrations were observed to soften the nail to clinically unacceptable levels (Table 1). Labrasol and N-acetyl-L-cysteine were used as enhancers in the synthesis of nPEVs. The nail penetration enhancer (N-acetyl-L-cysteine) was found to increase flux across the nail plate by diminishing disulfide linkages in the keratin of the nail, which was linked to pore formation and subsequent swelling and softening of the nail plate, resulting in a reduction in nail barrier integrity [10]. Because the nails are negatively charged at pH 7.4, the positive charge inducer stearylamine was added to help with transungual penetration [11]. Labrasol increases fluidity of the vesicles allowing greater deformability leading to greater penetration of vesicles through the pores [12] (Drug Delivery, 2017, 24(1), 98–108).

Table 1. Composition and characterization of ITZ-nPEVs Batches.

Batches	Component (% *w/v*)			Drug Content (mg/5 mL of nPEVs) *	% EE *	Particle Size (nm) *	PDI *	Zeta Potential (mV) *
	ITZ	Lipid	Cholesterol					
S1	1	4	-	95.36 ± 0.31	95.36 ± 0.51	196.55 ± 0.025	0.092 ± 0.03	+11.1 ± 0.52
S2	1	4	2	96.59 ± 0.44	96.59 ± 0.44	221.2 ± 0.056	0.19 ± 0.045	+17.2 ± 0.35
S3	**1**	**7**	**3**	98.43 ± 0.32	97.22 ± 0.46	240.33 ± 0.016	0.38 ± 0.01	+19.1 ± 0.87
S4	2	7	3	193.89 ± 0.8	96.94 ± 0.70	252.2 ±0.019	0.49 ± 0.011	+22.5 ± 0.28

* Each value represents mean, $n = 3 \pm$ SD.

2.3. Drug Content and % EE

The drug content and % EE of ITZ-nPEVs ranged from 95.36 ± 0.517 to 193.89 ± 0.83 mg/5 mL of nPEVs and 95.36 ± 0.517 and 96.94 ± 0.70%, respectively (Table 1). These high % EE values can be ascribed to ITZ's lipophilicity (log P = 5.66), which allows it to be effectively incorporated into lipid bilayers in the various formulations [13].

The drug content of ITZ-nPEVs of selected batch S3 was found to be 98.43 ± 0.32 mg in 5 mL of nPEVs and the % EE of selected batch S3 was found to be 97.22 ± 0.46%. It was observed that the selected batch S4 showed the maximum drug content and % EE due to increase in lipid and cholesterol ratio (2:7:3).

2.4. PS, PDI and ZP

The average particle size of ITZ-nPEVs varied from 196.55 ± 0.025 to 252.2 ± 0.019 nm, as reported in Table 1 and Figure S2a. The PDI values of ITZ-nPEVs did not exceed 0.4, indicating that the solution was homogeneous and monodisperse [14]. It was observed that the concentration of lipid increases, the particle size of formulated ITZ-nPEVs also increased. The particle size of S3 was found to be 240.33 ± 0.016 nm. Because of the presence of the positive charge inducer stearylamine, the zeta potential values varied from +11.1 to +22.5 mV (Figure S2b). The zeta potential of chosen batch S3 was found to be, 19.1 mV. According to Mohammed et al. (2021), the large magnitude of charge indicates good stability against vesicle aggregation and fusion [15].

The tiny particle size produced for all of the developed ITZ-nPEVs formulations (196.55 to 252.2 nm) is evident from Table 1. ITZ-nPEVs vesicles of this size have a significant interfacial surface area, which aids drug absorption and lymphatic transit [16]. For nanoformulations, relatively high polydispersity indices (>0.5) are considered typical. This is because the surfactant monolayer's interfacial tension is very low for nanostructures, so there is less of a penalty (more chance) for having a non-spherical shape, compared to normal emulsions, which typically have spherical structures due to high interfacial tensions favoring globule interfacial areas reduction (The sphere has the lowest interfacial area for a given volume).

2.5. Elasticity

The deformability index of S1- S4 ITZ-nPEVs were ranging from 1.35 to 0.200 $mL \cdot s^{-1}$ as shown in Table 2. The deformability index of selected batch S3 was found to be 0.449 $mL \cdot s^{-1}$. The S3 vesicles had a lower deformability index than S1 and S2 vesicles, which might be due to the lipid's lesser ability to interact with the penetration enhancer when compared to cholesterol. The deformability of nanovesicles was owing to the presence of labrasol within the membrane vesicles, which confers fluidity, flexibility, and the ability to create vesicles so that they can deform, according to Yusuf et al. (2014) [17]. However, the phenomenon is relevant up to a particular surfactant concentration limit, after which mixed vesicles develop, which are hard vesicles with little or no deformability.

Table 2. Deformability index and viscosity of ITZ-nPEVs and CMFG-ITZ-nPEVs formulations.

	ITZ-nPEVs			CMFG-ITZ-nPEVs			
Sr. No.	Batches	Deformability Index (mL·s^{-1})	Viscosity (cP) *	Batches	CMFG (*w*/*v*)	Chitosan (*w*/*v*)	Viscosity (cP) *
1	S1	1.35	0.98 ± 0.02	G1	1%	1%	155.7 ± 0.567
2	S2	0.556	1.32 ± 0.015	G2	0.5%	1%	116.1 ± 0.85
3	S3	0.449	1.41 ± 0.032	G3	1%	0.5%	132 ± 0.737
4	S4	0.200	1.72 ± 0.025				

* Each value represents mean, $n = 3 \pm$ SD.

2.6. Viscosity

As shown in Table 2, the viscosity of ITZ-nPEVs and CMFG-ITZ-nPEVs ranged from 0.98 ± 0.02 to 2.41 ± 0.131 cP. Because of the presence of vesicular lamellar structures with a large hydrodynamic volume, the ITZ-nPEVs dispersions had greater viscosity values than water [4]. S4 ITZ-nPEVs had a much greater viscosity (1.72 cP) than CMFG-ITZ-nPEVs (2.41 ± 0.131 cP), which was significantly less.

At increasing shear rates, however, the viscosity steadily rises, indicating shear thickening behavior. Because the creation of the interparticle structure was hampered by electrostatic repulsion at low shear rates, the viscosity was Newtonian. Almahfood and Bai (2021) explained that the shear rate was greater than 120 s^{-1}; however, the attraction of nanogel dispersions increased, causing the viscosity to steadily rise. Furthermore, when the shear rate increases, nanogel dispersions show an abrupt increase in viscosity values, which might be attributed to enhanced particle contact produced by the high rotating speed. Despite this, a larger concentration of nanogel dispersion did not follow the same pattern [18]. This might be explained by the microstructure of nanogel dispersions changing at greater shear rates.

2.7. ITZ- nPEVs Shape

The scanning electron microscopic (SEM) study was carried out on a selected batch (S3) of ITZ- nPEVs with drug, lipid, and surfactant ratio of 1:7:3 as shown in Figure 1. The border and core of well-identified vesicular structures with spherical shape may be seen in SEM of the nPEVs (Figure 1a). The structural appearance revealed a lighter core encompassed by a denser border that perfectly enclosed the center. When a thin lipid layer is hydrated, it develops enclosed vesicular network that supports in shape from spherical to circular in order to achieve thermodynamic stability by lowering the systems total free energy [19]. Even after applying various mechanical loads such as sonication and extrusion, no disturbances in vesicular structure proved vesicle integrity (Figure 1b).

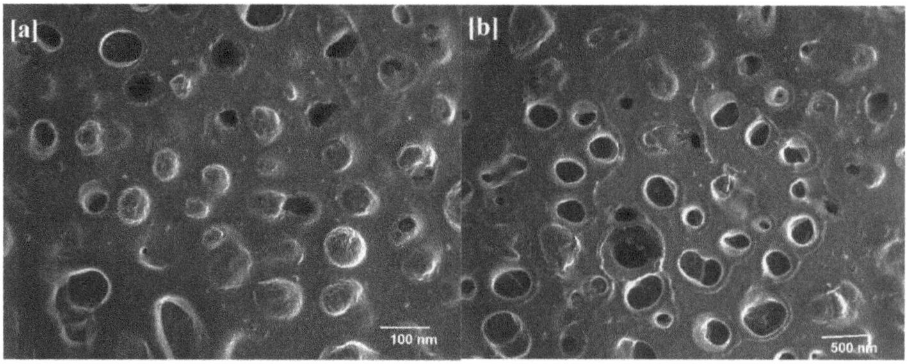

Figure 1. (**a**) SEM photograph of selected S3 and (**b**) size-measured vesicles.

2.8. In Vitro ITZ Release

The ITZ release of each batch and CMFG-ITZ-nPEVs was carried out by using dialysis membrane into the USP dissolution apparatus (Type II) for 12 h in phosphate buffer (pH 7.4). The cumulative ITZ release of all batches was in the range of 56.95 ± 0.21–98.75 ± 0.28 as shown in Figure 2a. The drug release of a selected batch S3 and CMFG-ITZ-nPEVs was found to be 98.75 ± 0.28% and 76.56 ± 2.77% for 12 h, as shown Figure 2b. The CMFG-ITZ-nPEVs have the ability to release the drug in controlled way, which is evident in the present investigation. Thus, constant/unhindered drug release over prolonged time could be achieved due to improvement in solubility of ITZ [17]. The slow ITZ release in case of free drug was because of its inherent poor aqueous solubility. ITZ belongs to the BCS II class [20].

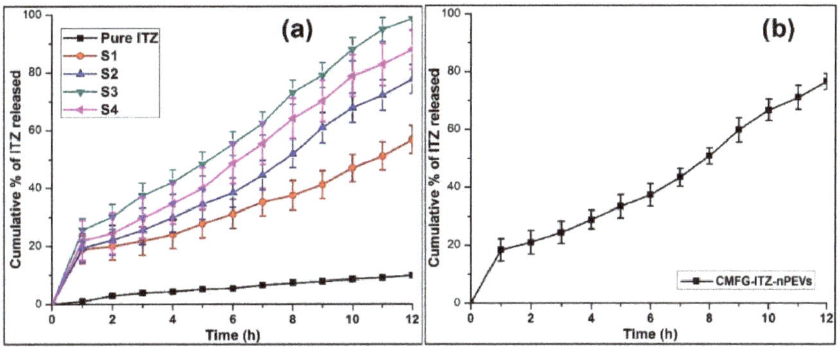

Figure 2. In vitro release of ITZ from (**a**) pure drug, S1-S4 ITZ-nPEVs, and (**b**) CMFG-ITZ-nPEVs (Mean ± SD).

Table 3 shows that the in vitro drug release was best described by Higuchi equation with the highest linearity (R^2 = 0.9789) for optimized batch S3. Slope of Korsemayer–Peppas equation greater than 0.5 and less than 0.85 which indicates non-Fickian diffusion, i.e., drug release occurred by both diffusion and erosion [21].

Table 3. In vitro release kinetics of ITZ with various nPEVs and CMFG-ITZ-PEVs (mean ± SD, *n* = 3).

	Correlation Coefficient (R^2)					
Formulation	**Zero-Order**	**First Order**	**Higuchi**	**Hixon Crowell**	**Korsmeyer-Peppas**	**Release Exponent (*n*)**
Pure ITZ	0.9612 ± 0.48	0.7433 ± 0.67	0.9715 ± 0.34	0.8920 ± 0.19	0.8912 ± 0.17	0.417 ± 0.35
S1	0.9766 ± 0.12	0.7466 ± 0.28	0.9726 ± 0.21	0.8707 ± 0.14	0.8865 ± 0.15	0.478 ± 0.38
S2	0.9874 ± 0.22	0.7762 ± 0.19	0.9614 ± 0.23	0.9101 ± 0.23	0.9244 ± 0.15	0.588 ± 0.18
S3	0.9895 ± 0.16	0.7492 ± 0.15	0.9788 ± 0.31	0.9189 ± 0.16	0.9779 ± 0.33	0.613 ± 0.43
S4	0.9924 ± 0.31	0.7756 ± 0.19	0.9732 ± 0.24	0.9134 ± 0.23	0.9584 ± 0.32	0.598 ± 0.31
CMFG-ITZ-PEVs	0.9912 ± 0.34	0.7652 ± 0.23	0.982 ± 0.16	0.9212 ± 0.31	0.9712 ± 0.25	0.591 ± 0.43

2.9. Nail Hydration/Transungual Drug Uptake of ITZ-nPEVs

The nail hydration average weight gain group 2 (S1–S4 batches) was found to be 62.0, 68.2, 75.6, and 72.7 mg, respectively. For, the groups I (control) and group 4 (Itrostred gel) were 49.2 and 52.65 mg, respectively. For chosen batch S3 and the marketed gel, the hydration enhancement factor HE24 values were 1.53 and 1.07, respectively (Table 4). The hydrophilic nature of formula S3 is likely to be responsible for the much larger weight gain seen when compared to Itrostred gel. In this instance, this was advantageous because water was considered to be the greatest nail plasticizer, resulting in greater drug flux across the nails [22].

Table 4. Nail hydration study of various formulation.

Sr. No.	Groups	Formulations	Weight of Nails before Hydration (mg)	Weight of Nails after Hydration (mg)	HE24 (h)
1	Control (group I)	Deionized water	50	49.2	-
2	Formulation (group II)	S1	50	62.0	1.26
		S2	50	68.2	1.38
		S3	50	75.6	1.53
		S4	50	72.7	1.47
3	CMFG-ITZ-nPEVs (group III)	-	50	81.11	1.92
3	Marketed gel (group IV)	Itrostred gel	50	52.65	1.07

The transungual uptake of ITZ was due to the effective partitioning of the drug into the nail clipping. The amount of ITZ taken up by the nail clippings exposed to S3 batch and Itrostred gel were 94.2% and 67.36%, respectively, the corresponding nail uptake enhancement factor EFnail for S3 batch was found to be 1.39 as compared to the marked gel [23].

Figure 3 illustrates ITZ's great affinity for nail clippings, as nPEVs allowed it to enter the nail in substantial numbers, allowing it to cure the deeply rooted onychomycosis infection.

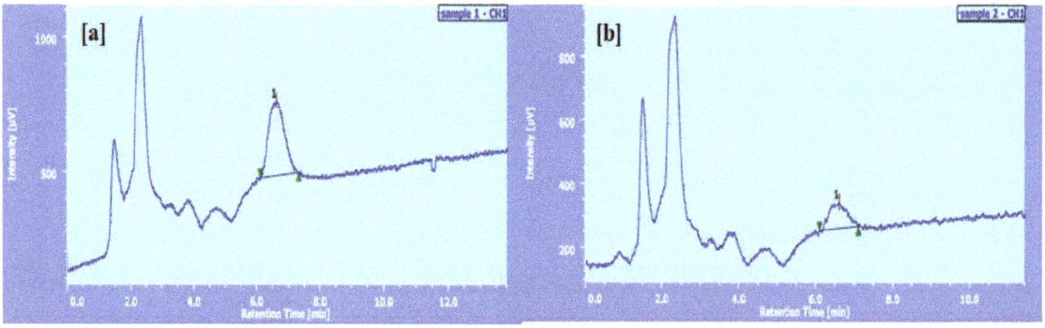

Figure 3. Chromatogram of (**a**) S3 batch and (**b**) Itrostred gel.

2.10. The Efficacy of ITZ-nPEVs for the Treatment of Onychomycosis

Several researchers suggested that *Candida albicans* (MTCC No. 227) be used to evaluate in vitro antifungal activity as it is the most common dermatophyte that causes onychomycosis [3,24]. ITZ is a fungistatic antifungal medication with a broad spectrum of activity (Table 5).

Table 5. Antifungal activity of various formulation.

Sr. No.	Formulations	Zone of Inhibition * (mm)
1	Control	5.1 ± 0.12
2	Optimized batch (S3) of nPEVs	27.0 ± 0.25
3	CMFG-ITZ-nPEVs gel	33.2 ± 0.11
4	Itrostred Gel	22.9 ± 0.44

* Each value represents mean, $n = 3 \pm$ SD.

The antifungal activity of the formulations, which included vesicular dispersion (S3), plain unmediated formula (control), ITZ-nPEVs loaded gel, and commercial product (Itrostred gel), was tested using the agar diffusion technique [25]. The "zones of inhibition" are the transparent rings that emerge around the dishes. The more efficient the formulation, the bigger the zone of inhibition. Surprisingly, against *Candida albicans*, the simple unmedicated formula (control) revealed a mean zone of inhibition (5.1 0 ± 0.12 mm). This might be explained by the fact that cysteine and its derivatives (N-acetyl-L-cysteine) have been found to have antifungal properties.

The mean zone of inhibition for Formula S3 was 27.0 ± 0.25 mm, while the mean zone of inhibition for CMFG-ITZ-nPEVs gel was 33.2 ± 0.09 mm, which was substantially bigger than the mean zone of inhibition for the commercial preparation Itrsostred gel (22.9 ± 0.44 mm). This might be due to the larger release and diffusion potential of formulation CMFG-ITZ-nPEVs gel, as well as the antifungal potential of N-acetyl-L-cysteine and CMFG gel compared to the commercial preparation, resulting in more partitioning of ITZ from the preparation [26]. The increase in the zone of inhibition with CMFG-ITZ-nPEVs gel compared to ITZ-nPEVs could be because of the inherent potent antifungal activity of fenugreek [27]. Note that vesicles have been successfully used in the topical treatment of onychomycosis employing transfersomal, liposomal, and ethosomal terbinafine [4,28]. The findings show that nail penetration enhancers with nanovesicles (nPEVs) are a potential ungual delivery mechanism that can be used in clinical trials on onychomycotic patients.

2.11. Stability Study

The CMFG-ITZ-nPEVs gel was kept for stability study and further characterization studies. From the results shown in Table 6, it was observed that CMFG-ITZ-nPEVs gel was stable for period of 6 months at 45 ± 0.5 °C and 60% ± 5% RH. Upon storage, only a slight increase in particle size and PDI was observed (349.33 ± 0.92 nm and 0.41, respectively). The drug content, % EE, zeta potential and in vitro drug release of ITZ after storage was the same as before storage 98.21 ± 0.12 mg/100 mg of drug in 5 mL of nPEVs, 98.21 ± 0.12%, 19.6 mV and 98.79 ± 0.44%, respectively. This indicates that CMFG-ITZ-nPEVs have high physical stability when stored at 4 °C [29].

Table 6. Stability study of CMFG-ITZ-nPEVs gel.

Parameters	0 Month	1 Month	3 Month	6 Month
Drug Content * (mg/ 5 mL of nPEVs)	98.43 ± 0.32	98.39 ± 0.25	98.35 ± 0.39	97.21 ± 0.12
% Entrapment Efficiency *	98.43 ± 0.32	98.39 ± 0.25	98.35 ± 0.39	98.21 ± 0.12
Particle size * (nm)	240.33 ± 0.016	241 ± 0.47	299.25 ± 0.29	349.33 ± 0.92
Zeta potential * (mV)	19.1	19.3	19.5	19.6

(* Each value represents mean, (n = 3) ± SD).

3. Materials and Methods

3.1. Reagents

Itraconazole (ITZ) was supplied as a gift from Glenmark Pharmaceutical Ltd., Nashik, India. Lecithin USP-NF (LECIVA-S75) was supplied as gift from VAV Life Sciences Pvt. Ltd., Mumbai, India. Labrasol was kindly provided by Gattefosse Pvt. Ltd., Mumbai, India. Stearylamine and Sabouraud dextrose agar (SDA) supplied from HiMedia Laboratories Pvt. Ltd., Mumbai, India and N-acetyl-L-cysteine, Cholesterol, Mono chloroacetic acid, HPLC grade methanol and water were supplied from LOBA chemical, Pvt Ltd., Mumbai, India. Itrostred gel containing 1% ITZ was purchased from Nisha Medicals, Tiruchirappalli, Tamil Nadu, India manufactured by Leeford Healthcare Ltd. Thana, Solan, India.

3.2. HPLC Analysis

Determination of ITZ was accomplished using a validated HPLC method (Model No. LC-10AD, Shimadzu, Kyoto, Japan). The mobile phase was a mixture of methanol: water containing (75:25 v/v). The flow rate of mobile phase was 1 mL/min and the injection volume was 10 μL [30]. Samples were injected into a C18 column (Hypersil, 250 × 4.6 i.d., particle size 5 μm) and the column effluent was monitored at 262 nm.

3.3. Preparation of ITZ-nPEVs

The self-emulsifying nanovesicles ITZ-nPEVs were made using a thin-film hydration approach followed by sonication, and the composition of the variously synthesized ITZ-nPEVs is presented in Table 1. Penetration enhancers such as Labrasol (200 mg), N-acetyl-L-cysteine (250 mg), and Stearylamine (20 mg) were carefully weighed and dissolved in a chloroform: methanol combination (2:1; v/v) in all of the manufactured ITZ-nPEVs. Under decreased pressure at 40 °C and 150 rpm, the organic solvent mixture was evaporated (Rotary evaporator, Model No. SB-1000, Tokyo Rikakikai Co., Ltd., Bunkyo-Ku, Japan) to form a thin layer of dry lipid containing the medicine on the inner wall of the flask [31]. Through portion-wise addition, the dry lipid film was hydrated with 5 mL of phosphate buffer (pH 7.4). The dispersion was mechanically rotated for 30 min at 40 °C, then sonicated for 15 min at a frequency of 33 KHz to minimize the size of the vesicles and stored at 4 °C (Model No. 1.5 L 50, PCI analytics, Mumbai, India).

3.4. Elimination of Unentrapped ITZ from ITZ-nPEVs

The unentrapped ITZ was removed from the nPEVs using Bseiso et al. (2015) exhaustive dialysis method. Briefly, the ITZ-nPEVs were integrated into dialysis tubing (MW. Cut off 12,000–14,000) and dialyzed against 1 L of double distilled water (pH 7.04) at room temperature for 24 h. Preliminary dialysis experiments guided the selection of these parameters [32].

3.5. Preparation of ITZ Self- Emulsifying Nanovesicles Gel (CMFG-ITZ- nPEVs)

3.5.1. Extraction and Purification of Fenugreek Gum (FG)

Fenugreek seeds were cleaned, washed, and air-dried and then soaked in water overnight and the seeds were boiled in hot water for 3 h at 80 °C to extract the gum and inactivate the enzymes, respectively. The solution was then allowed to cool to room temperature before being pressed through a cotton towel. With the addition of an equivalent volume of acetone, the crude gum was precipitated from the ensuing viscous solution. Gum was purified by washing it in ethanol and then in acetone [33]. The purified gum was dried overnight at 50–60 °C in an oven. The dried gum was pulverized and sieved through mesh #100 and stored at room temperature for further use.

3.5.2. Synthesis of Carboxymethyl Fenugreek Gum (CMFG)

The 1:1 ratio of FG and sodium bicarbonate mixed well in a mortar followed by the addition of ethanol (<0.01%) for the surface treatment of gel. The gel transferred to a flask fitted with a thermometer and mechanically stirred for 30 min. The solid mono-chloroacetic acid (1%) was added to the above gel in the presence of temperature 75 °C with continuous stirring for another 3 h. The reaction mixture was immediately cooled and neutralized to pH 7 using dilute acetic acid [34]. The gel was washed twice with methanol: water (80:20) followed by methanol washing and dried at 50–60 °C in oven an overnight.

3.5.3. Preparation of CMFG-ITZ-nPEVs Gel

In the dark, Chen and colleagues described the synthesis of nanogel using a simple diffusion and dialysis approach [35]. In a nutshell, 50–100 mg chitosan was dissolved in 5 mL acetic acid at pH 3.0, and 50–100 mg CMFG (kept overnight for hydration in purified water) was dissolved in 5 mL dimethylformamide (DMF) by vortex and sonication (Table 2). Dropwise addition of CMFG solution into the chitosan solution was done for 12 h at 30 rpm at room temperature, then dialyzed for 24 h with deionized water. The dialysis medium was refreshed at least five times after the free CMFG and DMF were completely removed from the solution. Finally, the solution was filtered through a 0.22 m syringe filter before being lyophilized (Christ, Alpha1-2 LD plus, Osterode am Harz, Germany) to obtain the CMFG-ITZ-nPEVs gel, which was kept at 4 °C for 24 h.

3.6. Characterization

3.6.1. Drug Content (DC)

After disrupting the dialyzed nPEVs with methanol, the quantity of ITZ entrapped in them was determined. To create a transparent solution, an aliquot of nPEVs was combined with an appropriate proportion of methanol and then covered with a parafilm to prevent methanol evaporation [17]. After adequate dilution, the concentration of ITZ was detected spectrophotometrically (Model No. UV 2401(PC), S.220 V, Shimadzu Corporation, Kyoto, Japan) at 262.4 nm. At this wavelength, there was no interference from blank nPEVs.

3.6.2. % EE

The entrapment efficiency was calculated according to the following equations-

$$\text{\% Entrapment efficiency} = (\text{Actual drug content in ITZ-nPEVs}) / (\text{Therotical drug content in ITZ-nPEVs}) \times 100 \quad (1)$$

3.6.3. Deformability Index

Extrusion was used to determine the deformability index of ITZ-nPEVs utilising a locally produced and approved Sartorius stainless steel pressure filter holder. The vesicles were computed using the following equation after being extruded through a membrane filter with a pore size of 50 nm at a constant pressure of 0.17 MPa [36].

$$D = j/t\,[rv/rp]^2 \quad (2)$$

where

D is the deformability index ($mL \cdot s^{-1}$),
j is the amount of vesicular dispersion extruded in mL,
t is the time of extrusion in second,
rv is the size of vesicles after extrusion (nm), and
rp is the pore size of the filter (nm).

3.6.4. Viscosity of nPEVs

The prepared ITZ-nPEVs and CMFG-ITZ-nPEVs gel kept overnight for hydration in milliQ water and viscosity of that preparations were determined using Brookfield viscometer (Model No. CAP2000+L, Brookfield Engineering Lab., Middleborough, MA, USA) at 100 rpm using spindle No. 1 at 37 ± 0.5 °C [4].

3.6.5. DLS

The practical size (PS; nm), polydispersity index (PDI) and zeta potential (ZP) of ITZ-nPEVs and CMFG-ITZ-nPEVs gel formulations was assessed by laser Doppler anemometry in triplicate by dynamic light scattering using zeta sizer (Model No. ZS90, Malvern Instruments Ltd., Worcestershire, UK). Light scattering was monitored at 25 °C and 90° angle after appropriate dilution [37,38].

3.6.6. Morphology

SEM analysis (Model No. S3700N, Hitachi, Japan) was carried out on the selected ITZ-nPEVs formula in order to characterize the shape and ultrastructure of the vesicles according to the previous method described by Moideen et al. (2020) [38].

3.6.7. In Vitro Drug Release and Kinetics

The in vitro drug diffusion study of ITZ-nPEVs formulation was evaluated using USP dissolution apparatus (Type II). A dialysis membrane (average diameter; 15.9 mm, average flat width; 25.27 mm, Himedia®, Mumbai, India) was hydrated with the phosphate buffer pH 7.4 for 12 h. Volume of ITZ-nPEVs formulation equivalent to 100 mg ITZ was dispersed in 5 mL of phosphate buffer and then placed in the bag of activated membrane which was sealed from both the ends. The dialysis bag then ties to the middle of the shaft of the USP apparatus (DA-3, Veego Scientific Mevices, Mumbai, India) and paddle was put into the jar containing 300 mL dissolution medium. The temperature of the study was controlled at 37 ± 0.5 °C under stirring at the speed of 50 rpm. A one milliliter aliquot was withdrawn at fixed time intervals and immediately replaced with an equal volume of fresh buffer to maintain the sink condition [3]. All samples were analyzed at 261.80 nm by UV Spectrophotometry (UV 2401(PC), S.220 V, Shimadzu Corporation, Kyoto, Japan). The experiment was done in triplicate to assess the drug diffusion characteristics from nPEVs formulation. Drug release was compared with plain ITZ for which 100 mg of ITZ was suspended in the 5 mL of buffer and study was carried out similar to ITZ-nPEVs. Drug release kinetics was assumed to reflect different release mechanism of controlled release drug delivery systems. Therefore, five kinetics model were applied to analyze the in vitro data to find the best fitting equation according to our previous study.

3.6.8. Nail Hydration Study

Nail clippings were collected with nail clippers from healthy human volunteers (males and females, 25–50 years old). The current investigation employed just the middle, index, and ring fingernails as an in vitro model for evaluating transungual administration [39]. Nail clippings were thoroughly cleaned by washing five times with distilled water, wiping with tissue paper, and drying at 37 °C for 24 h before being kept in airtight containers [40]. Fifty milligrams of nail clippings was inserted in separate glass vials for the nail hydration experiment. For this investigation, three groups were formed: group I (control group), in which the pre-weighed nail clippings were immersed in 1 mL deionized water (pH 7.04), group II (nPEVs formulation), group III (nPEVs CMFG gel) and group IV (marketed Itrostred gel), in which the nail clippings were immersed in marketed Itrostred gel, which is equivalent to the 1 mL of nPEVs. The nail clippings were reweighed after thorough tissue paper wiping to quantify weight growth after the glass vials were sealed and incubated at room temperature for 24 h [9]. The following calculation was used to compute the hydration enhancement factor (HE) after 24 h (HE24):

$$\text{HE 24} = \text{(Weight gain of nail clippings of groups II/III/IV)}/ \\ \text{(Weight gain of nail clippings of group I)} \tag{3}$$

3.6.9. Transungual Drug Uptake Study

The S3 (1:7:3) was the optimized formulation of ITZ-nPEVs from the in vitro drug release and nail hydration study. Groups 2 (optimized batch S3) and 3 (Itrostred gel) nail clippings were rinsed three times with methanol to eliminate any residues of medication on the surface, then dissolved in 1 M sodium hydroxide (1 mL) with continual overnight stirring [41]. The solutions were filtered through a 0.22 m syringe filter after full digestion of the nail clippings, and an aliquot was collected and diluted with methanol before HPLC analysis. The enhancement factor (EF nail) was computed using the following equation to represent the improvement in ITZ penetration into nPEV nail clippings as compared to marketed gel (Itrostred gel)

$$\text{EF nail} = \text{(Extracted drug percentage in nail clippings of group II/III)}/ \\ \text{(Extracted drug percentage in nail clippings of group IV)} \tag{4}$$

3.6.10. Anti-Microbiological Efficacy

The antifungal activity of the control, a chosen batch of nPEVs formula (S3), nPEVs loaded into the gel formulation, and the commercial preparation (Itrostred gel) was tested against *Candida albicans* (MTCC No. 227). One milliliter of the fungal culture suspension was combined with 9.9 mL liquid broth (without agar) and inoculated for 24 h at 25 degrees Celsius in an incubator (Remi instruments cooling incubator, Mumbai, India). 1 mL of inoculated liquid broth containing fungal culture suspension was poured to the sterile petri dishes containing solidified agar growth medium, and the inoculum was dispersed equally across the solid agar surface by turning the plate clockwise and anticlockwise.

With the use of a sterile cork-borer, wells were formed in the centre of the plates, and each well (6 mm internal diameter) was accurately filled with either 0.1 mL of control, ITZ-nPEVs, CMGF-ITZ-nPEVs gel, or Itrostred gel corresponding to ITZ dosage in the 0.1 mL ITZ-nPEVs. The plates were then incubated in the incubator for three days at 25 °C to allow for fungal development [42]. The antifungal activity was determined by measuring fungal growth inhibition zones around the formulations. They were measured on mm scale, and a comprehensive antifungal analysis was performed in an aseptic environment.

3.6.11. Stability Study

The physical and chemical stability study of an ideal formulation of CMFG-ITZ-nPEVs at 45 $\pm$ 0.5 °C and 60 $\pm$ 5% RH for 3 months in stability chamber (Model No. HTC-3003, Wadegati TM Labe Quip (P) Ltd., Andheri (E), Mumbai, India). At an interval of 1 month, CMFG-ITZ-nPEVs gels analyzed for physical changes, drug content, particle size, zeta potential and in-vitro drug release.

4. Conclusions

The combination of the penetration enhancer labrasol, the nail penetration enhancer N-acetyl-L-cysteine, and the positive charge inducer stearylamine in aqueous deformable-natured nanovesicles (nPEVs) was proven to be a viable combination for improving ITZ transungual administration. The prepared CMGF-ITZ-nPEVs gel satisfy best attributes for topical application such as it spreads easily, exhibiting maximum slip and drag. This nanosized formulations enhance permeability of drug extend retention at the site of action and the CMGF-ITZ-nPEVs gel shown greater antifungal activity than the marketed gel. The ITZ-nPEVs revealed here provide a novel therapy option for nail-related illnesses such onychomycosis. Clinical trials to determine the effectiveness of ITZ-nPEVs in patients with onychomycosis are presently underway.

Supplementary Materials: The following supporting information can be downloaded at: https://www.mdpi.com/article/10.3390/polym14020325/s1, Figure S1: (**A**) Quantification chromatogram of ITZ, and (**B**) standard calibration curve of ITZ; Figure S2. (**a**) PS and PDI, (**b**) ZP of S3; Table S1: Peak area of ITZ at different concentration.

Author Contributions: Conceptualization, Investigation, Methodology, Writing—original draft made by B.R., S.K. and J.M.M.M. Funding acquisition, Software, Resources and Visualization done by A.A. (Ali Alqahtani), A.A.F., T.A. and A.A. (Ali Alamri). Formal analysis, Data curation, writing—review and editing, statistical analysis and validation carried out by F.A. and V.K. All authors have read and agreed to the published version of the manuscript.

Funding: The authors are grateful to the King Khalid University's Deanship of Scientific Research for sponsoring this study through the Large Research Group Project, under grant number of RGP2/186/42.

Institutional Review Board Statement: Not applicable.

Informed Consent Statement: Not applicable.

Data Availability Statement: Data sharing not applicable.

Acknowledgments: The authors are grateful to the King Khalid University's Deanship of Scientific Research for sponsoring this study through the Large Research Group Project, under grant number of RGP2/186/42.

Conflicts of Interest: The authors declare no conflict of interest.

References

1. Nouripour-Sisakht, S.; Mirhendi, H.; Shidfar, M.R.; Ahmadi, B.; Rezaei-Matehkolaei, A.; Geramishoar, M.; Zarei, F.; Jalalizand, N. Aspergillus species as emerging causative agents of onychomycosis. *J. Mycol. Med.* **2015**, *25*, 101–107. [CrossRef] [PubMed]
2. Jayatilake, J.A.; Tilakaratne, W.M.; Panagoda, G.J. Candidal onychomycosis: A mini-review. *Mycopathologia* **2009**, *168*, 165–173. [CrossRef] [PubMed]
3. Sigurgeirsson, B.; Ghannoum, M. Therapeutic potential of TDT 067 (terbinafine in Transfersome): A carrier-based dosage form of terbinafine for onychomycosis. *Expert Opin. Investig. Drugs* **2012**, *21*, 1549–1562. [CrossRef] [PubMed]
4. Bsieso, E.A.; Nasr, M.; Moftah, N.H.; Sammour, O.A.; Abd-El-Gawad, N.A. Could nanovesicles containing a penetration enhancer clinically improve the therapeutic outcome in skin fungal diseases? *Nanomedicine* **2015**, *10*, 2017–2031. [CrossRef]
5. Tiwary, A.K.; Sapra, B. High failure rate of transungal drug delivery: Need for new strategies. *Ther. Deliv.* **2017**, *8*, 239–242. [CrossRef]
6. Dhamoon, R.K.; Harvinder Popli, H.; Madhu Gupta, M. Novel Drug Delivery Strategies for the Treatment of Onychomycosis. *Pharm. Nanotechnol.* **2019**, *7*, 24–38. [CrossRef]
7. Wang, F.; Yang, P.; Choi, J.S.; Antovski, P.; Zhu, Y.; Xu, X.; Kuo, T.H.; Lin, L.E.; Kim, D.N.H.; Huang, P.C.; et al. Cross-Linked Fluorescent Supramolecular Nanoparticles for Intradermal Controlled Release of Antifungal Drug-A Therapeutic Approach for Onychomycosis. *ACS Nano* **2018**, *24*, 6851–6859. [CrossRef]
8. Elsherif, N.I.; Shamma, R.N.; Abdelbary, G. Terbinafine hydrochloride trans-ungual delivery via nanovesicular systems: In vitro characterization and ex vivo evaluation. *AAPS PharmSciTech* **2017**, *18*, 551–562. [CrossRef]
9. Palliyil, B.; Lebo, D.B.; Patel, P.R. A preformulation strategy for the selection of penetration enhancers for a transungual formulation. *AAPS PharmSciTech* **2013**, *14*, 682–691. [CrossRef]
10. Miron, D.; Cornelio, R.; Troleis, J.; Mariath, J.; Zimmer, A.R.; Mayorga, P.; Schapoval, E.E. Influence of penetration enhancers and molecular weight in antifungals permeation through bovine hoof membranes and prediction of efficacy in human nails. *Eur. J. Pharm. Sci.* **2014**, *51*, 20–25. [CrossRef]
11. Hao, J.; Li, S.K. Mechanistic study of electroosmotic transport across hydrated nail plates: Effects of pH and ionic strength. *J. Pharm. Sci.* **2008**, *97*, 5186–5197. [CrossRef]
12. Neamtu, I.; Rusu, A.G.; Diaconu, A.; Nita, L.E.; Chiriac, A.P. Basic concepts and recent advances in nanogels as carriers for medical applications. *Drug Deliv.* **2017**, *24*, 539–557. [CrossRef]
13. Muthu, M.J.M.; Kavitha, K.; Ruckmani, K.; Shanmuganathan, S. Skimmed milk powder and pectin decorated solid lipid nanoparticle containing soluble curcumin used for the treatment of colorectal cancer. *J. Food Process Eng.* **2019**, *43*, 1–15.
14. Mohamed, J.M.M.; Alqahtani, A.; Al Fatease, A.; Alqahtani, T.; Khan, B.A.; Ashmitha, B.; Vijaya, R. Human Hair Keratin Composite Scaffold: Characterisation and Biocompatibility Study on NIH 3T3 Fibroblast Cells. *Pharmaceuticals* **2021**, *14*, 781. [CrossRef]
15. Mohamed, J.M.M.; Alqahtani, A.; Khan, B.A.; Al Fatease, A.; Alqahtani, T.; Venkatesan, K.; Ahmad, F.; Alzghoul, B.I.; Alamri, A. Preparation of Soluble Complex of Curcumin for the Potential Antagonistic Effects on Human Colorectal Adenocarcinoma Cells. *Pharmaceuticals* **2021**, *14*, 939. [CrossRef]
16. Fagir, W.; Hathout, R.M.; Sammour, O.A.; ElShafeey, A.H. Self-microemulsifying systems of Finasteride with enhanced oral bioavailability: Multivariate statistical evaluation, characterization, spray-drying and in vivo studies in human volunteers. *Nanomedicine* **2015**, *10*, 3373–3389. [CrossRef]
17. Yusuf, M.; Sharma, V.; Pathak, K. Nanovesicles for transdermal delivery of felodipine: Development, characterization, and pharmacokinetics. *Int. J. Pharm. Investig.* **2014**, *4*, 119–130.
18. Almahfood, M.; Bai, B. Characterization and oil recovery enhancement by a polymeric nanogel combined with surfactant for sandstone reservoirs. *Pet. Sci.* **2021**, *18*, 123–135. [CrossRef]
19. Mohamed, J.M.; Alqahtani, A.; Ahmad, F.; Krishnaraju, V.; Kalpana, K. Stoichiometrically Governed Curcumin Solid Dispersion and Its Cytotoxic Evaluation on Colorectal Adenocarcinoma Cells. *Drug Des. Devel. Ther.* **2020**, *14*, 4639–4658. [CrossRef]
20. Neeraj Kumar, N.; Goindi, S.; Bansal, G. Physicochemical evaluation and in vitro release studies on itraconazolium sulfate salt. *Asian J. Pharm. Sci.* **2014**, *9*, 8–16. [CrossRef]
21. Mohamed, J.M.; Kavitha, K.; Chitra Karthikeyini, S.C.; Nanthineeswari, S. Soluble curcumin prepared using four different carriers by solid dispersions: Phase solubility, molecular modelling and physicochemical characterization. *Trop. J. Pharm. Res.* **2019**, *18*, 1581–1588.
22. Hafeez, F.; Hui, X.; Chiang, A.; Hornby, S.; Maibach, H. Transungual delivery of ketoconazole using novel lacquer formulation. *Int. J. Pharm.* **2013**, *456*, 357–361. [CrossRef]
23. Shahin, M.; Hady, S.A.; Hammad, M.; Mortada, N. Novel jojoba oilbased emulsion gel formulations for clotrimazole delivery. *AAPS PharmSciTech.* **2011**, *12*, 239–247. [CrossRef]

24. Abobakr, F.E.; Fayez, S.M.; Elwazzan, V.S.; Sakran, W. Effect of Different Nail Penetration Enhancers in Solid Lipid Nanoparticles Containing Terbinafine Hydrochloride for Treatment of Onychomycosis. *AAPS PharmSciTech* **2021**, *22*, 33. [CrossRef] [PubMed]
25. Devi, M.; Kumar, S.M.; Mahadevan, N. Amphotericin-B loaded vesicular systems for the treatment of topical fungal infection. *Int. J. Rec. Adv. Pharm. Res.* **2011**, *4*, 37–46.
26. Lin, T.-K.; Zhong, L.; Santiago, J.L. Anti-Inflammatory and Skin Barrier Repair Effects of Topical Application of Some Plant Oils. *Int. J. Mol. Sci.* **2018**, *19*, 70. [CrossRef]
27. Sudan, P.; Goswami, M.; Singh, J. Antifungal potential of Fenugreek seeds (*Trigonella foenum-graecum*) crude extracts against Microsporum gypseum. *Int. J. Pharm. Sci. Res.* **2020**, *11*, 646–649. [CrossRef]
28. Tanrıverdi, S.T.; Özer, Ö. Novel topical formulations of Terbinafine-HCl for treatment of onychomycosis. *Eur. J. Pharm. Sci.* **2013**, *48*, 628–636. [CrossRef]
29. Mohamed, J.M.; Ahmad, F.; Al-Subaie, A.M. Soluble 1:1 stoichiometry curcumin binary complex for potential apoptosis in human colorectal adenocarcinoma cells (SW480 and Caco-2 cells). *Res. J. Pharm. Tech.* **2021**, *14*, 21–29.
30. Shivakumar, H.N.; Juluri, A.; Desai, B.G.; Murthy, S.N. Ungual and transungual drug delivery. *Drug Dev. Ind. Pharm.* **2012**, *38*, 901–911. [CrossRef]
31. Skupin-Mrugalska, A.; Zalewski, T.; Elvang, P.A.; Nowaczyk, G.; Czajkowski, M.; Piotrowska-Kempisty, H. Insight into theranostic nanovesicles prepared by thin lipid hydration and microfluidic method. *Colloids Surf. B Biointer.* **2021**, *205*, 111871. [CrossRef] [PubMed]
32. Nasr, M.; Mansour, S.; Mortada, N.D.; El Shamy, A.A. Lipospheres as carriers for topical delivery of aceclofenac: Preparation, characterization and in vivo evaluation. *AAPS PharmSciTech* **2008**, *9*, 154–162. [CrossRef] [PubMed]
33. El-Mahdy, A.R. Preliminary studies on the mucilages extracted from Okra fruits, Taro tubers, Jew's mellow leaves and Fenugreek seeds. *Food Chem.* **1984**, *14*, 237–249. [CrossRef]
34. Parvathy, K.S.; Susheelamma, N.S.; Tharanathan, R.N.; Gaonkar, A.K. A simple non-aqueous method for carboxymethylation of galactomannans. *Carbohydr. Polym.* **2005**, *62*, 137–141. [CrossRef]
35. Chen, J.; Ding, J.; Xu, W.; Sun, T.; Xiao, H.; Zhuang, X.; Chen, X. Receptor and microenvironment dual-recognizable nanogel for targeted chemotherapy of highly metastatic malignancy. *Nano Lett.* **2017**, *17*, 4526–4533. [CrossRef] [PubMed]
36. Wang, Y.; Pang, L.; Wu, M.; Ou, N.A. validated LC-MS/MS method for determination of sertaconazole nitrate in human plasma. *J. Chromatogr. B Analyt. Technol. Biomed. Life Sci.* **2009**, *877*, 4047–4050. [CrossRef] [PubMed]
37. Mohamed, J.M.; Alqahtani, A.; Ahmad, F.; Krishnaraju, V.; Kalpana, K. Pectin co-functionalized dual layered solid lipid nanoparticle made by soluble curcumin for the targeted potential treatment of colorectal cancer. *Carbohydr. Polym.* **2020**, *252*, 117180. [CrossRef]
38. Moideen, M.M.J.; Alqahtani, A.; Venkatesan, K.; Ahmad, F.; Krisharaju, K.; Gayasuddin, M.; Shaik, R.A.; Ibraheem, K.M.M.; Salama, M.E.M.; Abed, S.Y. Application of the Box–Behnken design for the production of soluble curcumin: Skimmed milk powder inclusion complex for improving the treatment of colorectal cancer. *Food Sci. Nutr.* **2020**, *8*, 6643–6659. [CrossRef]
39. Pal, P.; Thakur, R.S.; Ray, S.; Mazumder, B. Design and development of a safer non-invasive transungual drug delivery system for topical treatment of onychomycosis. *Drug Dev. Ind. Pharm.* **2015**, *41*, 1095–1099. [CrossRef]
40. Chouhan, P.; Saini, T.R. Hydration of nail plate: A novel screening model for transungual drug permeation enhancers. *Int. J. Pharm.* **2012**, *436*, 179–182. [CrossRef]
41. Farhana, A.R.N.; Amin, I.; Hassan, A.S.S.; Shuhaimi, M. Gel formation of pectin from okra (*Abelmoschus esculentus* L. Moench) leaves, pulp and seeds. *Int. Food Res. J.* **2017**, *24*, 2161–2169.
42. Sahoo, S.; Pani, N.R.; Sahoo, S.K. Effect of microemulsion in topical sertaconazole hydrogel: In vitro and in vivo study. *Drug Deliv.* **2016**, *23*, 338–345. [CrossRef]

polymers

MDPI

Article

Blends of Carbohydrate Polymers for the Co-Microencapsulation of *Bacillus clausii* and Quercetin as Active Ingredients of a Functional Food

María Z. Saavedra-Leos [1], Manuel Román-Aguirre [2], Alberto Toxqui-Terán [3], Vicente Espinosa-Solís [4], Avelina Franco-Vega [5] and César Leyva-Porras [2,*]

1 Coordinación Académica Región Altiplano (COARA), Universidad Autónoma de San Luis Potosí, Matehuala, San Luis Potosi 78700, Mexico; zenaida.saavedra@uaslp.mx

2 Centro de Investigación en Materiales Avanzados S.C., CIMAV, Miguel de Cervantes No. 120, Complejo Industrial Chihuahua, Chihuahua 31136, Mexico; manuel.roman@cimav.edu.mx

3 Centro de Investigación en Materiales Avanzados S.C., Unidad Monterrey, Alianza Norte No. 202, Parque de Investigación e Innovación Tecnológica, Apodaca 66600, Mexico; alberto.toxqui@cimav.edu.mx

4 Coordinación Académica Región Huasteca Sur, Universidad Autónoma de San Luis Potosí, Carretera Tamazunchale-San Martin Km. 5. Tamazunchale, San Luis Potosi 79960, Mexico; vicente.espinosa@uaslp.mx

5 Facultad de Ciencias Químicas, Universidad Autónoma de San Luis Potosí, San Luis Potosi 78210, Mexico; avelina.franco@uaslp.mx

* Correspondence: cesar.leyva@cimav.edu.mx; Tel.: +52-61-4439-1100 (ext. 2011)

Citation: Saavedra-Leos, M.Z.; Román-Aguirre, M.; Toxqui-Terán, A.; Espinosa-Solís, V.; Franco-Vega, A.; Leyva-Porras, C. Blends of Carbohydrate Polymers for the Co-Microencapsulation of *Bacillus clausii* and Quercetin as Active Ingredients of a Functional Food. *Polymers* **2022**, *14*, 236. https://doi.org/10.3390/polym14020236

Academic Editors: Faisal Raza, Sergio Torres-Giner and Bramasta Nugraha

Received: 15 November 2021
Accepted: 2 January 2022
Published: 7 January 2022

Abstract: A functional food based on blends of carbohydrate polymers and active ingredients was prepared by spray drying. Inulin (IN) and maltodextrin (MX) were used as carrying agents to co-microencapsulate quercetin as an antioxidant and *Bacillus clausii* (Bc) as a probiotic. Through a reduced design of experiments, eleven runs were conducted and characterized by scanning electron microscopy (SEM), X-ray diffraction (XRD), and modulated differential scanning calorimetry (MDSC). The physical characterizations showed fine and non-aggregated powders, composed of pseudo-spherical particles with micrometric sizes. The observation of rod-like particles suggested that microorganisms were microencapsulated in these particles. The microstructure of the powders was amorphous, observing diffraction peaks attributed to the crystallization of the antioxidant. The glass transition temperature (Tg) of the blends was above the room temperature, which may promote a higher stability during storage. The antioxidant activity (AA) values increased for the IN-MX blends, while the viability of the microorganisms increased with the addition of MX. By a surface response plot (SRP) the yield showed a major dependency with the drying temperature and then with the concentration of IN. The work contributes to the use of carbohydrate polymers blends, and to the co-microencapsulation of active ingredients.

Keywords: carbohydrate polymers blends; functional food; antioxidant activity; co-microencapsulation; spray drying; bacteria viability (*Bacillus clausii*); probiotics

1. Introduction

Functional foods are defined as those products consumed as part of a normal diet with additionall health benefits beyond the traditional nutrients [1], reducing the risk of suffering from chronic diseases [2]. The incorporation of active compounds such as probiotics and antioxidants is currently one of the different strategies used to generate these type of foods, [3]. Functional foods contain bioactive compounds in low concentrations, such as antioxidants, glutamine, fatty acids, and even live microorganisms as probiotics. Probiotics are defined as live strains of strictly selected microorganisms, that when consumed in adequate amounts, confer a beneficial effect to the health [4]. The effects of probiotics can vary depending on the dose, the strain used and the components which the final product was formulated. These products can contain one or more strains, such as *Lactobacillus*, *Bifidobacterium*, *Lactococcus*, *Streptococcus*, *Enterococcus*, Gram-positive strains of the genus *Bacillus*, and yeasts of the genus *Saccharomyces* [5]. Another type of bioactive compounds are antioxidants that have demonstrated the ability to protect, delay cellular aging, and strengthen the immune system [6,7]. Antioxidants are compounds that inhibit unstable free radicals that lead to a chain reaction of cellular damage, causing cellular aging and chronic degenerative diseases. However, the use of these antioxidants in the food industry is limited, since they exhibit high sensitivity to environmental conditions such as light, oxygen, humidity and exposure to heat, causing a decrease or loss of their functional properties. In order to overcome these drawbacks, it is necessary implementing technologies to minimize the loss of functional and nutritional properties of these compounds. Microencapsulation is one of the strategies employed to preserve and extend the shelf life of foods containing bioactive ingredients [8]. Microencapsulation consists of mechanical and physicochemical processes that trap the functional substance or bioactive compound within the walls of another material acting as a protective barrier. Among the encapsulation techniques, spray drying is one of the simplest, cheapest, and fastest methodologies used by both the pharmaceutical and food industries. Dry products typically exhibit high quality, low levels of degradation, and excellent stability properties.

Carbohydrate polymers are naturally occurring molecules that exhibit similar behavior to synthetic polymers, i.e., with properties such as glass transition temperature (Tg), melting temperature (Tm), and molecular weight distribution (MWD). These polymers are mainly based on polysaccharides composed of glucose, sucrose, dextrose, arabinose and galactose; examples of these include starch, chitosan, maltodextrins (MX), inulin (IN), and gum Arabic (GA). Polysaccharides have been widely used individually as carrier agents for the conservation and microencapsulation of active ingredients in food and pharmaceutical products. For example, chitosan has been used in the preservation of meat products [9] and as a protective barrier in edible films [10]. MXs with different MWD have been compared as carrier agents in the yield, and content of natural antioxidants such as quercetin and resveratrol [11,12]. IN has also been employed as a carrying agent in the spray-drying preparation of a functional food based on orange juice [13]. MX and IN were compared in the conservation of antioxidants from blueberry juice, showing that low molecular MXs presented a higher retention value than IN [14]. Recently, the performance of IN and lactose as carrying agents in the co-microencapsulation of *Bacillus clausii* (Bc) and resveratrol as active ingredients of a functional food was reported [15]. The results showed higher antioxidant activity for IN, and similar cell viability for both wall materials.

Regarding the use of blends of carrying agents, most of the works are based on polysaccharide-protein complexes coacervates [16]. Bordón et al. [17] reported a higher encapsulation efficiency of chia oil when using soy protein isolate and GA blends at a ratio of 2:1. Guo et al. [18] employed a surfactant (Rhamnolipid) to fabricate complexes of pea protein isolate (PPI) and high methoxyl pectin (HMP) and studied its effect on the releasing of curcumin and resveratrol. They concluded that the use of the surfactant improved the encapsulation efficiency, enhanced the solubility in water and delayed the delivery of the antioxidants. Kumar and Saini [19] prepared edible bi-layer coatings for prolonging the shelf life of tomatoes, employing whey protein isolate (WPI), xanthan gum and clove oil. They found that the decrease in the total phenolic content was considerably lower on the coated fruits than on those uncoated. Sharifi et al. [20] reported the improvement in cell viability of *Lactobacillus plantarum* when adding phytosterols to a blend of WPI and GA.

Conversely, other works have reported the synergistic effect of using two or more polysaccharide components. Maisuthisakul and Gordon [21] studied the combination of GA, MX, and alginate (AL) on the encapsulation efficiency of phenolic compounds and the storage properties of mango seed kernel emulsions. The optimal mixture for these properties was composed of 5.95% of GA, 23.9% of MX, and 0.11% of AL. de Barros Fernandes, Vilela Borges, and Alvarenga Botrel [22] tested the replacement of GA by modified starch (MS), MX, and IN on the microencapsulation properties of rosemary essential oil. The highest oil retention (60%) was obtained when employing a 1:1 mixture of MS and MX. Silva and Hubinger [23] employed mixtures of MS or GA with MX at a ratio of 75:25 for the microencapsulation of green coffee oil. The highest encapsulation efficiency of 87.6% was achieved with the MS-MX blend. Damodharan et al. [24] employed AL and two gums to test the viability of microencapsulated bacteria. The composition of 1% AL, 0.5% Fenugreek gel and 0.5% Locust bean gum was selected based on the viscosity of the mixture, because this property directly affects the spray drying process. For this mixture, the survival rate of the bacteria was greater than 85% and 97% in simulated gastrointestinal and colonic fluids, respectively. Poletto et al. [25] compared the use of IN, rice bran, and starch (Hi-maize) on the encapsulation of *L. acidophilus* as a probiotic. The highest microencapsulation efficiency (96%) was presented by the blend containing 2% of AL and 10% of IN. Colín-Cruz et al. [26] employed GA, MX and whey protein concentrate (WPC) to prepare 50–50% blends. They found that the GA-MX blend increased the encapsulation efficiency of the phenolic compounds and anthocyanins to 98.4% and 99%, respectively, while the single WPC showed a higher encapsulation efficiency for the probiotic bacteria.

Determining the effects of the processing conditions on the physicochemical and functional performance of powder products containing microencapsulated active ingredients is essential for novel foods and pharmaceutical products development. Active ingredients, such as quercetin and *Bacillus claussi* microorganisms are sensitive to degradation by environmental conditions including temperature, humidity, and exposure to light and oxygen. Therefore, the co-microencapsulation of these ingredients is essential to maintain the antioxidant and probiotic properties during the storage of the powder product.

Derived from the above, the present work aims to obtain a functional food powder, with probiotic and antioxidant properties, based on mixtures of carbohydrate polymers such as MX and IN. For this purpose, a reduced design of experiments was developed to study the effect of the spray drying inlet temperature, and the concentration of the polysaccharides on the morphology, microstructure and Tg of the obtained powders, as well as their antioxidant activity and cell viability. In this sense, herein is demonstrated the beneficial use of blends of carbohydrate polymers, and how these polysaccharides affect the studied properties. The work contributes to the technological application of carbohydrate polymers as functional food matrices, the co-microencapsulation and conservation of active ingredients, and the preparation of a functional food powder.

2. Materials and Methods

2.1. Materials

The following reagents were purchased from the specified vendor. Commercial maltodextrin (MX) extracted from cornstarch, and inulin (IN) (Ingredion, Guadalajara, Mexico). The dextrose equivalent (DE) of MX was 10, corresponding to a molecular weight of 1625 g/mole and a degree of polymerization (DP) of 2–16 units of glucose. *Bacillus* bacteria (Bc) strain (*Bacillus clausii*) in Sunuberase solution (Sanofi-Aventis, Coyoacán, CDMX, Mexico). Quercetin 3-D-Galactoside (99%, Química Farmacéutica Esteroidal, Tláhuac, CDMX, México). Analytical grade 2,2-diphenyl-1-picrylhydrazyl (DPPH), (±)-6-hydroxy-2,5,7,8-tetramethylchromane-2-carboxylic acid (Trolox), gallic acid, sodium carbonate (Na_2CO_3), and Folin–Ciocalteu reagent (Sigma–Aldrich Chemical Co., Toluca, Mexico).

2.2. Preparation of Spray-Dried Powders

Spray drying process was employed in the microencapsulation of Bc and quercetin in the form of powders. Typically, the preparation of the feeding solutions consisted of mixing 20 g of the corresponding carrying agent (inulin, maltodextrin or the blend), 1 g of quercetin, 5 mL of the commercial solution with bacteria (equivalent to a concentration of 2×10^{12} CFU), and distilled water for obtaining a total volume of 100 mL of solution. Microencapsulation was carried out in a Mini Spray Dryer B290 (BÜCHI, Labortechnik AG, Flawil, Switzerland) at the following operation conditions: feed temperature of 40 °C, feeding flow of 7 cm^3/min, hot airflow of 28 m^3/h, aspiration of 70%, and pressure of

1.5 bar. The inlet temperatures were varied in the range of 150–220 °C. This range of temperatures was selected to avoid the collapse of the microstructure and other unwanted characteristics such as stickiness and agglomeration of the powders.

A reduced design of experiments was carried out to test the effect of the inlet temperature and the concentration of the carrying agents in the blends. Through the coding of parameters ranging from –1 for the lowest value, and 1 for the highest value, robustness and reliability are obtained in the acquired data. The experiment design contains points outside the surface (±1.4) as control points to carry out interpolations of the variables, verify the reliability and establish inflection points. Table 1 shows the run number and the corresponding experimental conditions. Once the powders were obtained, these were individually placed in airtight bags and stored in darkness at 4 °C. Each sample was labeled as INMX_x, where IN and MX stand for the carbohydrate polymer employed as the carrying agent in the blend, and x stands for the run number.

Table 1. Reduced experimental design.

Run	Order	Temperature	Carrying Agent	Temperature (°C)	MD (%)	IN (%)
1	1	−1.000	−1.000	150	20	0
2	9	0.000	0.000	180	10	10
3	6	1.414	0.000	234	10	10
4	8	0.000	1.414	180	0	28.8
5	10	0.000	0.000	180	10	10
6	7	0.000	−1.414	180	28.8	0
7	5	−1.414	0.000	126	10	10
8	3	−1.000	1.000	150	0	20
9	11	0.000	0.000	180	10	10
10	2	1.000	−1.000	210	20	0
11	4	1.000	1.000	210	0	20

2.3. Scanning Electron Microscopy (SEM)

Morphological characterization was conducted using a scanning electron microscope (SEM) (JSM-7401F, JEOL, Tokyo, Japan) operated at an accelerating voltage of 2 kV. Powder samples were first dispersed on a double-side copper conductive tape, then covered with a thin layer of gold utilizing a sputtering to reduce charging effects (Denton Desk II sputter coater, Denton, TX, USA).

2.4. X-ray Diffraction (XRD)

Microstructural characterization was determined by x-ray diffraction (XRD) analysis in a D8 Advance ECO diffractometer (Bruker, Karlsruhe, Germany) equipped with Cu-K radiation (l = 1.5406 Å) operated at 45 kV, 40 mA and a detector in a Bragg–Brentano geometry. Scans were performed in the 2θ range of 5–50°, with a step size of 0.016° and 20 s per step.

2.5. Thermal Analysis

A modulated differential scanning calorimeter (MDSC) Q200 (TA Instruments, New Castle, DE, USA) equipped with an RCS90 cooling system was employed for determining the Tg. The instrument was calibrated with indium for melting temperature and enthalpy, while sapphire was used as the standard for heat capacity (Cp). Samples about 10 mg were encapsulated in Tzero aluminum pans. Thermograms were acquired at a temperature range of −50 to 250 °C, with a modulation period of 40 s and amplitude of 1.5 °C.

2.6. Determination of Water Activity

For each of the microencapsulated powders, water activity (aw) was determined into an Aqualab Series 3 Water Activity Meter (Meter Group, Inc. Pullman, WA, USA). According to the AOAC, the method requires drying the sample in an oven at 110 °C for 2 h, and calculating the ratio of the final and initial masses.

2.7. Radical Scavenging Activity of the Functional Food

The antioxidant capacity of microencapsulated quercetin was determined according to the methodology reported in [15,27]. The microencapsulated powders were dissolved in ethanol at concentrations of 5, 10 and 30 μg/mL. Then, 1.7 mL of each solution was mixed with 1.7 mL of DPPH* ethanol solution (0.1 mmol/L). The initial powder concentration in solution were 2.5, 5 and 15 μg/mL, while the DPPH* solution concentration decreased to 0.05 mmol/L. The mixed solution (3.4 mL) was poured into a 10 mm thick quartz cell. The antioxidant capacity was evaluated as the decrease in the initial concentration of DPPH* scavenged by quercetin after 30 min of preparation. The variation in the absorbance intensity of DPPH* was measured at a wavelength of 517 nm in a UV-Vis spectrophotometer Evolution 220 (Thermo Scientific, Waltham, MA, US). The scavenging activity (%DPPH*) was calculated according to Equation (1):

$$\text{Scavenging Activity (\% DPPH)} = \frac{A_0 - A_{30}}{A_0} \times 100 \quad (1)$$

where A_0 is the initial absorbance of DPPH*, and A_{30} is the absorbance of the DPPH* after 30 min of adding the microencapsulated antioxidant.

2.8. Viability of Bacillus Clausii in the Microencapsulated

The number of available Bc bacteria cells was evaluated by means of the plate extension technique, with Trypticase-Soy Agar (TSA) (Becton Dickinson, Franklin Lakes, NJ, US), using serial dilutions of the encapsulated samples from 1×10^{-1} to 1×10^{-7}. Growing conditions were aerobic, with an incubation period of 48 h at 37 °C in an incubator (Novatech, Jalisco, GDL, Mexico). To determine the number of colony-forming units per gram (CFU/g), the concentrations exhibiting between 300 and 30 CFU (1×10^{-4} and 1×10^{-5}) were selected. Equation (2) was employed for the quantification of culturability. All experiments were performed by triplicate, and the reported values represent the average of the calculated values.

$$\frac{\text{CFU}}{\text{g}} = \left[\frac{\text{N}^\circ \text{ plate colonies} \times \text{dilution factor}}{\text{mL sample seeded}}\right] \quad (2)$$

2.9. Powder Yield

Yield percentage (%) was calculated according to Equation (3), by the ratio of the masses of the collected powder (W_P), and the liquid (W_L) fed into the spray dryer.

$$Y(\%) = \frac{W_P}{W_L} \times 100 \quad (3)$$

2.10. Encapsulation Efficiency (EE)

The total phenolic content (TPC) and the surface phenolic content (SPC) were determined by the modified Folin–Ciocalteu method [28]. For TPC, 50 mg of microcapsules were weighed and dissolved in a 1 mL solution of ethanol-acetic acid-water (50:8:42 *v*/*v*). For SPC 50 mg of microcapsules were dispersed with a 1 mL solution of ethanol-methanol (1:1 *v*/*v*). Both mixtures were agitated using magnetic stirring for 1 min and centrifuged at 11,000 rpm by 15 min at 10 °C. Absorption at 750 nm was measured using a UV/VIS spectrometer. Calibration curves were prepared with different quercetin concentrations in ethanol-acetic acid-water solution, or ethanol-methanol solution. TPC and SPC were expressed as quercetin equivalents (QE) in milligrams per gram of microencapsulates.

The encapsulation efficiency (EE) was expressed as the ratio of encapsulated phenolic content (EPC) to total phenolic content (TPC). EPC was determined as the difference between TPC and SPC. The encapsulation efficiency of microcapsules was calculated according to Equation (4).

$$EE(\%) = \left(\frac{TPC - SPC}{TPC}\right) \times 100 \tag{4}$$

2.11. Statistical Analysis

All experiments were performed by triplicate, reporting mean values and standard deviations. A one-way analysis of variance (ANOVA) was performed to establish a significance level of 0.05, and the Tukey's honestly significant difference (HSD) post hoc test was used to determine the difference between the means. The statistical analyses were conducted using the IBM SPSS statistics version 21.0 software (SPSS Inc., Chicago, IL, USA).

3. Results and Discussion

3.1. Morphological Characterization

The overall appearance of the spray-dried powders was a yellowish color composed of fine non-aggregated particles, suggesting that the processing conditions were adequate to avoid the collapse of the microstructure and the appearance of undesired drying characteristics such as agglomeration, stickiness, and crystallization [29].

Figure 1 shows SEM micrographs acquired at 1000× of the spray-dried powders. By comparing the prepared blends (samples INMX_1–11 in Figure 1A) against the single MX and IN blank samples (Figure 1B), is possible to observe the following features. (i) The morphology of the particles was in general pseudo-spherical, but at some processing conditions, the shape was spheroidal and irregular as deflate balls. In some cases, a third morphology composed of elongated fiber-like or rod-like particles was observed. (ii) The particle size was in the order of the micrometers with at least two size distributions: large particles of a few tens of microns, and small particles below 5 microns. (iii) The surface of the particles was smooth at some processing conditions and wrinkled at others. (iv) Bacteria were not observed on the particles or in between, suggesting that they were completely microencapsulated or fully eliminated by thermal degradation during the spray drying process.

By relating the processing conditions with the above-mentioned observations, it seems that the morphology of IN particles was deformed with the increase in the drying temperature (INMX_8, 4, and 11). On the other hand, the MX particles were relatively stable at the intermediate and higher drying temperatures (INMX_1, 6, and 10), since at these temperatures (180 and 210 °C) the morphology of the particles was relatively more regular than at 150 °C. The observed surface appearance of deflated balls or wrinkle surfaces is caused by the rapid removal of water during drying. Additionally, the lack of surface cracks on the particles is important to reduce gas permeability and, to promote the conservation of the active ingredients within the walls of the particles [22], and it indicates the complete coverage of the active materials by the polysaccharides [23]. Araujo-Díaz et al. [14] showed the variation in the morphology of particles with the adsorption of moisture of spray-dried MX and IN powders. They found that the morphology of the particles was initially spherical, while after the powders were exposed to different water activities, the particles started to coalesce and grow with irregular morphologies.

Although in some studies, the decrease in the size of the particle has been related to the addition of a second carrier agent [26], in the present work the size of the particles increased with the addition of the two polysaccharides. For example, at the same drying temperature (180 °C) the average sizes and standard deviations of the IN, MX and blend samples (INMX_4, 6 and 2) were 3.2 ± 2.57 µm, 4.1 ± 2.95 µm, and 8.1 ± 5.05 µm, respectively.

Related to whether or not bacteria are present in the functional powdered food, by comparing the morphology of the particles in the micrographs, in the blank samples (Figure 1B) is observed the presence of spherical and pseudo-spherical particles, and the absence of particles with elongated rod-like morphologies. This suggests that the *Bacilus claussi* microorganisms were microencapsulated with the corresponding polysaccharide in the 11 runs (Figure 1A), and formed this type of elongated particles. Conversely, several studies where the organisms were not observed either, have reported that the morphology of the particles was not modified with the addition of bacteria [15,20]. However, in these works, these powders showed significant bacterial activity.

The morphological characterization suggested that the obtained powders herein were fully dried and that the active ingredients, i.e., antioxidant and microorganisms were successfully microencapsulated within the pseudo-spherical particles and the rod-like particles, respectively.

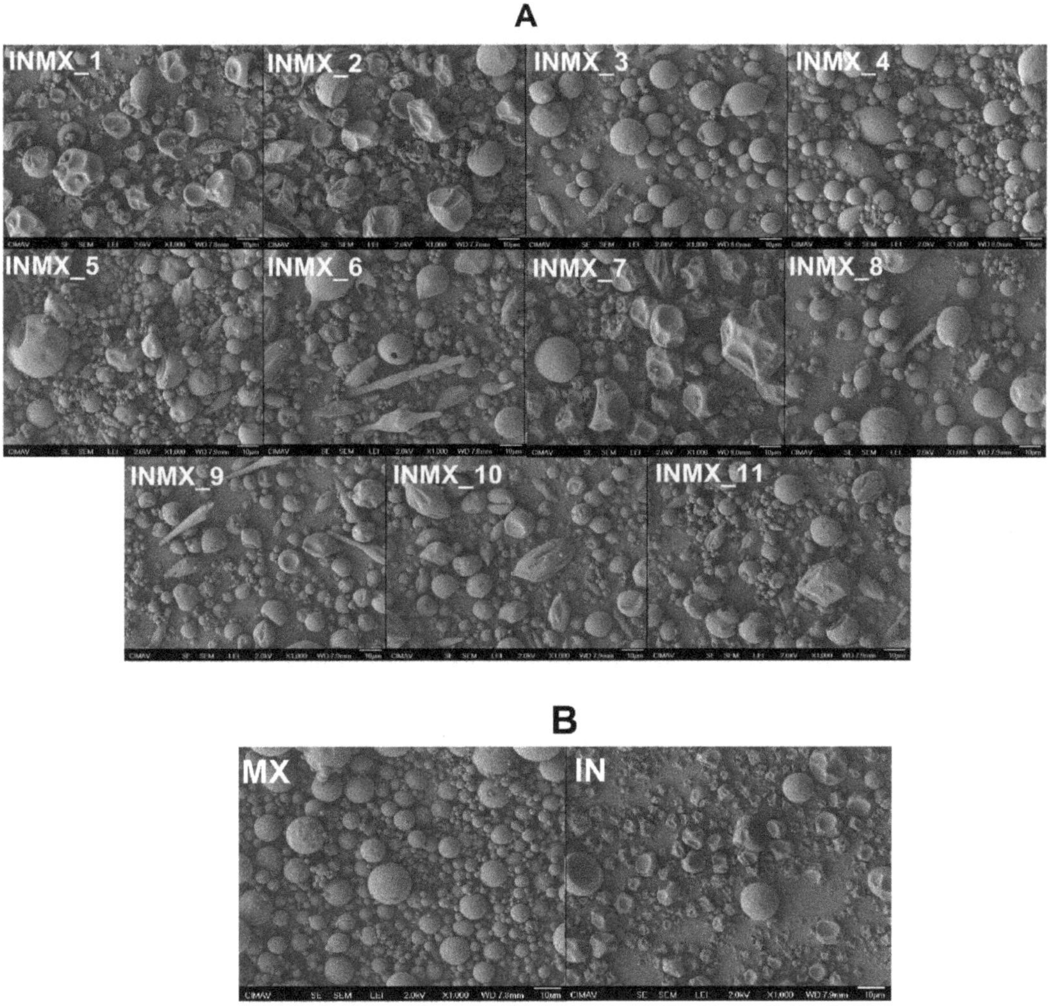

Figure 1. Acquired SEM micrographs at 1000× of the spray-dried powders: (**A**) carbohydrate polymers blends, and (**B**) blank samples.

3.2. Microstructural Characterization

The microstructure of the powdered functional food was studied by XRD. Figure 2 shows the X-rays diffractograms of the spray-dried powders containing the active ingredients and the blank samples. The diffractograms of the blank samples (MX and IN) showed a single low intensity and broad peak about an angle 2θ of 18°, and the absence of other diffraction peaks. This indicated that in both polysaccharides the microstructure was completely amorphous after the spray drying process. MX and IN are based on carbohydrate polymers composed of chains of glucose and fructose, respectively. In consequence, their microstructure and properties are different. For example, when these polysaccharides are individually subjected to the adsorption of moisture, the MX powder does not crystallize, but just changes its microstructure from the amorphous into the rubbery state at low and intermediate water activities, and into a liquid state at high water activities [30]. Meanwhile IN modifies its microstructure from the amorphous state into a crystallized matrix, showing a corresponding increase in the intensity of the diffraction peaks at 2θ of 12, 16, 18.5, and 23° [29].

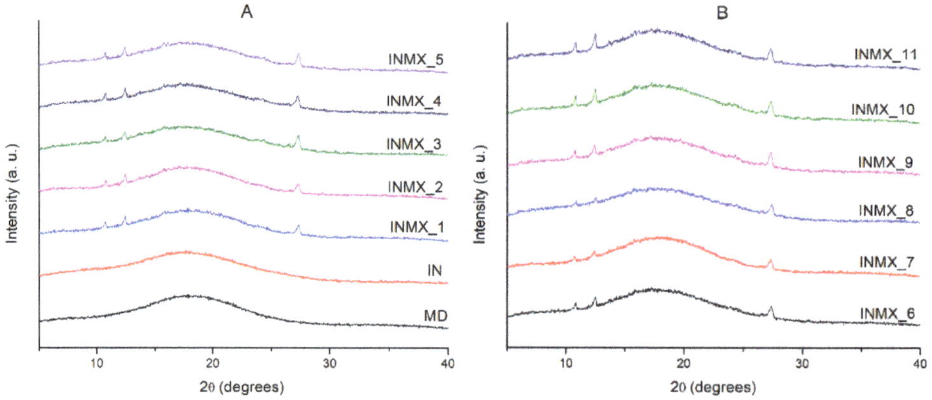

Figure 2. X-rays diffractograms of the spray-dried powders containing the active ingredients: (**A**) IN and MX blanks, and blends INMX_1–5. (**B**) Blends INMX_6–11.

On the other hand, the samples containing the active ingredients (INMX_1–11) besides the amorphous broad peak at 18°, presented three notable diffraction peaks at 2θ angles of 10.8, 12.4 and 27.3°. This observation is interesting because it could suggest the crystallization of the carrying agents during the spray drying. However, according to the design of experiments (Table 1) several of the samples were prepared as a mixture of two polysaccharides, while others contained only one carrying agent. Therefore, from these observations it can be deduced that some of the active ingredients are crystallizing during the drying. Recently, Klitou et al. [31] reported the simulated and experimental XRD diffractograms of quercetin crystallized in dimethyl sulfoxide (DMSO), identifying characteristic diffraction peaks at 2θ angles of 10.5, 12.9, 16.3, 17.1, 18.3, 19.5, 20.4, 23.2, 27.2, and 27.8°. Morphological observations from SEM could suggested that the peaks in diffractograms are caused either by the non-spherical shaped particles such as elongated fiber-like particles or by the crystallization of quercetin.

3.3. Thermal Analysis

The determination of Tg is very important because this value indicates the transition from the vitreous state into the rubber state. Commonly, the powders obtained by spray drying are in the vitreous state, in which the mobility of polysaccharides chains is restricted, limiting the diffusion phenomena of water molecules. Macroscopically, this is observed as a well-dispersed and fine powder i.e., without forming aggregates or caking. Additionally, the Tg values have been related to the stability during storage of food products [32], in such a way that carrying agents with higher Tg produce powders with greater stability during processing and storage. When the Tg value is close or below the ambient temperature, the system may experience a thermodynamic imbalance, modifying its microstructure from the amorphous into an intermediate rubber or crystalline state. Thus, the selection of carrier agents is important since the final Tg of the mixture will depend on factors such as molecular weight, water content, and chemical compatibility [22]. Figure 3 shows the MDSC thermograms of selected spray-dried powders containing the active ingredients

(INMX_3, 7 and 9) and the blank samples (MX and IN). In each graph are plotted three curves: on top (blue color) the total heat flow curve, in the middle (black color) the reversible heat flow curve, and on the bottom (red color) the non-reversible heat flow curve. Additionally, on each curve are indicated the beginning (T_i), the peak value, and the ending (T_f) of the identified thermal event.

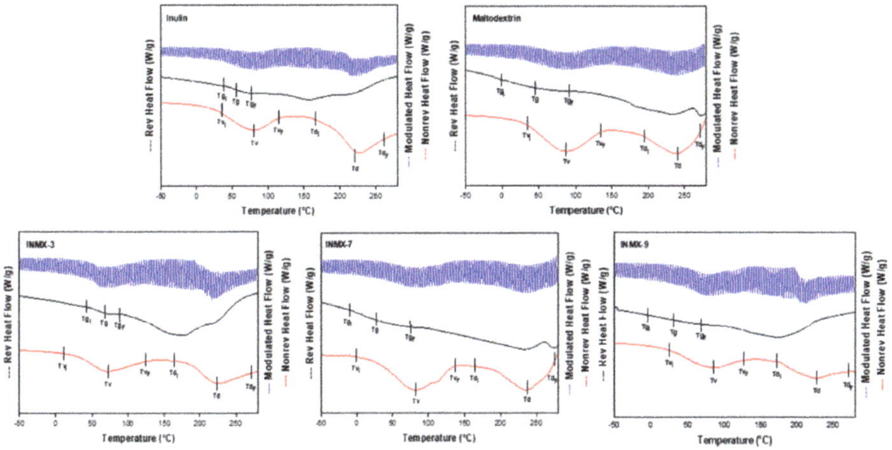

Figure 3. MDSC thermograms of selected spray-dried powders containing the active ingredients (INMX_3, 7, and 9) and the blank samples (MX and IN).

The summary of the Tg values is presented in Table 2. The Tg values were determined in the range of 15.9–110.2 °C, while a_w was 2.02–5.50. In all cases, the Tg decreased monotonically with increasing a_w. These results are very similar to those reported by Vera Lavelli et al. [33] who obtained encapsulated phenols from grape skin with maltodextrin (GPS) with different aw values. They observed the formation of lumps at 19% of moisture and a_w of 0.75, and a viscous liquid at 12% of moisture and a_w of 0.56. Bordón et al. [17] reported a similar behavior for blends of SPI-GA prepared at 1:1 and 2:1 ratios. From the prepared powders, the blend dried at 234 °C (INMX_3) showed the highest Tg value (60.7 °C), while the rest of the blends presented values below 30 °C. Thus, if the functional food is to be stored at room temperature (25 °C), it is probable that the blend dried at 234 °C may present the greatest stability than the rest of the tested blends. The maximum stability of food occurs when the storage temperature is lower than the Tg. Colín-Cruz showed that the addition of other carbohydrate polymers increased the Tg from 46.1 °C to 51.6 °C for WPC and GA-WPC, respectively [26].

Table 2. Summary of the results of the spray-dried powders containing the active ingredients.

Run	Tg (°C)	a_w	AA (%)	*Bc* (Log_{10} CFU/g)	Yield (%)	EE (%)
1	35.2	2.42	8.3 ± 2.13	6.90845 ± 0.007	51.09	7.48 ± 0.16
2	28.1.8	2.77	16.48 ± 1.12	8.01671 ± 0.088	48.95	29.50 ± 0.42
3	60.7	2.41	23.11 ± 2.6	6.95422 ± 0.006	52.09	96.49 ± 0.64
4	110.2	4.48	27.03 ± 2.63	4.30049 ± 0.03	49.1	80.71 ± 0.12
5	24.3	4.48	20.08 ± 1.98	7.62276 ± 0.029	48.19	17.84 ± 0.77
6	39.7	2.45	15.61 ± 3.6	8.10206 ± 0.144	47.09	46.34 ± 0.14
7	15.9	5.22	6.91 ± 1.07	8.63241 ± 0.042	41.14	93.26 ± 0.68
8	51.1	4.81	14.52 ± 1.85	4.75257 ± 0.075	49.28	83.02 ± 0.42
9	25.9	4.01	13.39 ± 2.68	7.65051 ± 0.068	49.66	29.21 ± 0.57
10	40.1	2.02	17.36 ± 0.74	7.80211 ± 0.033	61.28	43.25 ± 0.47
11	38.4	5.50	18.24 ± 0.83	8.20749 ± 0.293	50.71	26.62 ± 0.34

(Tg) glass transition temperature, (a_w) water activity, (AA) antioxidant activity, (*Bc*) viability of *Bc* bacteria, and (EE) encapsulation efficiency.

From the previous physical characterization, it is evident that the spray drying process promoted the obtaining of a powder functional food with particle size and morphology for avoiding particle aggregation, an amorphous microstructure to retain and preserve the active ingredients, and different Tg values to tailor different stabilities during storage.

3.4. Antioxidant Activity

The antioxidant activity (AA) was determined in terms of radical-scavenging using the stable DPPH radical. Reduction of DPPH• by an antioxidant (DPPH• + A → DPPH-H + A•) or by a radical species (DPPH• + R• → DPPH-R) results in a loss of absorbance at 515 nm [34]. The AA was determined at concentrations of 2.5, 5 and 15 μg/mL. The results showed a noticeable increase in the AA at 15 μg/mL for all the samples. Figure 4 shows the DDPH scavenging activity (%) of the spray-dried powders containing the active ingredients (INMX_1–11). The observed antioxidant activity was related to the content of quercetin released after 30 min of exposition. Evidently, the ability to scavenge free radicals increased with the amount of quercetin released. The AA values are presented in Table 2. Run 7 (INMX_7) showed the lowest AA value of 6.91%, while run 4 (INMX_4) had the highest value of 27.03%. These experiments corresponding to the 50-50 blend of IN-MX dried at 126 °C, and to the IN dried at 180 °C with the highest concentration of solids (28%), respectively. By comparing the single carrying agents, IN showed a higher AA than MX at all the drying temperatures. This suggested a tight binding between MX and quercetin, that retains quercetin bioactivity from interacting with free DPPH radicals.

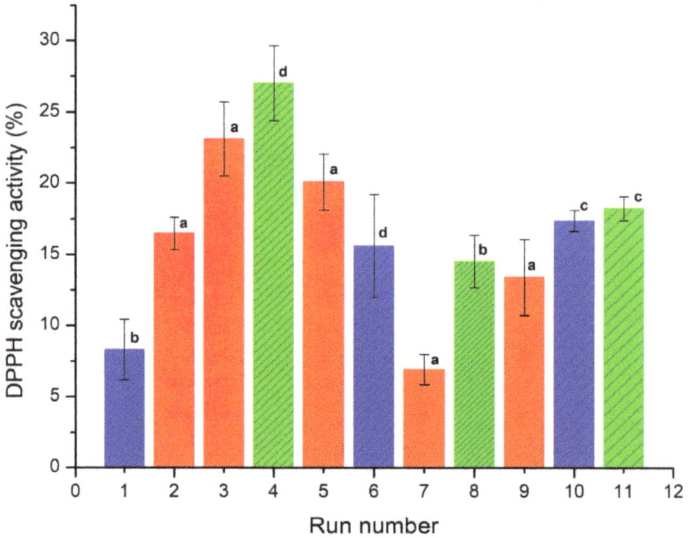

Figure 4. DDPH scavenging capacity (%) of the spray-dried powders containing the active ingredients (INMX_1–11) at 30 min of exposition. Bar color indicates the polysaccharide group (blue for MX, green for IN, and red for blends). Pattern thickness indicates the drying temperature (dense for low temperature, medium for intermediate temperature, and sparse for high temperature). Lowercase letters indicate the Tukey's test results at significance level of 0.05. a: significance difference, effect of drying temperature; b: significance difference, effect of composition at 150 °C; c: no significance difference, effect of composition at 210 °C; d: significance difference, effect of composition at 180 °C and 28.4% solids.

For the microencapsulates prepared with carbohydrate blends (INMX_2, 3, 5, 7, and 9) the AA values varied in the range of 6.91–23.11%, increasing with the drying temperature, and with the content of IN.

IN microencapsulates at the highest concentration (28%) produced the highest antioxidant activity, while at the concentration of 20% (INMX_8 and 11) the AA values were 14.52 and 18.24%. This behavior resulted from the number of dissolved solids in the solution, where quercetin was mixed with the polysaccharide. However, when comparing the samples with the same concentration of solids, i.e., 20%, it is observed that blends INMX_3 and 5 presented higher AA values than those of single IN. Additionally, the IN presents a cost in the market approximately four times higher than the MX. Therefore, reducing the IN content in the food product while maintaining the AA at a high level is beneficial. These observations suggested a synergistic effect on the microencapsulation and conservation of antioxidants when mixing two polysaccharides such as IN and MX.

3.5. Culturability of *B. clausii* after the Spray-Drying Process

Figure 5 shows the results obtained for the survival rate of *B. clausii* microencapsulated after the spray drying process. Each treatment was inoculated with a population of 10.32 log CFU/g of lactobacillus. All treatments presented at least one log reduction cycle due to the spray drying process. Equal to our results, Paim et al. [35] reported that spray drying caused a reduction near of 1 log cycle in *Bifidobacterium* spp. Lactis encapsulated at temperatures similar to those employed in this work.

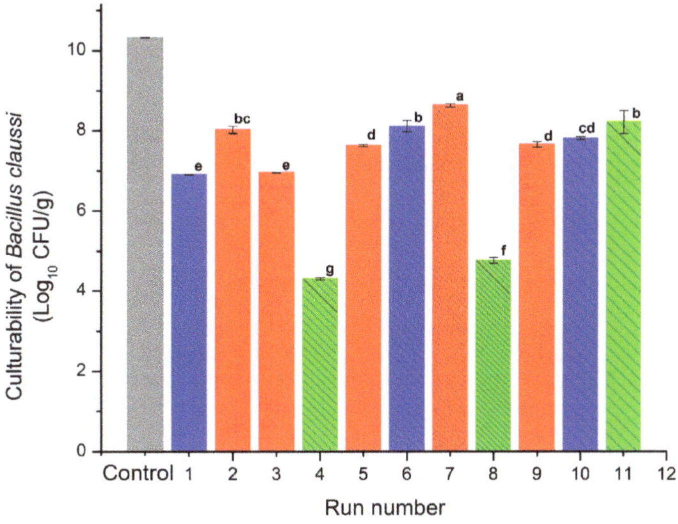

Figure 5. Culturability of *B. clausii* of the spray-dried powders containing the active ingredients (INMX_1–11). Bar color indicates the polysaccharide group (blue for MX, green for IN, and red for blends). Pattern thickness indicates the drying temperature (dense for low temperature, medium for intermediate temperature, and sparse for high temperature). Lowercase letters (a–g) indicate the Tukey's test results at significance level of 0.05.

The blends presented similar viability values in the range of 7–8.6 log CFU/g. The highest viability value was presented by the sample dried at the lowest temperature (INMX_7). Except for sample INMX_8 with a viability value of 8.3 log CFU/g, the other samples containing only IN (INMX_4 and 11) presented the lowest cell viability values of 4.2 and 4.6 log CFU/g, respectively. On the other hand, the samples containing only MX presented values between 6.9–8 log CFU/g.

These observations indicated that at low drying temperatures, i.e., 150 °C, IN is more efficient as a microencapsulating agent for the microorganism. Meanwhile, MX performs well as a protective agent for microorganisms in a wide range of temperatures, for example 150–210 °C. In the case of the blends, the addition of MX was beneficial, since it promoted the microencapsulation and conservation of the microorganism in the presence of IN, maintaining relatively high viability throughout the entire range of temperatures tested.

Pandey and Mishra [36] encapsulated *L. plantarum* by spray drying in a matrix composed of inulin, dextran, and maltodextrin. They obtained an optimum composition of 0.4%, 4.6%, and 8.4% of inulin, dextran, and maltodextrin, respectively. Although inulin provides favorable conditions for the growth and viability of probiotics, the *Bc* microorganisms did not efficiently metabolize the long carbohydrate chains composing the microstructure of IN, and consequently did not increase their viability.

Based on the cell viability results, all of the spray-dried samples prepared in this work (with exception of runs INMX_4 and 11) may be considered as powders with probiotic properties. The powders presented viabilities higher than 6 log CFU/g, which is recommended by FAO/WHO (2003) as the minimum value required to produce therapeutic benefits. Although the use of inulin as single microencapsulating material is not adequate for the survival of the lactobacillus, its addition in the blend may be beneficial as an aid in the spray drying, increasing the overall Tg of the powder and reducing processing problems such as stickiness [37,38].

3.6. Effect of the Processing Conditions on the Yield

A surface response plot (SRP) is a graphical representation of the effect of two experimental variables on a given response variable. These plots have been employed to describe the behavior of polymeric systems under distinct processing conditions [11,39]. In this sense, a SRP was constructed to relate the effect of the spray drying temperature and concentration of IN on the yield (%) of powder obtained. The calculated values of the yield are included in Table 2, while Figure 6 presents the SRP for the yield of the spray-dried powders containing the active ingredients (INMX_1–11). In the *X*-axis is plotted the drying temperature, in the *Y*-axis the IN concentration, and in the *Z*-axis the yield. In the IN concentration axis, the concentration values of cero corresponds to the runs containing only MX (INMX_1, 6 and 10). The IN concentration value of 10% correspond to the blends (INMX_2, 3, 5, 7, and 9), while the concentration values of 20% and 28% belong to the runs containing only IN (INMX_4, 8 and 11). At the lowest concentration value, the yield increased almost linearly with the drying temperature. The highest yield value of 61% was obtained for the run INMX_10, processed at 210 °C and with 20% of MX. The blends showed an increase in the yield with the temperature, reaching a maximum value at the intermediate drying temperature (180 °C), observed as a flat region in the center of the surface. At the high IN concentrations, the yield remained almost unchanged with the temperature. Another noticeable feature observed in the SRP is the color of the fringes, which correspond to different yield values. These fringes are helpful to identify similar yield values obtained at distinct processing conditions. For example, at the temperature of 160 °C and single MX, or a temperature of 150 °C and IN concentration of 25%, either condition may be selected to obtain a yield of 48–49% (central green fringe).

The calculated predicting model derived from the non-linear surface fit is presented in Equation (5):

$$Y(\%) = 13.7401 + 0.26271T + 0.75803C - 2.5014 \times 10^{-4}T^2 + 0.01636C^2 - 0.0073T \times C \quad (5)$$

where Y is the predicted yield (%), T the drying temperature (°C), and C is the IN concentration (%). With this model is possible to predict the value of the yield at different processing conditions of T and C. However, the model is only valid within the values of the processing conditions tested herein.

The encapsulation efficiency (EE) of the encapsulated quercetin in INMX_1–11 blends is shown in Table 2. EE varied in the range of 7–96%, corresponding to a quercetin content of 0.53–12.47 mg of quercetin per g of powder. Single MX presented largest EE values at intermediate and highest drying temperatures, than single IN at the highest drying temperature. The INMX blends presented higher EE values than the single MX and IN powders. In addition, the INMX_3 and 7 showed the highest EE values, corresponding to the highest and lowest drying temperatures, respectively.

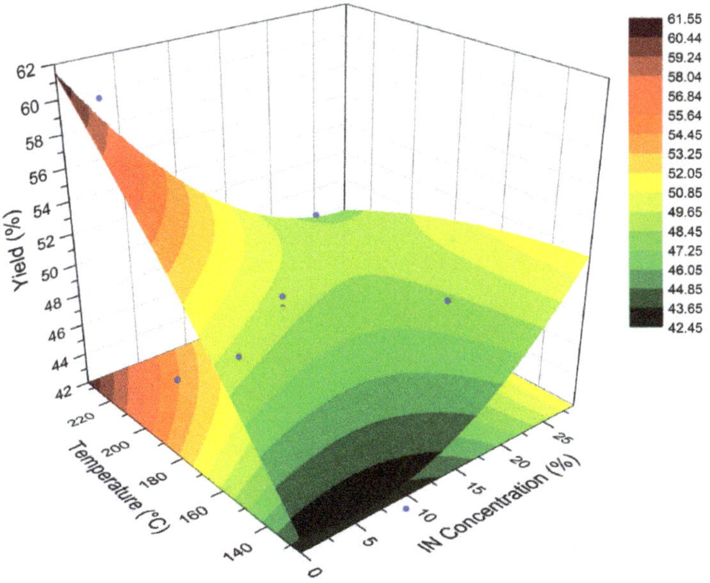

Figure 6. SRP for the yield of the spray-dried powders containing the active ingredients (INMX_1–11).

Cilek et al. [28] extracted and encapsulated the phenolic compounds from sour cherry pomace by freeze-dried. They employed MX and GA at ratios of 1:10 and 1:20, and 10% of solids concentration. The powders with only MX presented an EE of 69.38%, while for the blends, the EE increased up to 92.26% when increasing the GA content to a ratio of 6:4. The same behavior was observed in the current investigation, where higher EE was obtained when employing 1:1 blends of IN and MX.

Etzbach et al. [40] microencapsulated golden berry juice by spray drying using six different carrier agents and blends at 140 °C of inlet temperature and 20% of solids concentration. They determined carotenoid retention in the range of 16.4–77.2%, and attributed this behavior to different particle morphologies and drying rates caused by the viscosity of the feed suspension. The extent of the spray drying process depends on the viscosity of the feed suspension. During the spray drying, the first drying phase is formed at lower temperatures, while the second drying phase or crust is formed at higher temperatures. Highly viscous feed suspensions such as those containing AL and GA provoke circulation currents within the droplet, promoting a rapid crust formation of the first drying phase. Low viscous feed suspensions such as those containing MX reduce the exposure to high drying temperatures since the first drying phase of crust formation is extended.

4. Conclusions

A powdered functional food based on blends of carbohydrate polymers was prepared by spray drying. The resulting powders were composed of inulin (IN), maltodextrin (MX), and active ingredients with antioxidant and probiotic properties such as quercetin and *Bacillus clausii*, respectively. The physical characterization showed a non-aggregated powder with pseudo-spherical shape particles of micrometric sizes. The observation of rod-like particles in the blends and not in the single polysaccharides, suggested that the microorganisms were microencapsulated in these type of particles. An amorphous microstructure indicated the microencapsulation of the active ingredients within the particles, while the diffraction peaks suggested the crystallization of quercetin. The determined Tg values were above the room temperature, which may promote the stability of the powder during storage. The antioxidant activity and viability showed synergistic effects with the IN-MX blends. The antioxidant activity increased with the addition of IN, while the viability increased with the addition of MX. A response surface plot (RSP) was constructed for the yield of the functional food powder. The yield of the blends was slightly more affected by the drying temperature than by the IN concentration. This RSP was useful to identify regions of similar yield values at different processing conditions. The INMX blends presented higher encapsulation efficiency (EE) values than the single MX and IN powders.

This work showed the beneficial use of blends of carbohydrate polymers for the microencapsulation and preservation of active ingredients for food and pharmaceutical applications.

Author Contributions: Conceptualization, C.L.-P. and M.Z.S.-L.; methodology, M.R.-A., A.T.-T., V.E.-S. and A.F.-V.; software, C.L.-P. and M.Z.S.-L.; validation, C.L.-P. and M.Z.S.-L.; formal analysis, M.Z.S.-L., M.R.-A., A.T.-T., V.E.-S., A.F.-V. and C.L.-P.; investigation, C.L.-P. and M.Z.S.-L.; resources, M.Z.S.-L.; data curation, M.Z.S.-L., M.R.-A., A.T.-T., V.E.-S., A.F.-V. and C.L.-P. and M.Z.S.-L.; writing—original draft preparation, C.L.-P.; writing—review and editing, M.R.-A. and C.L.-P.; visualization, M.R.-A., A.T.-T. and V.E.-S.; supervision, M.Z.S.-L.; project administration, C.L.-P.; funding acquisition, C.L.-P. All authors have read and agreed to the published version of the manuscript.

Funding: This research was funded by the Centro de Investigación en Materiales Avanzados S.C. (CIMAV); grant number CCDPI-21/2021.

Institutional Review Board Statement: Not applicable.

Informed Consent Statement: Not applicable.

Data Availability Statement: Data are contained within the article.

Acknowledgments: The authors thank Andrés Isaak González Jacquez from CIMAV for the XRD analysis support, and the Laboratorio Nacional de Nanotecnología (Nanotech) for the use of the SEM. C.L.-P. thanks Andrea P. Balderrama-Aguilar for her support in the grammatical correction of the revised manuscript.

Conflicts of Interest: The authors declare no conflict of interest. The funders had no role in the design of the study; in the collection, analyses, or interpretation of data; in the writing of the manuscript, or in the decision to publish the results.

References

1. Milner, J. Functional foods and health promotion. *J. Nutr.* **1999**, *129*, 1395S–1397S. [CrossRef] [PubMed]
2. Konstantinidi, M.; Koutelidakis, A.E. Functional foods and bioactive compounds: A review of its possible role on weight management and obesity's metabolic consequences. *Medicines* **2019**, *6*, 94. [CrossRef] [PubMed]
3. Cederholm, T.; Barazzoni, R.; Austin, P.; Ballmer, P.; Biolo, G.; Bischoff, S.C.; Compher, C.; Correia, I.; Higashiguchi, T.; Holst, M. ESPEN guidelines on definitions and terminology of clinical nutrition. *Clin. Nutr.* **2017**, *36*, 49–64. [CrossRef] [PubMed]
4. Pandey, K.R.; Naik, S.R.; Vakil, B.V. Probiotics, prebiotics and synbiotics-a review. *J. Food Sci. Technol.* **2015**, *52*, 7577–7587. [CrossRef] [PubMed]
5. Tripathi, M.K.; Giri, S.K. Probiotic functional foods: Survival of probiotics during processing and storage. *J. Funct. Foods* **2014**, *9*, 225–241. [CrossRef]
6. Lee, L.; Choi, E.; Kim, C.; Sung, J.; Kim, Y.; Seo, D.; Choi, H.; Choi, Y.; Kum, J.; Park, J. Contribution of flavonoids to the antioxidant properties of common and tartary buckwheat. *J. Cereal Sci.* **2016**, *68*, 181–186. [CrossRef]
7. Masisi, K.; Beta, T.; Moghadasian, M.H. Antioxidant properties of diverse cereal grains: A review on in vitro and in vivo studies. *Food Chem.* **2016**, *196*, 90–97. [CrossRef]
8. Piñón-Balderrama, C.I.; Leyva-Porras, C.; Terán-Figueroa, Y.; Espinosa-Solís, V.; Álvarez-Salas, C.; Saavedra-Leos, M.Z. Encapsulation of active ingredients in food industry by spray-drying and nano spray-drying technologies. *Processes* **2020**, *8*, 889. [CrossRef]
9. Kanatt, S.R.; Chander, R.; Sharma, A. Chitosan and mint mixture: A new preservative for meat and meat products. *Food Chem.* **2008**, *107*, 845–852. [CrossRef]
10. Zhong, Q.; Xia, W. Physicochemical properties of edible and preservative films from chitosan/cassava starch/gelatin blend plasticized with glycerol. *Food Technol. Biotechnol.* **2008**, *46*, 262–269.
11. Saavedra-Leos, M.Z.; Leyva-Porras, C.; López-Martínez, L.A.; González-García, R.; Martínez, J.O.; Compeán Martínez, I.; Toxqui-Terán, A. Evaluation of the spray drying conditions of blueberry juice-maltodextrin on the yield, content, and retention of quercetin 3-d-galactoside. *Polymers* **2019**, *11*, 312. [CrossRef] [PubMed]

12. Leyva-Porras, C.; Saavedra-Leos, M.Z.; Cervantes-González, E.; Aguirre-Bañuelos, P.; Silva-Cázarez, M.B.; Álvarez-Salas, C. Spray drying of blueberry juice-maltodextrin mixtures: Evaluation of processing conditions on content of resveratrol. *Antioxidants* **2019**, *8*, 437. [CrossRef]
13. Saavedra-Leos, M.Z.; Leyva-Porras, C.; Martínez-Guerra, E.; Pérez-García, S.A.; Aguilar-Martínez, J.A.; Álvarez-Salas, C. Physical properties of inulin and inulin–orange juice: Physical characterization and technological application. *Carbohyd. Polym.* **2014**, *105*, 10–19. [CrossRef] [PubMed]
14. Araujo-Díaz, S.; Leyva-Porras, C.; Aguirre-Bañuelos, P.; Álvarez-Salas, C.; Saavedra-Leos, Z. Evaluation of the physical properties and conservation of the antioxidants content, employing inulin and maltodextrin in the spray drying of blueberry juice. *Carbohydr. Polym.* **2017**, *167*, 317–325. [CrossRef] [PubMed]
15. Vázquez-Maldonado, D.; Espinosa-Solis, V.; Leyva-Porras, C.; Aguirre-Bañuelos, P.; Martinez-Gutierrez, F.; Román-Aguirre, M.; Saavedra-Leos, M.Z. Preparation of spray-pried functional food: Effect of adding *Bacillus clausii* bacteria as a co-microencapsulating agent on the conservation of resveratrol. *Processes* **2020**, *8*, 849. [CrossRef]
16. Devi, N.; Sarmah, M.; Khatun, B.; Maji, T.K. Encapsulation of active ingredients in polysaccharide–protein complex coacervates. *Adv. Colloid Interface Sci.* **2017**, *239*, 136–145. [CrossRef]
17. Bordón, M.G.; Paredes, A.J.; Camacho, N.M.; Penci, M.C.; González, A.; Palma, S.D.; Ribotta, P.D.; Martinez, M.L. Formulation, spray-drying and physicochemical characterization of functional powders loaded with chia seed oil and prepared by complex coacervation. *Powder Technol.* **2021**, *391*, 479–493. [CrossRef]
18. Guo, Q.; Shu, X.; Hu, Y.; Su, J.; Chen, S.; Decker, E.A.; Gao, Y. Formulated protein-polysaccharide-surfactant ternary complexes for co-encapsulation of curcumin and resveratrol: Characterization, stability and in vitro digestibility. *Food Hydrocoll.* **2021**, *111*, 106265. [CrossRef]
19. Kumar, A.; Saini, C.S. Edible composite bi-layer coating based on whey protein isolate, xanthan gum and clove oil for prolonging shelf life of tomatoes. *Meas. Food* **2021**, *2*, 100005. [CrossRef]
20. Sharifi, S.; Rezazad-Bari, M.; Alizadeh, M.; Almasi, H.; Amiri, S. Use of whey protein isolate and gum Arabic for the co-encapsulation of probiotic *Lactobacillus plantarum* and phytosterols by complex coacervation: Enhanced viability of probiotic in Iranian white cheese. *Food Hydrocoll.* **2021**, *113*, 106496. [CrossRef]
21. Maisuthisakul, P.; Gordon, M.H. Influence of polysaccharides and storage during processing on the properties of mango seed kernel extract (microencapsulation). *Food Chem.* **2012**, *134*, 1453–1460. [CrossRef] [PubMed]
22. de Barros Fernandes, R.V.; Borges, S.V.; Botrel, D.A. Gum arabic/starch/maltodextrin/inulin as wall materials on the microencapsulation of rosemary essential oil. *Carbohydr. Polym.* **2014**, *101*, 524–532. [CrossRef] [PubMed]
23. Silva, V.; Vieira, G.; Hubinger, M. Influence of different combinations of wall materials and homogenisation pressure on the microencapsulation of green coffee oil by spray drying. *Food Res. Int.* **2014**, *61*, 132–143. [CrossRef]
24. Damodharan, K.; Palaniyandi, S.A.; Yang, S.H.; Suh, J.W. Co-encapsulation of lactic acid bacteria and prebiotic with alginate-fenugreek gum-locust bean gum matrix: Viability of encapsulated bacteria under simulated gastrointestinal condition and during storage time. *Biotechnol. Bioprocess Eng.* **2017**, *22*, 265–271. [CrossRef]
25. Poletto, G.; Raddatz, G.C.; Cichoski, A.J.; Zepka, L.Q.; Lopes, E.J.; Barin, J.S.; Wagner, R.; de Menezes, C.R. Study of viability and storage stability of Lactobacillus acidophillus when encapsulated with the prebiotics rice bran, inulin and Hi-maize. *Food Hydrocoll.* **2019**, *95*, 238–244. [CrossRef]
26. Colín-Cruz, M.; Pimentel-González, D.; Carrillo-Navas, H.; Alvarez-Ramírez, J.; Guadarrama-Lezama, A. Co-encapsulation of bioactive compounds from blackberry juice and probiotic bacteria in biopolymeric matrices. *LWT* **2019**, *110*, 94–101. [CrossRef]
27. Brand-Williams, W.; Cuvelier, M.; Berset, C. Use of a free radical method to evaluate antioxidant activity. *LWT* **1995**, *28*, 25–30. [CrossRef]
28. Cilek, B.; Luca, A.; Hasirci, V.; Sahin, S.; Sumnu, G. Microencapsulation of phenolic compounds extracted from sour cherry pomace: Effect of formulation, ultrasonication time and core to coating ratio. *Eur. Food Res. Technol.* **2012**, *235*, 587–596. [CrossRef]
29. Leyva-Porras, C.; López-Pablos, A.L.; Alvarez-Salas, C.; Pérez-Urizar, J.; Saavedra-Leos, Z. Physical properties of inulin and technological applications. In *Polysaccharides*; Ramawat, K.M.J., Ed.; Springer: New York, NY, USA, 2015; pp. 959–984.
30. Saavedra-Leos, Z.; Leyva-Porras, C.; Araujo-Díaz, S.B.; Toxqui-Terán, A.; Borrás-Enríquez, A.J. Technological application of maltodextrins according to the degree of polymerization. *Molecules* **2015**, *20*, 21067–21081. [CrossRef]
31. Klitou, P.; Pask, C.M.; Onoufriadi, L.; Rosbottom, I.; Simone, E. Solid-state characterization and role of solvent molecules on the crystal structure, packing, and physiochemical properties of different quercetin solvates. *Cryst. Growth Des.* **2020**, *20*, 6573–6584. [CrossRef]
32. Saavedra–Leos, M.Z.; Leyva-Porras, C.; Alvarez-Salas, C.; Longoria-Rodríguez, F.; López-Pablos, A.L.; González-García, R.; Pérez-Urizar, J.T. Obtaining orange juice–maltodextrin powders without structure collapse based on the glass transition temperature and degree of polymerization. *CyTA-J. Food* **2018**, *16*, 61–69. [CrossRef]
33. Lavelli, V.; Harsha, P.S.S.; Laureati, M.; Pagliarini, E. Degradation kinetics of encapsulated grape skin phenolics and micronized grape skins in various water activity environments and criteria to develop wide-ranging and tailor-made food applications. *Inn. Food Sci. Emerg. Technol.* **2017**, *39*, 156–164. [CrossRef]
34. Fukumoto, L.; Mazza, G. Assessing antioxidant and prooxidant activities of phenolic compounds. *J. Agric. Food Chem.* **2000**, *48*, 3597–3604. [CrossRef]

35. Paim, D.R.; Costa, S.D.; Walter, E.H.; Tonon, R.V. Microencapsulation of probiotic jussara (*Euterpe edulis* M.) juice by spray drying. *LWT* **2016**, *74*, 21–25. [CrossRef]
36. Pandey, P.; Mishra, H.N. Co-microencapsulation of γ-aminobutyric acid (GABA) and probiotic bacteria in thermostable and biocompatible exopolysaccharides matrix. *LWT* **2021**, *136*, 110293. [CrossRef]
37. Adhikari, B.; Howes, T.; Wood, B.; Bhandari, B. The effect of low molecular weight surfactants and proteins on surface stickiness of sucrose during powder formation through spray drying. *J. Food Eng.* **2009**, *94*, 135–143. [CrossRef]
38. Rajam, R.; Anandharamakrishnan, C. Microencapsulation of *Lactobacillus plantarum* (MTCC 5422) with fructooligosaccharide as wall material by spray drying. *LWT* **2015**, *60*, 773–780. [CrossRef]
39. Leyva-Porras, C.; Balderrama-Aguilar, A.; Estrada-Ávila, Y.; Espelosín-Gómez, I.; Mendoza-Duarte, M.; Piñón-Balderrama, C.; Saavedra-Leos, M.Z.; Estrada-Moreno, I. Injection molding of low-density polyethylene (LDPE) as a model polymer: Effect of molding parameters on the microstructure and crystallinity. *Polymers* **2021**, *13*, 3597. [CrossRef] [PubMed]
40. Etzbach, L.; Meinert, M.; Faber, T.; Klein, C.; Schieber, A.; Weber, F. Effects of carrier agents on powder properties, stability of carotenoids, and encapsulation efficiency of goldenberry (*Physalis peruviana* L.) powder produced by co-current spray drying. *Curr. Res. Food Sci.* **2020**, *3*, 73–81. [CrossRef] [PubMed]

polymers

Article

Chitosan Reinforced with Kenaf Nanocrystalline Cellulose as an Effective Carrier for the Delivery of Platelet Lysate in the Acceleration of Wound Healing

Payal Bhatnagar [1], Jia Xian Law [2,*] and Shiow-Fern Ng [1,*]

[1] Centre for Drug Delivery Technology, Faculty of Pharmacy, Universiti Kebangsaan Malaysia, Jalan Raja Muda Abdul Aziz, Kuala Lumpur 50300, Malaysia; payalbhatnagar2020@gmail.com

[2] Centre for Tissue Engineering & Regenerative Medicine, 12th Floor, Clinical Block, UKM Medical Centre, Jalan Yaa'cob Latif, Cheras, Kuala Lumpur 56000, Malaysia

* Correspondence: lawjx@ppukm.ukm.edu.my (J.X.L.); nsfern@ukm.edu.my (S.-F.N.); Tel.: +60-3-9145-7677 (J.X.L.); +60-3-9289-7977 (S.-F.N.); Fax: +60-3-9289-7060 (S.-F.N.)

Abstract: The clinical use of platelet lysate (PL) in the treatment of wounds is limited by its rapid degradation by proteases at the tissue site. This research aims to develop a chitosan (CS) and kenaf nanocrystalline cellulose (NCC) hydrogel composite, which intend to stabilize PL and control its release onto the wound site for prolonged action. NCC was synthesized from raw kenaf bast fibers and incorporated into the CS hydrogel. The physicochemical properties, in vitro cytocompatibility, cell proliferation, wound scratch assay, PL release, and CS stabilizing effect of the hydrogel composites were analyzed. The study of swelling ratio (>1000%) and moisture loss (60–90%) showed the excellent water retention capacity of the CS-NCC-PL hydrogels as compared with the commercial product. In vitro release PL study (flux = 0.165 mg/cm^2/h) indicated that NCC act as a nanofiller and provided the sustained release of PL compared with the CS hydrogel alone. The CS also showed the protective effect of growth factor (GF) present in PL, thereby promoting fast wound healing via the formulation. The CS-NCC hydrogels also augmented fibroblast proliferation in vitro and enhanced wound closures over 72 h. This study provides a new insight on CS with renewable source kenaf NCC as a nanofiller as a potential autologous PL wound therapy.

Keywords: chitosan; kenaf; nanocrystalline cellulose; platelet lysate; wound healing

Citation: Bhatnagar, P.; Law, J.X.; Ng, S.-F. Chitosan Reinforced with Kenaf Nanocrystalline Cellulose as an Effective Carrier for the Delivery of Platelet Lysate in the Acceleration of Wound Healing. *Polymers* **2021**, *13*, 4392. https://doi.org/10.3390/polym13244392

Academic Editors: Bramasta Nugraha and Faisal Raza

Received: 22 October 2021
Accepted: 30 November 2021
Published: 15 December 2021

1. Introduction

In the last decade, biopolymers have attracted substantial attention mainly because of their renewability, biocompatibility, biodegradability, and abundance. Nanocellulose, a biopolymer derived from plants, is a promising biomaterial in skin grafts, implants, tissue engineering, and wound healing. Nanocellulose are classified into nanocrystalline cellulose (NCC) and cellulose nanofibrils (CNF). NCC consists of amorphous and highly ordered crystalline cellulose structures. NCC exhibits overwhelming performance as a nanomaterial because of its dimensions 5–100 nm in diameter with lengths up to hundreds of nanometers (100–600 nm). NCC can be obtained from inexpensive biomass renewable resources, such as wood, shrubs, and herbs. Plant-derived NCC is highly beneficial for wound dressing applications because of its high capability to absorb liquids and form translucent films [1]. These properties are crucial for non-healing and chronic wounds, where exudates need to be managed adequately. In addition, the translucency of NCC allows the wound development to be evaluated without needing to remove the dressing. Agricultural waste is a valuable source of advanced biomaterials. Nanocellulose may be obtained from agro-waste and further used as reinforcement in biopolymers. Kenaf (*Hibiscus cannabinus* L.) is an important industrial crop with high economic and ecological importance in many tropical countries, including Malaysia. Kenaf plant components that are of industrial importance include bast and core fibers. Bast fibers are isolated from the outer layer of plant fibers (30% of dry weight), whereas the core refers to the inner fiber layer (70% of dry weight). Bast fibers have been extensively investigated for their excellent mechanical properties because of their high length-to-diameter ratio and superior crystallinity, allowing these fibers to be applied as a reinforcing agent with other natural or synthetic polymers for biomedical applications [2]. NCC isolated from kenaf waste has been extended to various scientific research for their special characteristics, such as sustainability, affordability, and well-established mechanical, thermal, and electrical properties, which attracted scientists to develop new promising materials with unique values [3]. Currently, the use of kenaf-derived nanocelluloses is limited to the packaging and paper industries. The use of kenaf-based NCC as wound dressing has yet to be researched and explored.

Platelet lysate (PL) derived from platelet-rich plasma (PRP) is an autologous source of therapeutic proteins that is extensively researched in hard-to-heal wounds and tissue regeneration [4–6]. PL is a rich source of growth factors (GFs), including epidermal growth factor (EGF), insulin-like growth factor (IGF), transforming growth factor beta (TGF-β), platelet-derived growth factor (PDGF), which are crucial in regulating cell proliferation, migration, and differentiation by binding to specific transmembrane receptors on target cells. EGF secreted during the hemostasis of inflammation by platelets exhibits chemotactic effect on keratinocytes by promoting re-epithelialization [7,8]. TGF-β has three isoforms (i.e., TGF-β; 1–3). TGF-β1 is highly produced during wound healing by platelets, neutrophils, macrophages, and fibroblasts and is responsible for the synthesis of extracellular matrix components. IGF is discharged by platelets at the beginning of hemostasis. It entices leukocytes and participates in cell inflammation and proliferation. Thus, IGF serves a regulatory function in fibroblast proliferation in tissues. The PL serves as the cellular induction of normal wound healing responses and PL therapy has clinical significance regardless of the wound etiology. Hence, PL applications have gained considerable popularity in tissue regeneration and wound healing. GFs are released quickly from PL; thus, their activity and clinical efficacy are easily lost [9]. As a result, hydrogels or carriers suitable for PL are highly sought after by researchers.

Chitosan (CS) is a polysaccharide which chemically exist as (1→4)-2 amino-2-deoxy-β-D-glucan; originated from chitin, a key constituent of crustacean outer skeletons commonly used as an antimicrobial agent for preventing and treating infections owing to its natural antimicrobial property [10]. CS shows unique hemostatic properties and promotes the infiltration and migration of neutrophils and macrophages in early stages of wound healing, making it a suitable biopolymer for wound dressing [11]. CS exists in the form of 3D hydrogel polymer networks that can absorb and retain a large quantity of moisture on account of the abundance of hydrophilic groups [12]. CS dressings provoke minimal adverse reactions with little or almost absent fibrous encapsulation and provide protection against bacterial infections [13]. Recently, CS and modified CS have been deemed suitable for the delivery of PRP or PL to wounds [6–15]. Rossi et al. demonstrated via PDGF evaluation that CS dressings maintain the platelet GF in unaltered active form [14]. CS fibers also tightly bind with major plasma proteins and at specific platelet surface proteins. The combination of CS with PL shows the sustained release of GFs and increases glycoprotein IIIa expression in platelets [16].

Despite the significant therapeutic potential of PL in wound repair, PL generally suffers clinical limitations, such as short half-life, instability, degradation by protease at the tissue site, and toxicity at high systemic dose [17]. An efficient delivery system has been sought to stabilize PL for its sustained release in wound healing. The applicability of NCC as a potential cell culture scaffold has been previously reported because it provides the desired 3D environments for the growth and differentiation of skin cells [18,19]. A successful PL delivery system from hydrogels could be developed by mimicking tissue regeneration in terms of endogenous release profiles of PL. This research aimed to develop a CS hydrogel reinforced with NCC and loaded with PL as a controlled-release vehicle for wound healing. CS with a 2% w/v was employed as a PL stabilizing agent and cell growth-promoting polymer and added with NCC 0.4% *w/v* to provide a nanocellulose network that can facilitate the loading and delivery of PL in wound healing.

2. Materials and Methods

2.1. Materials

Kenaf raw bast fiber was provided by the National Kenaf and Tobacco Board (Lembaga Kenaf dan Tembakau Negara, LKTN), Malaysia. Low-molecular-weight (LMW, analytical grade) CS (molecular weight of 50–190 kDa, 75–85% degree of deacetylation) was purchased from Sigma Aldrich (Dublin, Ireland), glacial acetic acid (GAA; 100%) was purchased from R.M Chemicals Pvt. Ltd. (Chandigarh, India), PL, cell culture media, and primary skin cells were received from Centre For Tissue Engineering and Regenerative Medicine (CTERM), UKM. Enzyme-linked immunosorbent assay (ELISA) kit was obtained from Insphiro Technology (Selangor, Malaysia). Alamar Blue was obtained from Invitrogen (Waltham, MA, USA). Dulbecco's phosphate-buffered saline (DPBS) and fetal bovine serum (FBS) were purchased from Biowest (Riverside, MO, USA). Collagenase type I was obtained from Worthington (Columbus, OH, USA), Dulbecco's modified Eagle's medium (F12: DMEM; 1:1), antibacterial–antimycotic, Glutamax, and 4-(2-hydroxyethyl)-1-piperazine ethane sulfonic acid (HEPES) were procured from Gibco (Grand Island, NY, USA). All chemicals, such as sodium hydroxide (NaOH), sodium chlorite ($NaClO_2$), and sulfuric acid (H_2SO_4), were analytical grade (Dublin, Ireland).

2.2. Preparation of Nanocrystalline Cellulose from Kenaf Bast Fibers

NCC was extracted from raw kenaf bast fibers adapted from previous method with slight modifications [20]. Briefly, the retting of raw bast fibers was carried out by soaking it in distilled water overnight and filtered several times with subsequent drying at 60 °C in the oven. The dried fibers were ground and sieved to obtain finer fibers. Thereafter, pulverization was carried out by treating the fibers with 5% (*w/v*) NaOH at 80 °C for 2 h, and this step was carried out thrice to accomplish delignification. The fibers were then thoroughly washed and filtered using distilled water to remove residual chemicals. Subsequently, the alkali-treated fibers were bleached using a combination of acetic acid and sodium chlorite to remove residual lignin and hemicellulose. The bleached pulp was filtered and washed numerous times after a series of bleaching procedures until the pH reached 7. The bleaching treatment was repeated five times at 80 °C for 3 h to obtain white fibers and thereafter stored in water swollen state. Finally, acid hydrolysis was commenced by immersing 4% (*w/w*) bleached kenaf bast fibers into 65% (*v/v*) sulfuric acid at a temperature of 45 °C for 30 min. The fiber suspension was constantly homogenized using a magnetic stirrer. Then, the fiber suspension was diluted by adding distilled water and allowed to cool. Afterwards, the acid was removed by centrifuging the fiber suspension at 12,000× *g* rpm for 30 min, and this process was repeated five times for complete removal of residual acid. Then, the fiber pellet was dispersed in distilled water and poured into a dialysis bag (MWCO 11 KDa; cellulose acetate) under slow stirring until complete neutralization. Subsequently, the suspension of tiny fibers was ultrasonicated for 5 min at a frequency of 20 kHz with an amplitude of 80%. This process was carried out under an ice box to prevent overheating. The resulting thick suspension containing the NCC was stored at 4 °C and freeze-dried for further characterization and hydrogel preparation.

2.3. PL Processing and Quantification of GFs

The PL was processed aseptically by freeze-thawing for one cycle and subsequently centrifuged at 5000× *g* rpm at 4 °C for 20 min. The resulting pellet containing cell debris was discarded and the processed PL was kept at −80 °C with the addition of 40 IU of LMW heparin as an anticoagulant until further use.

The concentrations of key GFs (EGF and TGF) were determined using ELISA based on Sandwich-ELISA using 96-well plates in accordance with the manufacturer's instructions.

Optical density (OD) were measured under 450 nm wavelength using a microplate reader Bio-Rad (Berkeley, CA, USA).

2.4. Preparation of CS Hydrogel and CS-NCC Composite Hydrogels

The porous CS hydrogels were prepared as previously described method with slight modifications [21]. In brief, 2% (*w*/*v*) CS solution was prepared by dissolving fine CS powder in 1% GAA, and pH was adjusted to 7.0 using 1 M NaOH. Subsequently, the solution was stirred on a magnetic stirrer for 1 h at room temperature. Afterward, CS solution was transferred into 24-well tissue-culture plates and frozen at −20 °C for 24 h, followed by freeze drying (Labconco, Topeka, KS, USA, Model no.117; weight-24 kg) at −80 °C for 4 days to ensure complete drying.

CS hydrogels containing PL (CS-PL) were made by mixing 1 mL of PL/gram of CS hydrogel (2% *w*/*v*) on a magnetic stirrer for 30 min at 20 °C. Then, the mixture was transferred to a 24-well tissue-culture plate for lyophilization at −80 °C for 4 days.

As for the CS-NCC composite hydrogel, NCC was dispersed in deionized water (DI) to produce a 0.4% (*w*/*v*) concentration [22]. Then, the slurry of NCC was added to the 2% (*w*/*v*) solution of CS. The resulting dispersion was ultra-sonicated at an amplitude of 40% for 5 min to homogenize NCC in CS solution and then allowed to mix for 1 h on a magnetic stirrer in a closed reactor. Then, acetic acid (1%) was added to solubilize the CS and the mixture was mechanically stirred for the next 5 h to obtain a complete dissolution of CS. Consequently, hydrogels were formed through the neutralization of the viscous suspension of CS by pouring it on a petri plate containing 1 M NaOH for 1 h. The prepared hydrogels were washed with distilled water until a neutral pH was obtained. Finally, the composite hydrogel of CS-NCC without using any specific cross-linkers were prepared and subsequently freeze-dried for further characterization. The CS-NCC-PL gel was prepared by thorough mixing of the CS-NCC gel with PL (1 mL/g). The CS-NCC gel was stored in the refrigerator at 4 °C. Upon use, PL (stored at −80 °C) was thawed to room temperature prior and added into the CS-NCC gel via simple mixing. The unused CS-NCC-PL hydrogel was stored at −20 °C but thawed to room temperature before tests.

2.5. Characterization of NCC and Hydrogels

2.5.1. Chemical Composition, Fiber Yield, and Zeta Potential

Chemical composition of NCC was determined in accordance with TAPPI standard methods T 222 (acid-insoluble lignin in wood and pulp) [23]. The fiber yield of NCC was calculated in terms of percentage (%) of the initial weight of bleached fibers after hydrolysis. The suspension of the fiber obtained after dialysis treatment was freeze-dried and compared with the initial weight of fiber. The final weight of NCC (*Mf*) and the initial weight of fiber (*Mi*) were measured to calculate the yield using Equation (1) [24]. Fiber yield was calculated using the following equation.

$$\text{Yield } (\%) = (Mf/Mi) \times 100 \quad (1)$$

The zeta-potential of NCC was determined using Zetasizer Nano-ZS (Malvern Instruments Ltd., Malvern, UK) to identify the electrical charges of NCC. The NCC samples were tested after acid hydrolysis of the fiber suspension.

2.5.2. X-ray Diffraction Characterization (XRD)

XRD patterns of bleached and NCC from kenaf bast fibers were performed on X-ray diffractometer (Empyrean PANalytical, Marvin, UK) to examine the changes in crystallinity before and after chemical treatment. The diffraction intensity of Cu Kα radiation (λ = 0.1542 nm; 40 kV and 40 mA) was measured in a 2θ range between 5° and 70° with scan rate of 0.5° per min. Peak analysis was performed using Diffrac.EvaV4.0 software. Meanwhile, the crystallinity index of fibers was calculated as previously described method [25] using the following Equation (2).

$$CrI\ (\%) = [I_{002} - I_{amorph}/I_{002}] \times 100 \quad (2)$$

where CrI is the crystallinity index is the maximum peak intensity at the (002) plane (around 22.5° for native cellulose) and I_{amorph} is the minimum intensity of the amorphous portion taken at 2θ = 18°

2.5.3. Scanning Electron Microscopy (SEM)

A SEM instrument (Carl Zeiss Merlin Compact-Germany, Oberkochen, Germany) was used to observe the surface morphology of NCC. The acceleration voltage was set up in the range of 5 to 20 kV, and dried samples were sputter-coated with gold to avoid the charging effect during SEM observations. The fiber diameter was measured by using Smart TIFF image viewer software.

2.5.4. Fourier Transform Infrared Spectroscopy-Attenuated Total Reflectance (FTIR-ATR) Spectroscopy

FTIR-ATR spectroscopy (Spectrum 100; Perkin Elmer, Walthman, MA, USA) was performed on raw fibers, bleached fibers, NCC, CS, PL, CS-NCC, CS-PL, and CS-NCC-PL hydrogels.

Infrared spectra of CS hydrogel control, PL, NCC, CS hydrogel-reinforced PL, and NCC were determined between 4000 and 650 cm^{-1} using FTIR-ATR spectrometer (Spectrum 100; Perkin Elmer, Walthman, MA, USA). The spectra were acquired using 32 scans and a 4 cm^{-1} resolution.

2.5.5. Swelling Behavior of Hydrogels

The swelling behavior of freeze-dried samples of CS, CS-NCC, CS-NCC-PL, CS-PL hydrogel, and Intrasite™ gel as positive control were tested in DI at 37 °C for 3, 6, and 24 h. The dried samples were weighed and placed in 20 mL of DI, and the hydrogels were allowed to reach their swelling equilibrium. The weights of the hydrogels (W2) were measured at 3, 6, and 24 h of duration. All formulations were run in triplicates, and average values were presented. The swelling ratio was calculated using the following Equation (3).

$$\text{Swelling ratio}\ (\%) = (W2 - W1)/(W1) \times 100 \quad (3)$$

where W1 is the weight before swelling and W2 is the weight after swelling

2.5.6. Moisture Loss Study

The moisture retention capacity of the hydrogels was evaluated using the desiccant method of Standard Test Method for Water Vapour Transmission of Materials (ASTM E96/E96M-16, 2015) [26]. Hydrogel samples (0.5 g, triplicates) were spread in thin layers in a 2 cm-diameter crucible. The samples were then placed into airtight containers lined with a bed of silica gel as a desiccant. After 24 h, the crucibles containing the samples were re-weighed and percentage of moisture loss was calculated using the following Equation (4).

$$\text{Moisture Loss}\ (\%) = (W2/W1) \times 100 \quad (4)$$

where W1 is the weight of the crucible before drying and W2 is the weight of the crucible after drying. Moisture loss was the water loss from the exposed surface of hydrogels over 24 h. The test was conducted on the CS, CS-NCC, CS-PL, CS-NCC-PL hydrogels. Intrasite™ gel served as the positive control.

2.5.7. In Vitro Protein Release Assessment

The in vitro release profile of PL was investigated on two hydrogel preparations: CS-PL and CS-NCC-PL. Protein release was studied using Franz diffusion cell (Permegear

Inc., Hellertown, PA, USA) in triplicates. All samples were prepared by mixing 5 mg/g of PL in hydrogel, and the proteins were incorporated into the hydrogel overnight at −10 °C. The release study was conducted using a cellulose acetate membrane with a mesh size of 0.45 µm. DI at pH 7.0 was used as the receptor medium. The receptor chamber was filled with DI until the mark of the sampling port was reached. The cellulose acetate membrane was then placed on top of the receptor chamber opening (0.7855 cm^2). The receptor chamber was maintained at 37 ± 1 °C in a circulating water bath. The hydrogel weighing 1 g was placed on top of the cellulose acetate membrane, and all of the compartments were held together with a clamp. Samples (1 mL) were withdrawn at predetermined time intervals at 3, 6, and 24 h. The receptor medium was replaced with an equal volume of DI to maintain the sink conditions. The released proteins in the media were added with a few drops of Bradford reagent and assayed using a UV-Vis spectrophotometer (Shimadzu, Kyoto, Japan) at 280 nm. DI served as a blank. The absorbance of each sample was determined and recorded. The concentration of unknown proteins was then calculated by plotting the calibration curve. The cumulative amount of proteins that permeated out of the membrane was calculated and plotted against time (h). This experiment was repeated in triplicates for the in vitro release and characterization of therapeutic proteins present in PL that were incorporated in the hydrogel. A validated UV spectrophotometric method was used to quantify the PL loaded in the hydrogel systems at 280 nm to determine the concentration of proteins released at 3, 6, and 24 h.

2.6. *Cytocompatibility Studies*

2.6.1. Isolation of Human Dermal Fibroblast (HDF)

This study was approved by the Universiti Kebangsaan Malaysia Research Ethics Committee (UKM PPI/111/8/JEP-2021-052). Redundant abdominoplasty skin tissue samples were received from the patient with written informed consent and processed within 48 h with the ISO protocol followed at CTERM. The skin was completely rinsed in DPBS, cut into small pieces (1–2 cm^2), and immersed overnight in 10 mL of serum-free Epilife medium containing 25.3 mg of Dispase at 2–8 °C to isolate the epidermis from the dermis layers. On the next day, the epidermis layer was separated from the dermis layer. Thereafter, the dermis was chopped into smaller pieces and digested with 0.6% collagenase type I (Worthington, Columbus, OH, USA) for 4–8 h in an incubator shaker maintained at 37 °C. The cell suspension was centrifuged at 5000× *g* rpm for 5 min at 37 °C, and the cell pellet was rinsed with DPBS after trypsinization with TE-EDTA (0.05%). Finally, the cell pellet was re-suspended in F12: DMEM (1:1) supplemented with 10% FBS, 1% antibacterial–antimycotic, 1% Glutamax, and 2% HEPES. Cells were cultured at 37 °C in 5% CO_2 with the medium changed every 2–3 days.

2.6.2. Cell Culture

HDFs were used to study the cytocompatibility of the hydrogels. Cells with the passage of P1-3 were cultured in F12: DMEM supplemented with 10% FBS at 37 °C in an incubator supplemented with 5% CO_2. PL (10%) was used alone, as well as in all hydrogel formulations. The culture medium was replenished every 2–3 days and subsequently trypsinized once more than 90% confluence was achieved and transferred to T75 flasks for further assay.

2.6.3. Cell Viability

The cytotoxic effect of the fabricated hydrogels (CS, CS-NCC, and CS-NCC-PL) on skin cells was investigated. Cell viability assay was performed indirectly using primary HDFs (CTERM, UKM Medical Centre, Kuala Lumpur, Malaysia) cultured in DMEM by utilizing Alamar Blue. All cells were maintained at 37 °C in humidified 5% CO_2 atmosphere. In this study, all hydrogel samples were washed with sterile DPBS and then incubated in a culture medium for 24 h to obtain the leachates (membrane sterilized 0.22 µm) from the hydrogel. HDFs with passage number P2 were seeded onto a 96-well plate at a density of 10^4 cells/well and incubated in fresh media for 24 h at 37 °C to ensure cell attachment and proliferation. Leachates from the hydrogels were sterilized by membrane filtration (0.45 μm). Afterward, the culture medium was replaced with leachates of the hydrogels of volume 200 μL in each well. The microplate was then incubated for 24, 48, and 72 h, and 10% of Alamar Blue was added at the end of each time points and incubated for 4 h in the dark. Finally, OD was measured at 570 nm using a microplate reader (BioTek PowerWave XS, Winooski, VT, USA). The results were calculated as percentage cell viability relative to the control group (cells without hydrogel treatment) from Equation (5).

$$\text{Cell viability (\%)} = [\text{OD of treated/OD of control}] \times 100 \quad (5)$$

2.6.4. Cell Proliferation

All hydrogel samples were placed in a micro well plate and washed with sterile DPBS prior to analysis. Thereafter, culture media were added and then incubated for 24 h to retrieve the extract from the hydrogels indirectly as previously mentioned in cell viability assay. HDFs (1×10^4) were seeded in a 96-well plate for 24 h and subsequently treated with sterile hydrogel extracts. DMEM was used as control and incubated for 24, 48, and 72 h. Alamar Blue cell proliferation assay was carried out as per the manufacturer's protocol in accordance with previous work [27]. Alamar Blue (10%) was added into each well containing the control and treatment groups and incubated at 37 °C for 4 h in the dark. Absorbance was recorded using a spectrophotometer (BioTek, PowerWave XS, USA) at 570 and 600 nm. The percent reduction in Alamar Blue was calculated from following [Equation (6)].

$$\text{Percent reduction (\%)} = [(\varepsilon OX)\ \lambda 2A\lambda 1 - (\varepsilon OX)\ \lambda 1A\lambda 2]/[(\varepsilon RED)\ \lambda 1A'\lambda 2 - (\varepsilon RED)\ \lambda 2A'\lambda 1] \times 100 \quad (6)$$

where (εOX) λ2 = 117,216, (εOX) λ1 = 80,586, (εRED) λ1 = 155,677, (εRED) λ2 = 14,652. Aλ1 and Aλ2 = Observed absorbance reading for the test well at 570 nm and 600 nm, respectively. A'λ1 and A'λ2 = Observed absorbance reading for control well at 570 and 600 nm, respectively.

2.6.5. Scratch Wound Assay

The in vitro wound scratch assay is an economic and fast method to predict the wound healing ability of compounds by assessing their migration rate on the skin cells. In this work, the migration rate of the HDFs was calculated via scratch assay to ensure that the hydrogel formulations do not interfere in wound healing. The HDFs were seeded in a 12-well plate (Greiner Bio-One, Kremstest, Austria) and then incubated at 37 °C in humidified 5% CO_2 atmosphere until 100% confluence. The spent culture was discarded, and a scratch was made at the middle of each well on a cell monolayer using a sterile 10 μL pipette tip. Afterward, the cells were rinsed with DPBS by slight swirling the microplate, and different hydrogel extracts were subsequently added to the scratched cells. Cells without treatment served as the control group. Wound closure was observed through live imaging by acquiring images every 60 min for 72 h at three spots per well using a Nikon A1R-A1 CLSM. Cell migration rate was calculated for 24 h. The tissue-culture plate inclosing cells was fixed inside the Chamlide Incubator System (Live Cell Instrument, Seoul, Korea) at 37 °C and 5% CO_2. The images were analyzed by NIS Elements AR 3.1 (Nikon). The migration rate of the cells was calculated from following [Equation (7)].

$$\text{Cell migration rate} = (\text{measurement at 0 h} - \text{measurement at 24 h})/24\text{ h} \quad (7)$$

2.6.6. LIVE/DEAD® Cell Viability Assay

This assay was conducted to evaluate the functional status of the cells by identifying cytoplasmic esterase activity using the LIVE/DEAD™ Viability/Cytotoxicity kit for mammalian cells (Invitrogen). The kit comprises of calcein, which fluoresces green in living cells, and ethidium bromide, which fluoresces red in dead cells. In brief, the HDFs were plated at the same seeding density as per cell viability and proliferation assay and maintained as above prior to treatment with samples. The cells were treated with calcein and ethidium bromide for 30 min as per the manufacturer's instructions. Later, the cells were rinsed with DBPS and observed using a Nikon A1R fluorescence microscope (Nikon, Tokyo, Japan).

2.6.7. CS Stabilizing Effect on PL

A cell proliferation assay was carried out using protease degradation and heat treatment approaches to establish the protective effect of CS on PL.

Protease Degradation Test

Cell proliferation assay was conducted to determine the protective effect of CS against proteases on GF. In brief, all PL-loaded CS hydrogels and PL alone (10%) were subjected to 0.05% trypsin treatment at 37 °C for 1 h. Then, the HDFs (P2, 2×10^4) were incubated with trypsin-treated PL and CS hydrogel for 24 h followed by Alamar Blue addition to the cells and incubated for the next 4 h. Then, absorbance was recorded at 570 and 600 nm. Cell proliferation was calculated by percentage reduction in Resazurin. Cells without treatment served as control.

Heat Treatment Test

PL (10%) and CS hydrogels containing PL were exposed to 0, 25 °C, 37 °C, and 45 °C for 24 h to examine the stabilizing effect of CS on PL. Then, extracts of both heat-treated groups were added to the HDFs (P3, 2×10^4) as per above method, and cell proliferation was determined.

2.7. Statistical Analysis

Experiments were performed in triplicates and mean ± SD was reported. Data were analyzed using one-way analysis of variance and Tukey's multiple comparisons test, by using GraphPad Prism version 5.00 (GraphPad Software, La Jolla, CA, USA). The level of significance was set at $p < 0.05$.

3. Results

3.1. Quantification of GFs in PL

The concentrations of TGF-β and EGF from PL were measured using ELISA. ELISA was performed for standard and sample as per manual instructions, and concentrations were determined as 477.26 pg/mL and 150 ng/mL for EGF and TGF-β, respectively, from the calibration curves. The level of TGF-β was threefold higher than that of EGF, which is consistent with reported literature [28].

3.2. Chemical Composition, Fiber Yield, Zeta Potential, and Crystallinity of NCC

After various stages of chemical treatment on raw, alkali-treated, and bleached fibers, chemical composition of the fibers was determined as previously described by Tuerxun Duolikun (2018). The results are presented in Table 1. After a series of chemical treatment on the kenaf biomass fibers, cellulose content significantly increased from raw to bleached to 30% to 84%, whereas hemicellulose and lignin contents declined to 5% and 3%, respectively [29].

Table 1. Chemical composition of kenaf fibers after chemical treatments.

Material	Chemical Composition (%)		
	Cellulose	**Hemicellulose**	**Lignin**
Raw	30	31	30
Alkali-Treated	70	20	15
Bleached	84	5	3

The fiber yield of the NCC after acid hydrolysis was 40% (of initial weight), which is consistent with the fiber yield of NCC from other plant sources, such as sisal (30%) and mengkuang leaves (28%) [30]. In general, fiber yield is dependent on pre-treatment methods and hydrolysis environment. The low fiber yield of NCC might be caused by sulfuric acid treatment during production, which caused the degradation and removal of amorphous and other non-cellulosic regions of the fibers that result in weight loss.

The zeta potential of the NCC suspension was recorded as (-10.9 ± 5.47 mV). The NCC becomes crystalline and possesses a negative charge on the surface of the cellulose chain. They become more stable through electrostatic repulsion among the negatively charged groups on the polymer chains [31]. The anionic NCC is found suitable to form composite hydrogels with cationic CS polymer. The abundance of hydroxyl groups in NCC cellulose is responsible for the negative charges that bonded with CS via the electrostatic interaction of protonation of NH_2 on CS and hydroxyl groups. Platelets also carry negative charges onto their surfaces due to the presence of sialic acid (N-acetyl-neuraminic acid) and amino acids such as glutamate and aspartate [32]. PL was loaded into NCC-reinforced CS hydrogel and associated by non-covalent bonding and subsequently stabilized by CS through protein bindings that promote fibrin gel formation and thus retained GF functionality for a long time [9].

Cellulose naturally comprises of crystalline and amorphous portions. The amorphous region (contains impurities of lignin, hemicellulose etc.) needs to be eliminated to make cellulose highly pure and crystalline with desirable properties. Therefore, chemical treatment including sulfuric acid hydrolysis was carried out to obtain an extremely crystalline and purified form of cellulose by hydrolyzing the amorphous region.

To investigate the crystallinity of the bleached fibers and effect of acid treatment on the resulting NCC, X-ray, diffractometry (XRD) was carried out. Figure 1 presents the obtained XRD patterns for kenaf bast fibers for bleached and acid treated fibers. The crystallinity index of both fibers were calculated using Diffrac.EvaV4.0 software. Diffraction peaks at 2θ value of 14.5°, 16.5°, and 22.5° at plane of 101, 10-1, and 002, respectively, were observed. From the diffraction pattern it could be noticed that cellulose was present in the form of cellulose [33,34]. Crystallinity index was calculated for the bleached fibers and NCC. For the kenaf biomass, the crystallinity index values of the bleached fibers and NCC were reported as 56% and 71.6%, respectively, in consistence with similar findings [35]. The higher crystallinity of NCC than the bleached fibers could be due to the removal of amorphous cellulosic region by acid hydrolysis. The XRD result suggested that the amorphous region of the bleached fibers degraded during extraction, whereas the crystalline region remained unaffected. The high crystallinity of NCC was related to the high tensile strength of the fibers. Therefore, the mechanical properties of the nanocomposite can be improved by using NCC as a reinforcing agent.

3.3. Scanning Electron Microscopy

Surface morphological analysis was performed on the bleached fibers and kenaf NCC. The SEM images are depicted in the Figure 2 at different magnifications. As shown in Figure 2a,c the bleached fiber bark structures were apparent. Meanwhile, NCC microphotographs in Figure 2b,d revealed that the surface of the NCC became smooth and the fibers appeared as a web-like network with diameters approximately 40–90 nm in consistent with similar SEM surface morphologies [24]. After a series of chemical treatments, impurities such as pectin, hemicellulose, and lignin were removed from the structure of the bleached fibers, as can be implied from the FTIR findings. The small diameter of NCC was because of acid hydrolysis, which significantly removed the amorphous portion from the crystalline part, which is in accordance with previous similar finding [34].

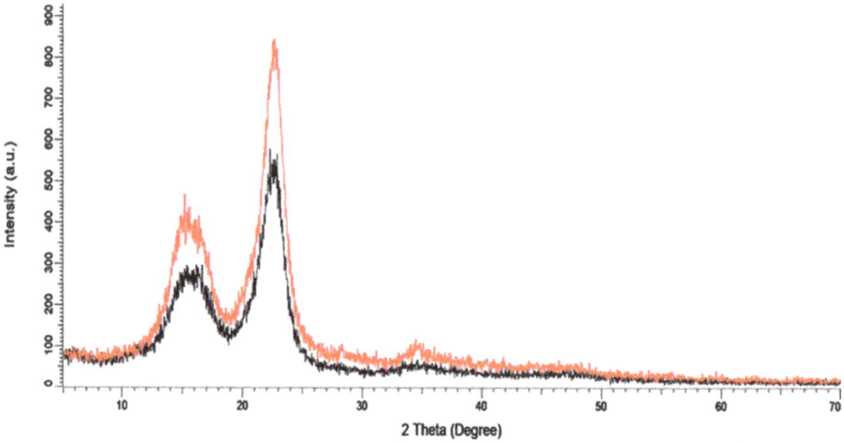

Figure 1. The XRD patterns of both NCC (Red) and (Bleached fibers (Black) from kenaf bast fiber.

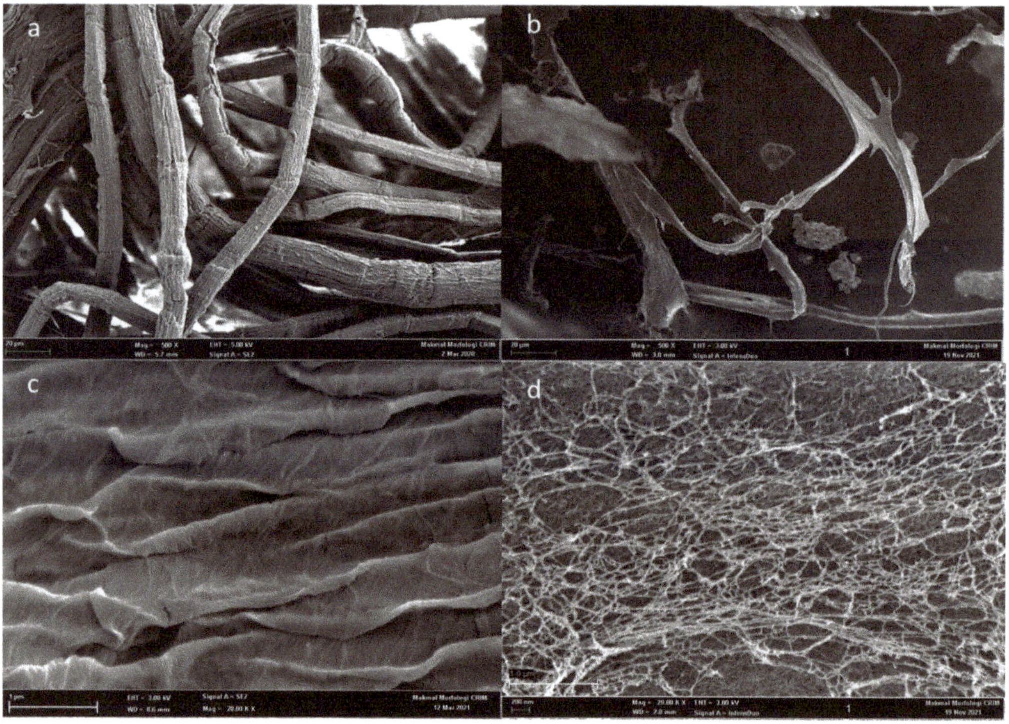

Figure 2. Photographs of SEM images of (**a**) bleached fibers (**b**) NCC at 500X (**c**) bleached fibers (**d**) NCC at 20KX.

3.4. FTIR-ATR Spectroscopic Analysis of NCC

FTIR was carried out on raw fibers, bleached fibers, and NCC to determine their chemical composition after chemical and mechanical treatment. The results are shown in Figure 3a and Table 2. All spectra detected a broad and intense peak at 3300 cm^{-1} region which is attributed to the characteristic of polysaccharides hydroxyl bonds [36]. C–H symmetrical stretching and CH2 symmetrical stretching at 2900–2800 cm^{-1} revealed polysaccharide, wax, and oil content of the fibers [36]. Another peak was observed in the spectra of the raw fibers at 1242 cm^{-1}, which was associated with C-O stretching of the aryl group present in lignin. The disappearance of this peak in bleached and NCC suggested the separation of lignin by chemical treatment [36].The vibration peak in the fibers at 1326–1340 cm^{-1} was linked to bending of the C-H and C-O bonds in polysaccharide aromatic rings [36]. Absorption peak was shown in all samples at 1023–1030 cm^{-1}, which were associated with C-O and C-N vibrations [36]. The absorption peak at 1634 cm^{-1} in NCC was due to adsorbed water, which was suggestive of NCC [36].

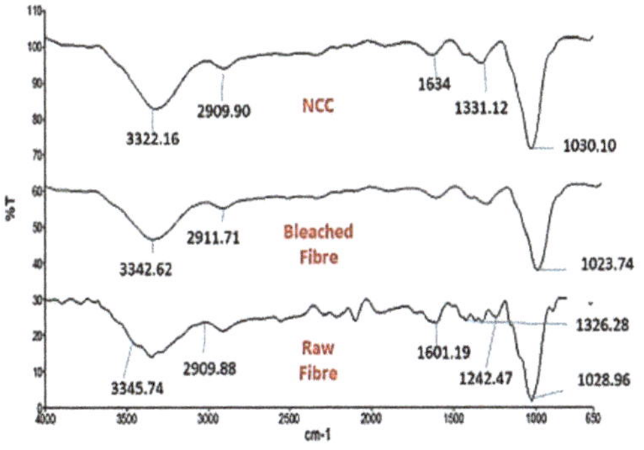

(a)

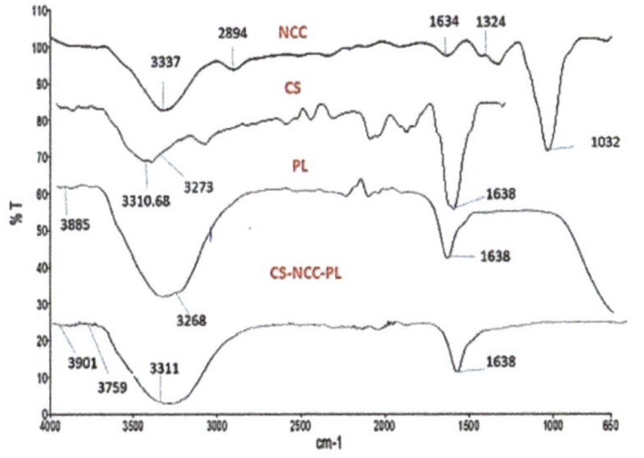

(b)

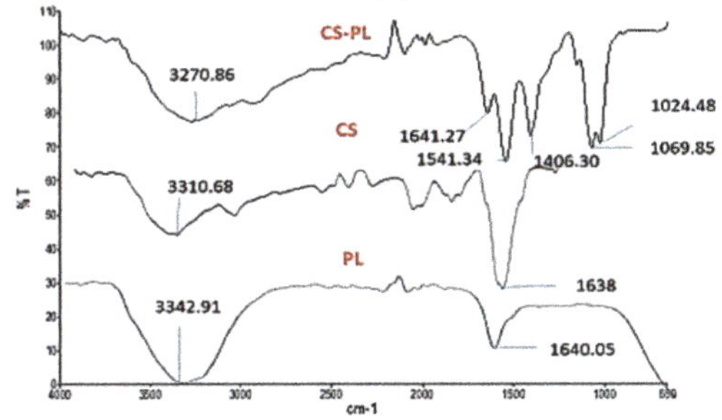

(c)

Figure 3. FTIR analysis comparison of (**a**) NCC, bleached fiber and raw fiber (**b**) NCC, CS, PL, and CS-NCC-PL (**c**) CS-PL, CS and PL alone.

Table 2. FTIR characteristic peaks of Kenaf raw fibers, bleached fibers, and NCC.

Raw Fibers Peak (cm^{-1})	Bleached Fibers Peak (cm^{-1})	NCC Peak (cm^{-1})	Peak Assignment
3345.74	3342.62	3322.16	O–H stretching
2909.88	2911.71	2909.90	C–H symmetrical stretching and CH2 symmetrical stretching
1326.28	-	-	C–O aromatic ring
1242.47	-	-	C–O stretching
1601.19	-	-	C=C groups
-	-	1634	Adsorbed water
1028.96	1023.74	1030.10	C-O and O-H groups stretching

FTIR was conducted to investigate the possible interaction of functional group between PL and CS hydrogel, as presented in Figure 3b. CS showed a broad band at 3500–3200 cm^{-1}, which can be attributed to the O–H and N–H stretching vibrations of functional groups in hydrogen bonds. Characteristic absorption bands at 1634 cm^{-1} corresponded to C=O stretching in the amide I vibration. The absorption band at 1540 cm^{-1} appeared due to N–H bending in amide II vibration. The spectra at 1069 and 1024 cm^{-1} corresponded to C–O stretching vibrations, which were characteristics of CS structure. Association of PL in CS hydrogel was confirmed by displacement of characteristic bands at 3219–3270 cm^{-1} due to O-H stretching and 1634–1641 cm^{-1} due to NH vibrations [37]. These modifications suggested a possible interaction between PL and CS.

FTIR spectra of NCC, CS, PL, and CS-NCC-PL are represented in Figure 3c. A characteristic peak of CS was observed at 3310 cm^{-1} owing to the O-H group. CS-NCC was observed by shifting of the peak from 3337 cm^{-1} to 3759 cm^{-1}, which indicated possible overlapping of hydrogen bonds. PL with a characteristic peak at 3885 cm^{-1} was due to O-H stretching that shifted slightly toward 3901 cm^{-1}. Thus, CS incorporated with NCC and PL possessed two extra peaks, which corresponded to NCC and PL as compared with control CS hydrogel. These results indicate that NCC was prepared and successfully incorporated in CS hydrogel along with PL.

3.5. Swelling Study

Freeze drying allows the nucleation of ice crystals from solution and further growth along the lines of thermal gradients. Exclusion of the CS acetate salt from the ice crystal phase and subsequent ice removal by lyophilization generate a porous material [38]. Freeze drying is usually employed to produce porous CS hydrogels to assess their water swelling behavior effectively.

An ideal dressing must be capable of absorbing the wound exudates that could potentially cause bacterial infection at the wound bed. Swelling properties determines the moisture absorption capacity of a dressing, which is a crucial action for absorbing pus and exudates from weeping wounds. The swelling ratios over time of the freeze-dried hydrogels are shown in Figure 4. All hydrogels swelled at different rates, and equilibriums were achieved up to 1000 times of their initial weight within 24 h of water imbibition. During the initial swelling, water was absorbed via capillaries located in the internal structure of the hydrogels. As 3D networks, porous structures provide channels for the molecules to enter and escape. The hydrophilic groups (-OH/-COOH/-COO-) present in CS were bound with water molecules by hydrogen bonds that created a hydration layer. This phenomenon may explain why all hydrogels showed the fastest swelling at the beginning (<3 h). The addition of PL in the CS hydrogels reduced the swelling ratio (~500% reduction). The addition of PL may decrease availability of CS hydrophilic groups to bind with water. The swelling ratio also decreased further (~300% reduction) when NCC was added into CS. This behavior could be ascribed to the fact that NCC lodges the free space volume in the CS polymeric matrix, thereby restricting the volume available for swelling and causing the formation of a rigid hydrogel structure that cannot be easily penetrated by water molecules. Hence, the water absorption decreased, which consequently decreased the swelling ratio [39]. However, the addition of PL to the CS-NCC hydrogel increased the swelling ratio owing to its large hydrophilic groups in molecular chains, which promoted the establishment of hydration layers [40]. The higher water holding capacities (>1000%) of the hydrogels indicate that the formulated hydrogels are suitable for medium to heavy suppurating wounds. This is a crucial property for a dressing in minimizing infection. At the same time, the hydrogels maintain a moist local microenvironment for tissue repair process to take place.

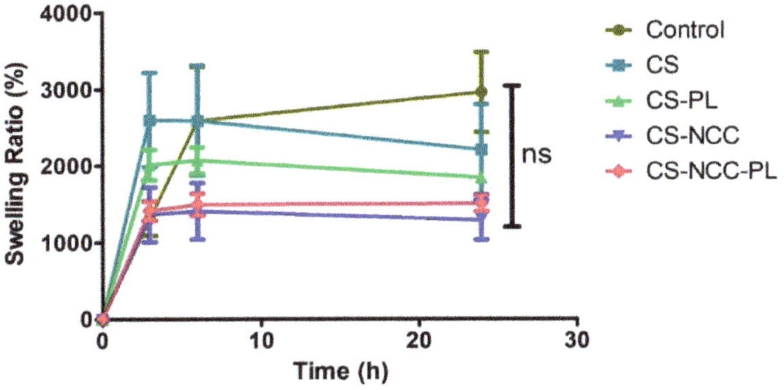

Figure 4. Swelling ratio of Control (Intrasite Gel), CS hydrogel, CS-NCC hydrogel, CS-PL hydrogel and CS-NCC-PL hydrogel over 24 h. The error bars showed standard deviation based on triplicated samples at each time point.

3.6. Moisture Loss Study

Moisture retention capacity is an important characteristic for a wound dressing. Hydrogels should provide a moist environment to the wound to accelerate healing [40]. Moisture loss from the different hydrogels was evaluated by employing the desiccation method. Moisture loss was expressed in percentage and calculated after 24 h of hydrogel drying. As shown in Figure 5, Intrasite™ hydrogel lost almost 80% of moisture after 24 h, followed by PL, which lost 90% of moisture. Meanwhile, the CS-PL hydrogel lost approximately 42% of moisture as compared with the CS hydrogel. The PL entrapped within the network of polymer and prevented moisture loss. Therefore, the hydrogels under investigation held moisture for a longer period as compared with the commercial hydrogel. The CS-NCC-PL hydrogel can maintain a moist environment on chronic wounds for an extended time.

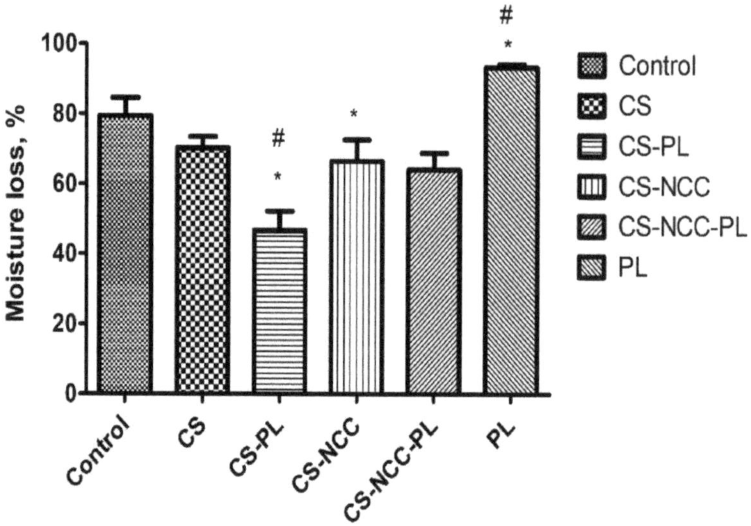

Figure 5. Moisture loss profile of formulated hydrogels over 24 h (expressed in mean ±SD, $n = 3$). The asterisks (*) represent significant difference ($p < 0.05$) compared to control. The hashtag (#) represent significant difference ($p < 0.05$) between the groups.

3.7. *In Vitro Protein Release Assay*

The cumulative release profiles of PL from the CS-PL and CS-NCC-PL hydrogels are represented in Figure 6. The PL released from the CS-PL hydrogel showed faster release at the first 3 h compared with that from CS-NCC. Thereafter, the PL release increased gradually (PL flux = 0.165 mg/cm^2/h) and reached the maximum release of 5.22 $\pm$ 1.47 mg/cm^2 at 24 h. During this time, proteins permeated from the inside matrix of the hydrogel via swelling and diffusion mechanism. In the CS-NCC-PL hydrogel, the rate of PL release was significantly decreased and much controlled throughout the test duration (PL flux = 0.075 mg/cm^2/h). This phenomenon suggested that NCC might act as a nanofiller and provide sustained release because of its capacity to retain the proteins within the hydrogel matrix for a long period of time (maximum PL release of 3.00 $\pm$ 1.11 mg/cm^2 at 24 h). For chronic wound healing, hydrogel comprises of platelet proteins, and a cocktail of various GFs is desired for tissue proliferation. The CS-NCC hydrogel composite is successful in controlling the PL release and is a promising vehicle for PL in wound healing.

3.7.1. Cell Viability

The cytotoxic effect of hydrogel formulations on HDFs was tested by Alamar Blue assay. The results of cell viability are presented in Figure 7. This experiment revealed that the cell viability of the CS-PL and CS-NCC-PL hydrogels was higher than that of PL alone for 24, 48, and 72 h. This hike in cell viability of the PL-loaded hydrogels is probably due to the protective effect of CS-NCC on PL. As mentioned previously, CS can stabilize PL and protect it from degradation. Overall, the cytotoxic effect of hydrogels in this study with or without PL was negligible ($p < 0.05$, one-way ANOVA, Tukey's multiple comparison test). Therefore, the hydrogel formulations are non-toxic and safe to be applied onto wounds.

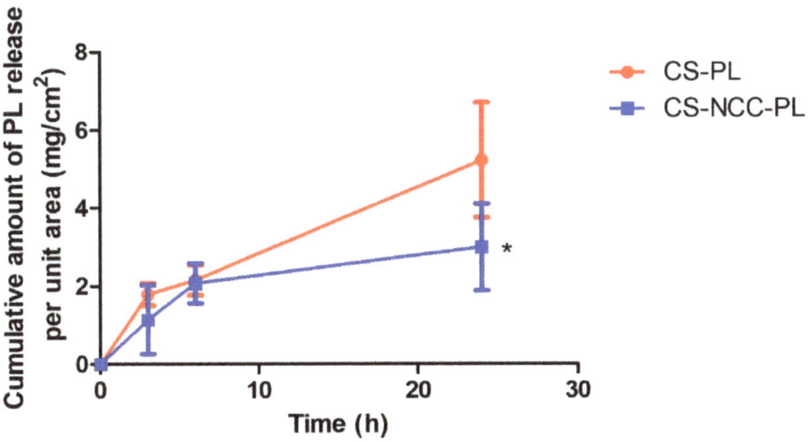

Figure 6. In vitro cumulative release profile of PL from CS-PL and CS-NCC-PL. (*) means significant difference ($p < 0.05$) compared to CS-PL.

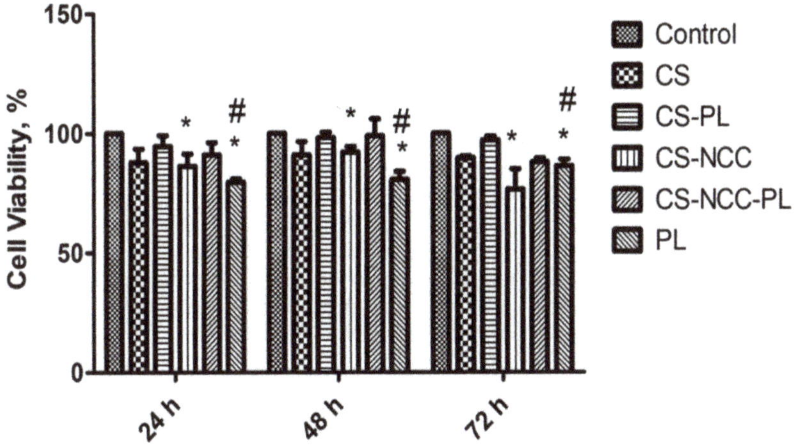

Figure 7. Percentage cell viability of hydrogels on Human dermal fibroblast (HDF) at different time points using Alamar blue assay, $n = 3$, The asterisks (*) represents statistically significant difference compared to control ($p < 0.05$) and hashtag (#) represent significant difference ($p < 0.05$) between groups.

3.7.2. Cell Proliferation

Cell proliferation was analyzed through Alamar Blue assay to ascertain any change in cell proportion. In this study, CS-NCC-PL hydrogels were tested by treating HDFs (1×10^4) with sterile hydrogel leachates in the microplates for 24, 48, and 72 h. The results of cell proliferation are provided in Figure 8. PL alone showed low proliferation with an increasing trend over 3 days. The hydrogels enhanced the HDF proliferation from 24 h to 48 h, demonstrating the growth and proliferation of the HDFs. The PL-loaded hydrogels significantly augmented fibroblast proliferation (>100% viability) compared with the blank hydrogels or PL alone, indicating fast wound closure without causing any cell toxicity. Higher cell proliferation induced by combination of chitosan with PL is also in agreement with similar study where it showed that platelet-rich plasma with chitosan-induced growth factor enrichment can stimulate the growth of fibroblasts [41]. This dictates the feasibility and safety of autologous PL in wound healing and complications in patients with intractable diseases such as diabetic ulcers and decubitus [41].

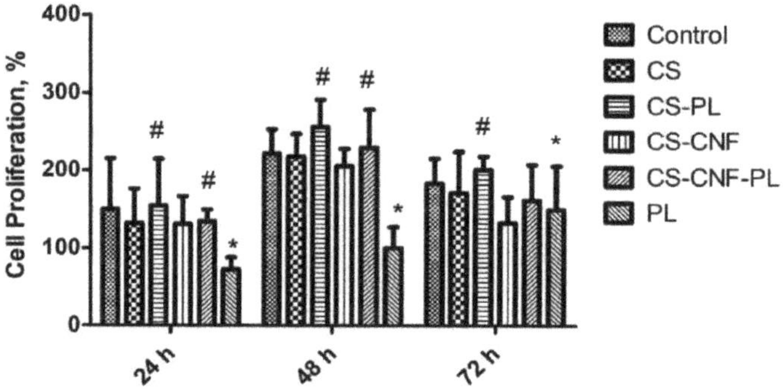

Figure 8. Cell proliferation study of hydrogels on human dermal fibroblast (HDF) at different time points using Alamar blue assay, $n = 3$, The asterisks (*) represent statistically significant different ($p < 0.05$) compared to control, the hashtag (#) means statistically significant different ($p < 0.05$) between groups.

3.8. Wound Scratch Assay

Cell migration across the provisional gap was carried out to assess the healing potential of the hydrogels. The results in Figure 9 show the effect of hydrogels on the migration rate of the HDFs for 24 h. All hydrogel groups showed significant migration of cells as compared with the control group ($p < 0.05$, one-way ANOVA followed by Tukey's multiple comparison test). The migration rates of the HDFs after being treated with the CS-PL hydrogels was significantly higher than CS alone ($p < 0.05$). This indicates the PL stimulates the cell migration rate. The addition of NCC does not affect the migration rate as CS-NCC-PL and CS-PL group ($p > 0.05$). The wound area-time plot and micrographs (Figures 10 and 11) indicated that all wounds were nearly closed in less than 48 h despite of the differences in the migration rates of the control and treatment groups. The HDFs were managed to occupy the free space within a span of 48 h, indicating that the hydrogels efficiently healed the HDFs.

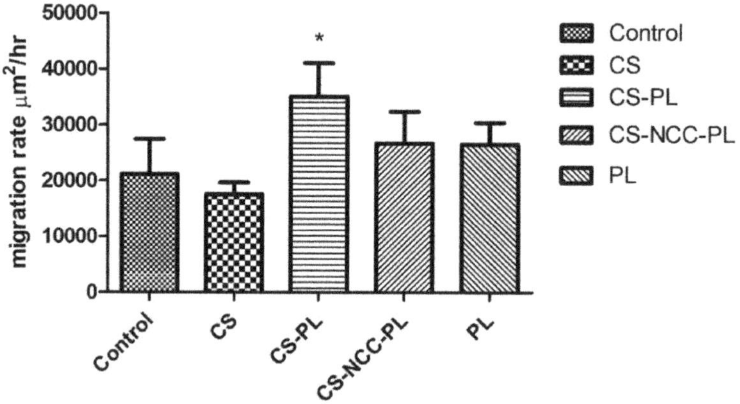

Figure 9. Rate of cell migration of HDFs treated with different hydrogels; $n = 3$, *—statistically significant different ($p < 0.05$) compared to CS and control.

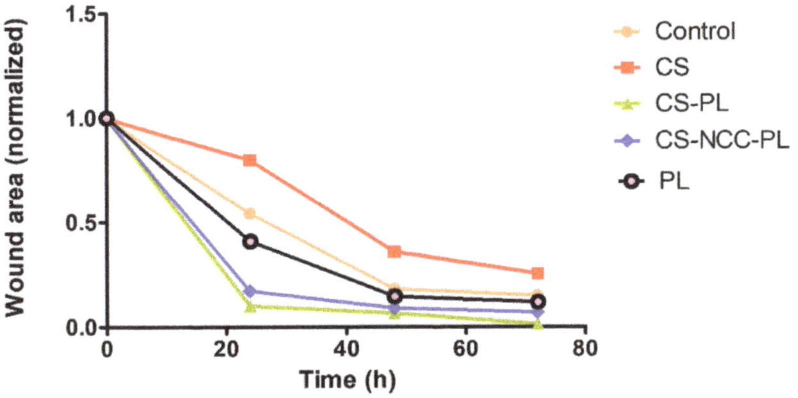

Figure 10. Wound area closure at different time points; $n = 3$.

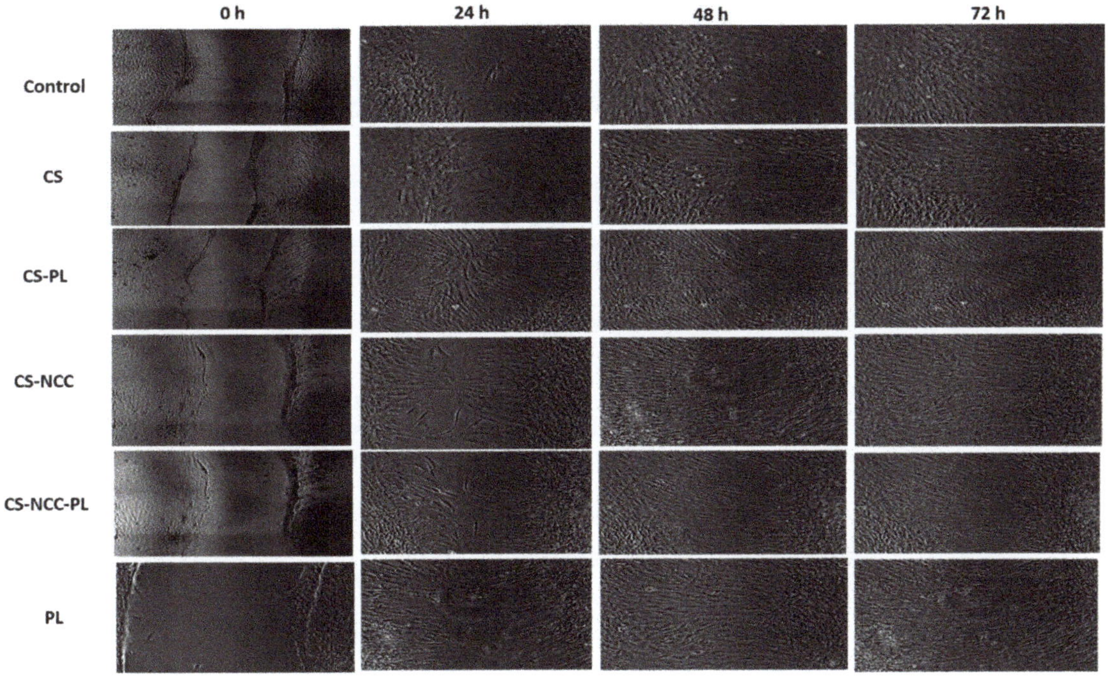

Figure 11. Migration of HDFs treated with hydrogels for 24, 48, and 72 h.

3.9. *LIVE/DEAD® Cell Viability Assay*

Cytotoxic effect of hydrogel formulations was further investigated using LIVE/DEAD™ Cell Viability Assay. This assay gives qualitative aspect of cell viability. The control and cells treated with the hydrogels lacked dead cells (stained red), as shown in Figure 12. Control and chitosan hydrogels with different combinations exhibited favorable cell viability after 24 h of incubation (captured in green color cells). In addition, after 48 h, cells continue to grow and become elongated for further maturation and differentiation. Additionally, these results comply with the results of Alamar Blue™ assay, suggesting the non-toxicity of the hydrogel after 24 and 72 h of treatment. Cell number and cell viability increased over the period of 72 h.

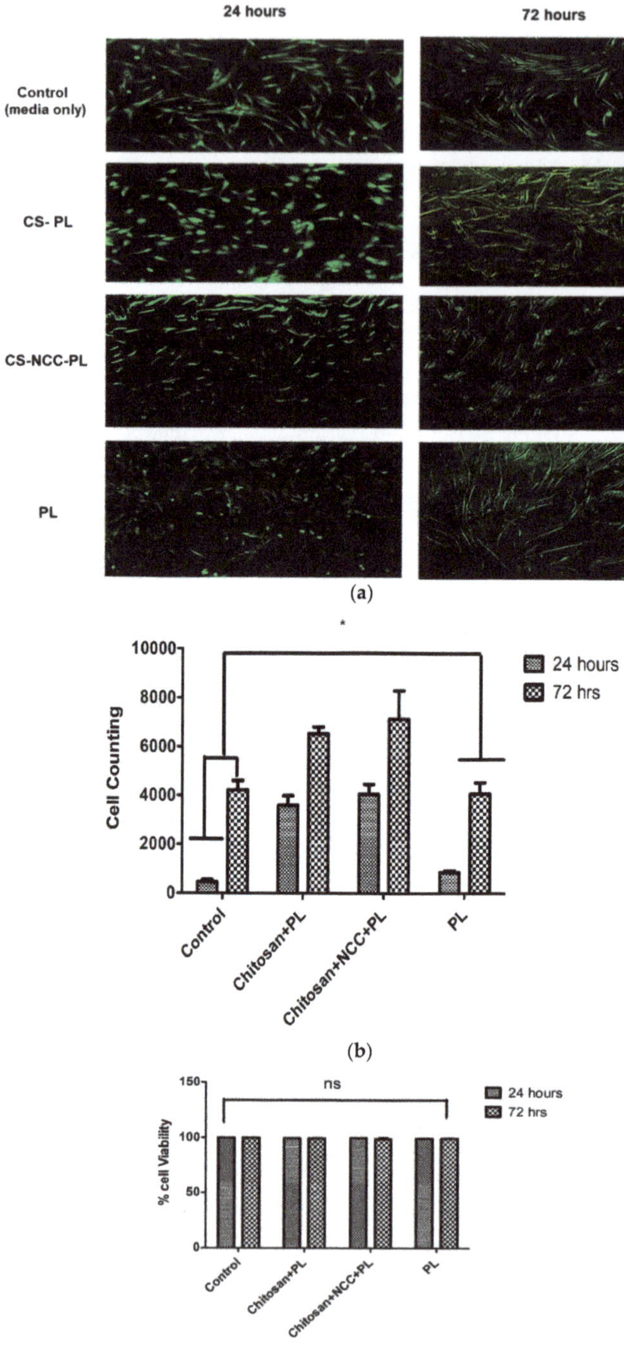

Figure 12. (**a**) Live Dead cell viability Assay at 200X magnification, (**b**) Cell counting treated with different hydrogels at 24 h and 72 h (**c**) % cell viability compared to control. $n = 3$. The asterisks (*)—statistically significant different ($p < 0.05$); ns—non-significant from control (untreated cells).

3.10. CS Stabilizing Effect on PL

Cell proliferation assay was carried out to assess the protective effect of CS on GF present in PL. CS along with NCC hydrogel with and without PL and PL alone groups were subjected to heat treatment and protease digestion. Afterward, the HDFs were subjected to these treatments for 24, 48, and 72 h. Results of these findings are provided in Figure 13a,b. All data show the significant protective effect of CS on PL for proteases and heat treatment. The PL loaded with CS or CS-NCC over 72 h had significantly higher proliferation than those unprotected PL. This protective effect of chitosan is supported with similar work carried out by Fisher et al., that proposed the mechanism where chitosan fibers tightly bind with major plasma proteins and a specific sub-set of platelet surface proteins which results in the acceleration of fibrin gel formation when platelet integrins contact with plasma proteins. This result indicates that CS can protect the GF present in PL, thereby promoting fast wound healing.

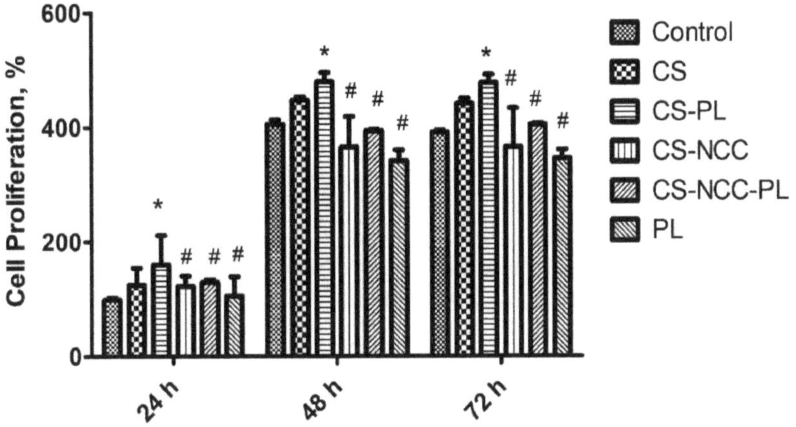

(a)

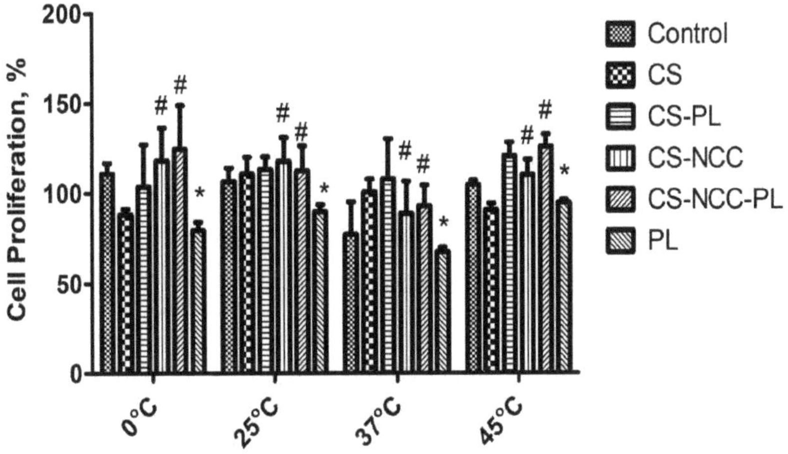

(b)

Figure 13. Chitosan stability studies on GF present in PL by cell proliferation study using Alamar blue assay (**a**) Effect of proteases treatment (**b**) Effect of heat treatment, $n = 3$, The asterisks (*) — statistically significant different compared to PL alone ($p < 0.05$); The hashtag (#) means statistically significant different ($p < 0.05$) between groups.

4. Conclusions

In general, GFs in PL suffer clinical limitations because of rapid degradation by proteases at the tissue site. To address the challenges related to PL instability, we developed a CS hydrogel combined with kenaf-derived NCC. It can stabilize PL and control the release of PL onto the wound site for prolonged action. Kenaf biomass-derived NCC at 0.4% concentration acted as the nanofiller for CS hydrogel and controlled PL release at a slower rate (maximum PL release of 3.00 ± 1.11 mg/cm^2 at 24 h) compared with the CS hydrogel alone. FTIR study confirmed the presence of NCCs and PL in the CS matrix. Swelling data revealed that NCC incorporation in the PL-loaded CS hydrogel possesses high swelling ratio and water retention capacity (>1000 times at less than 3 h), thereby benefiting the healing of high exudate wounds. In vitro study revealed that the hydrogels are non-toxic to host tissues (>100% HDF cell viability) and are able to close wounds at a faster rate compared with the controls. The protective effect of CS upon GFs in PL was also demonstrated via protease and heat treatment of the hydrogels. Thus, NCC-reinforced CS hydrogel emerged as a promising PL vehicle especially for autologous wound therapy for chronic wounds. This new hydrogel PL carrier may be extended to other autologous PRP therapies, such as rheumatoid arthritis, bone regeneration, low-grade musculoskeletal injuries, and dental applications.

Author Contributions: Conceptualization and methodology, S.-F.N.; writing—original draft preparation, S.-F.N. and P.B.; review and editing, J.X.L. and S.-F.N. funding acquisition, S.-F.N. All authors have read and agreed to the published version of the manuscript.

Funding: This research is financially supported by the Dana Impak Perdana (DIP) grant (DIP-2018-028), Universiti Kebangsaan Malaysia (UKM).

Institutional Review Board Statement: Not applicable.

Informed Consent Statement: Not applicable.

Data Availability Statement: The data presented in this study are available on request from the corresponding author.

Acknowledgments: Hydrogel formulation work and facilities was provided by the Faculty of Pharmacy, UKM and special thanks to Centre for Tissue Engineering and Regenerative Medicine (CTERM) for supporting the cell work.

Conflicts of Interest: The authors declare that they have no known competing financial interest or personal relationships that could have appeared to influence the work reported in this paper.

References

1. Tang, J.; Grishkewich, N.; Tam, K.C. Functionalization of cellulose nanocrystals for advanced applications. *J. Colloid Int. Sci.* **2017**, *494*, 397–409. [CrossRef] [PubMed]
2. Sulaiman, S.; Mokhtar, M.N.; Naim, M.N.; Baharuddin, A.S.; Salleh, M.A.M.; Sulaiman, A. Penghasilan nano-gentian selulosa (CNF) diperolehi daripada gentian kulit kenaf dan potensinya sebagai penyokong pemegunan enzim. *Malay. J. Anal. Sci.* **2016**, *20*, 309–317. [CrossRef]
3. Davoudpour, Y.; Hossain, M.S.; Abdul Khalil, H.P.S.; Mohamad Haafiz, M.K.; Mohd Ishak, Z.A.; Hassan, A.; Sarker, Z.I. Optimization of high pressure homogenization parameters for the isolation of cellulosic nanofibers using response surface methodology. *Ind. Crop. Prod.* **2015**, *74*, 381–387. [CrossRef]
4. Law, J.X.; Chowdhury, S.R.; Saim, A.; Idrus, R.B.H. Platelet-rich plasma with keratinocytes and fibroblasts enhance healing of full-thickness wounds. *J. Tissue Viability* **2017**, *26*, 208–215. [CrossRef]
5. Tsai, H.C.; Lehman, C.W.; Chen, C.M. Use of platelet-rich plasma and platelet-derived patches to treat chronic wounds. *J. Wound Care* **2019**, *28*, 15–21. [CrossRef]
6. Han, D.; He, Z.; Zhong, R.; Zhang, X.; Wang, H. Preparation and characterization of a hemostatic porous platelet-rich plasma chitosan/silk fibroin wound dressing. *Chin. J. Biotechnol.* **2020**, *36*, 332–340. [CrossRef]
7. Seeger, A.; Paller, S. The roles of growth factors in keratinocyte migration. *Adv. Wound Care* **2015**, *4*, 213–224. [CrossRef]
8. Stolzenburg-Veeser, L.; Golubnitschaja, O. Mini-encyclopaedia of the wound healing—Opportunities for integrating multi-omic approaches into medical practice. *J. Proteom.* **2018**, *188*, 71–84. [CrossRef]
9. Busilacchi, A.; Gigante, A.; Mattioli-Belmonte, M.; Manzotti, S.; Muzzarelli, R.A.A. Chitosan stabilizes platelet growth factors and modulates stem cell differentiation toward tissue regeneration. *Carbohydr. Polym.* **2013**, *98*, 665–676. [CrossRef] [PubMed]

10. Dai, T.; Tanaka, M.; Huang, Y.Y.; Hamblin, M.R. Chitosan preparations for wounds and burns: Antimicrobial and wound-healing effects. *Exp. Rev. Anti-Inf. Ther.* **2011**, *309*, 857–879. [CrossRef] [PubMed]
11. Dash, M.; Chiellini, F.; Ottenbrite, R.M.; Chiellini, E. Chitosan—A versatile semi-synthetic polymer in biomedical applications. *Prog. Polym. Sci.* **2011**, *36*, 981–1014. [CrossRef]
12. Giri, T.K.; Thakur, A.; Alexander, A.; Ajazuddin; Badwaik, H.; Tripathi, D.K. Modified chitosan hydrogels as drug delivery and tissue engineering systems: Present status and applications. *Acta Pharm. Sin. B* **2012**, *2*, 439–449. [CrossRef]
13. Patrulea, V.; Ostafe, V.; Borchard, G.; Jordan, O. Chitosan as a starting material for wound healing applications. *Eur. J. Pharm. Biopharm.* **2015**, *97*, 417–426. [CrossRef]
14. Rossi, S.; Faccendini, M.C.; Bonferoni, F.; Ferrari, G.; Sandri, C.; Caramella, C.M. "Sponge-like" dressings based on biopolymers for the delivery of platelet lysate to skin chronic wounds. *Int. J. Pharm.* **2013**, *440*, 207–215. [CrossRef] [PubMed]
15. Mohammadi, R.; Mehrtash, M.; Mehrtash, M.; Hassani, N.; Hassanpour, A. effect of platelet rich plasma combined with chitosan biodegradable film on full-thickness wound healing in rat model. *Bull. Emerg. Traum.* **2016**, *4*, 29.
16. Fischer, T.H.; Thatte, H.S.; Nichols, T.C.; Bender-Neal, D.E.; Bellinger, D.A.; Vournakis, J.N. Synergistic platelet integrin signaling and factor XII activation in poly-N-acetyl glucosamine fiber-mediated hemostasis. *Biomaterials* **2005**, *26*, 5433–5443. [CrossRef]
17. Wang, Z.; Lu, W.W.; Zhen, W.; Yang, D.S. Novel biomaterial strategies for controlled growth factor delivery for biomedical applications. *NPG Asia Mater.* **2017**, *9*, e435. [CrossRef]
18. Dorishetty, P.; Balu, R.; Athukoralalage, S.S.; Greaves, T.L.; Mata, J.; de Campo, L.; Saha, N.; Zannettino, A.C.W.; Dutta, N.K.; Choudhury, N.R. Tunable biomimetic hydrogels from silk fibroin and nanocellulose. *ACS Sustain. Chem. Eng.* **2020**, *8*, 2375–2389. [CrossRef]
19. Liu, J.; Cheng, F.; Grénman, H.; Spoljaric, S.; Seppälä, J.; Eriksson, J.E.; Willför, S.; Xu, C. Development of nanocellulose scaffolds with tunable structures to support 3D cell culture. *Carbohydr. Polym.* **2016**, *148*, 259–271. [CrossRef] [PubMed]
20. Song, K.; Zhu, X.; Zhu, W.; Li, X. Preparation and characterization of cellulose nanocrystal extracted from *Calotropis procera* biomass. *Bioresour. Bioprocess.* **2019**, *45*, 1–8. [CrossRef]
21. Kutlu, B.; Tiğli Aydin, R.S.; Akman, A.C.; Gümüşderelioglu, M.; Nohutcu, R.M. Platelet-rich plasma-loaded chitosan scaffolds: Preparation and growth factor release kinetics. *J. Biomed. Mater. Res. Part B Appl. Biomater.* **2013**, *101B*, 28–35. [CrossRef] [PubMed]
22. Doench, I.; Tran, T.A.; David, L.; Montembault, A.; Viguier, E.; Gorzelanny, C.G.; Sudre, T.; Cachon, M.; Louback-Mohamed, M.; Horbelt, N.; et al. Cellulose nanofiber-reinforced chitosan hydrogel composites for intervertebral disc tissue repair. *Biomimetics* **2019**, *4*, 19. [CrossRef]
23. Tuerxun, D.; Pulingam, T.; Nordin, N.I.; Chen, Y.W.; Bin Kamaldin, J.; Julkapli, N.B.M.; Lee, H.V.; Leo, B.F.; Bin Johan, M.R. Synthesis, characterization and cytotoxicity studies of nanocrystalline cellulose from the production waste of rubber-wood and kenaf-bast fibers. *Eur. Polym. J.* **2019**, *116*, 352–360. [CrossRef]
24. Sri Aprilia, N.A.; Arahman, N. Properties of nanocrystalline cellulose from pineapple crown leaf waste. In *IOP Conference Series: Materials Science and Engineering*; IOP Publishing: Bristol, UK, 2020; Volume 796. [CrossRef]
25. Maache, M.; Bezazi, A.; Amroune, S.; Scarpa, F.; Dufresne, A. Characterization of a novel natural cellulosic fiber from *Juncus effusus* L. *Carbohydr. Polym.* **2017**, *171*, 163–172. [CrossRef] [PubMed]
26. Lai, J.C.Y.; Lai, H.Y.; Rao, N.K.; Ng, S.F. Treatment for diabetic ulcer wounds using a fern tannin optimized hydrogel formulation with antibacterial and antioxidative properties. *J. Ethnopharmacol.* **2016**, *189*, 277–289. [CrossRef]
27. Xi Loh, E.Y.; Fauzi, M.B.; Ng, M.H.; Ng, P.Y.; Ng, S.F.; Ariffin, H.; Mohd Amin, M.C.I. Cellular and molecular interaction of human dermal fibroblasts with bacterial nanocellulose composite hydrogel for tissue regeneration. *ACS Appl. Mater. Interfaces* **2018**, *10*, 39532–39543. [CrossRef]
28. Nishimoto, S.; Fujita, K.; Sotsuka, Y.; Kinoshita, M.; Fujiwara, T.; Kawai, K.; Kakibuchi, M. Growth factor measurement and histological analysis in platelet rich fibrin: A pilot study. *J. Maxillofac. Oral Surg.* **2015**, *14*, 907–913. [CrossRef]
29. Jonoobi, M.; Khazaeian, A.; Tahir, P.M.; Azry, S.S.; Oksman, K. Characteristics of cellulose nanofibers isolated from rubberwood and empty fruit bunches of oil palm using chemo-mechanical process. *Cellulose* **2011**, *18*, 1085–1095. [CrossRef]
30. Garcia de Rodriguez, N.L.; Thielemans, W.A. Dufresne, Sisal cellulose whiskers reinforced polyvinyl acetate nanocomposites. *Cellulose* **2006**, *13*, 261–270. [CrossRef]
31. Ilyas, R.A.; Sapuan, S.M.; Ishak, M.R. Isolation and characterization of nanocrystalline cellulose from sugar palm fibres (*Arenga Pinnata*). *Carbohydr. Polym.* **2018**, *181*, 1038–1051. [CrossRef] [PubMed]
32. Karagkiozaki, V.; Logothetidis, S.; Lousinian, S.; Giannoglo, G. Impact of surface electric properties of carbon-based thin films on platelets activation for nano-medical and nano-sensing applications. *Int. J. Nanomed.* **2008**, *3*, 461. [CrossRef]
33. Karimi, S.; Tahir, P.M.; Karimi, A.; Dufresne, A.; Abdulkhani, A. Kenaf bast cellulosic fibers hierarchy: A comprehensive approach from micro to nano. *Carbohydr. Polym.* **2014**, *101*, 878–885. [CrossRef] [PubMed]
34. Khan, A.; Jawaid, M.; Kia Kian, L.; Khan, A.A.P.; Asiri, A.M. Isolation and production of nanocrystalline cellulose from conocarpus fiber. *Polymers* **2021**, *13*, 1835. [CrossRef]
35. Lv, W.; Xia, Z.; Song, Y.; Wang, P.; Liu, S.; Zhang, Y.; Ben, H.; Han, G.; Jiang, W. Using microwave assisted organic acid treatment to separate cellulose fiber and lignin from kenaf bast. *Ind. Crop. Prod.* **2021**, *171*, 113934. [CrossRef]
36. Le Troedec, M.; Sedan, D.; Peyratout, C.; Bonnet, J.P.; Smith, A.; Guinebretiere, R.; Gloaguen, V.; Krausz, P. Influence of various chemical treatments on the composition and structure of hemp fibres. *Compos. Part A Appl. Sci. Manuf.* **2008**, *39*, 514–522. [CrossRef]

37. Nacos, M.K.; Katapodis, P.; Pappas, C.; Daferera, D.; Tarantilis, P.A.; Christakopoulos, P.; Polissiou, M. Kenaf xylan—A source of biologically active acidic oligosaccharides. *Carbohydr. Polym.* **2006**, *66*, 126–134. [CrossRef]
38. Tang, Y.; Zhang, H.; Wei, Q.; Tang, X.; Zhuang, W. Biocompatible chitosan-collagen-hydroxyapatite nanofibers coated with platelet-rich plasma for regenerative engineering of the rotator cuff of the shoulder. *RSC Adv.* **2019**, *9*, 27013–27020. [CrossRef]
39. Song, W.; Xu, J.; Gao, L.; Zhang, Q.; Tong, J. Preparation of Freeze-Dried Porous Chitosan Microspheres for the Removal of Hexavalent Chromium. *Appl. Sci.* **2021**, *11*, 4217. [CrossRef]
40. Sampath, U.G.T.M.; Ching, Y.C.; Chuah, C.H.; Singh, R.; Lin, P.-C. Preparation and characterization of nanocellulose reinforced semi-interpenetrating polymer network of chitosan hydrogel. *Cellulose* **2017**, *24*, 2215–2228. [CrossRef]
41. Hattori, H.; Ishihara, M. Feasibility of improving platelet-rich plasma therapy by using chitosan with high platelet activation ability. *Exp. Ther. Med.* **2017**, *13*, 1176–1180. [CrossRef]

polymers

MDPI

Article

The Effect of Different Cleaning Methods on Protein Deposition and Optical Characteristics of Orthokeratology Lenses

Chen-Ying Su [1,†], Lung-Kun Yeh [2,3,†], Yi-Fei Tsao [1], Wen-Pin Lin [4,5], Chiun-Ho Hou [2,3], Hsueh-Fang Huang [4], Chi-Chun Lai [2,3] and Hsu-Wei Fang [1,6,*]

1 Department of Chemical Engineering and Biotechnology, National Taipei University of Technology, 1, Sec. 3, Zhongxiao E. Rd., Taipei 10608, Taiwan; chenying.su@ntut.edu.tw (C.-Y.S.); susan84103086@gmail.com (Y.-F.T.)
2 Department of Ophthalmology, Chang Gung Memorial Hospital, Linkou, No. 5, Fuxing St., Taoyuan 333, Taiwan; yehlungkun@gmail.com (L.-K.Y.); chiunho@cgmh.org.tw (C.-H.H.); chichun.lai@gmail.com (C.-C.L.)
3 College of Medicine, Chang Gung University, No.259, Wenhua 1st Rd., Taoyuan 333, Taiwan
4 Research and Development Center, Brighten Optix Co., 6F-1, No. 150, Sec. 4, Chengde Rd., Shilin Dist., Taipei 111, Taiwan; benson.lin@brightenoptix.com (W.-P.L.); sherry.huang@brightenoptix.com (H.-F.H.)
5 Department of Optometry, University of Kang Ning, No. 137, Alley 75, Sec. 3, Kang Ning Road, Neihu District, Taipei 11485, Taiwan
6 Institute of Biomedical Engineering and Nanomedicine, National Health Research Institutes, No. 35, Keyan Road, Zhunan Town, Miaoli County 35053, Taiwan
* Correspondence: hwfang@ntut.edu.tw
† These authors contributed equally to this work.

Citation: Su, C.-Y.; Yeh, L.-K.; Tsao, Y.-F.; Lin, W.-P.; Hou, C.-H.; Huang, H.-F.; Lai, C.-C.; Fang, H.-W. The Effect of Different Cleaning Methods on Protein Deposition and Optical Characteristics of Orthokeratology Lenses. *Polymers* **2021**, *13*, 4318. https://doi.org/10.3390/polym13244318

Academic Editors: Bramasta Nugraha and Faisal Raza

Received: 29 October 2021
Accepted: 7 December 2021
Published: 9 December 2021

Abstract: Orthokeratology lenses are commonly used for myopia control, especially in children. Tear lipids and proteins are immediately adsorbed when the lens is put on the cornea, and protein deposition may cause discomfort or infection. Therefore, we established an in vitro protein deposition analysis by mimicking the current cleaning methods for orthokeratology lens wearers for both short-term and long-term period. The results showed that the amounts of tear proteins accumulated daily and achieved a balance after 14 days when the lens was rubbed to clean or not. Protein deposition also affected the optical characteristics of the lens regardless of cleaning methods. Our results provided an in vitro analysis for protein deposition on the lens, and they may provide a potential effective method for developing care solutions or methods that can more effectively remove tear components from orthokeratology lenses.

Keywords: orthokeratology lens; protein deposition; optical characteristics; rubbing

1. Introduction

Orthokeratology (ortho-k) lenses have been used for affecting vision since 1945, when the corneal contact lens was made with plastic [1]. Modern ortho-k lens can be worn overnight to reshape the anterior cornea by the designs of reverse geometry; thus, patients with myopia do not need to wear glasses for vision correction during the daytime [2]. The safety of wearing ortho-k lenses has been monitored by several long-term clinical follow-ups, and complications still arise, although the majority was not immediate adverse events [3]. The major complications are microbial keratitis and superficial corneal staining, while microbial keratitis is a potentially vision-threating complication [4]. The possible cause of microbial keratitis might due to lack of eye movements which usually help to disrupt the bacterial glycocalyx, resulting in less spreading of lysozyme over the surface of eye tissue and making eyes being more susceptible to the infection [5]. In addition, microbial keratitis might be non-compliance, including inappropriate lens care and wearing continuously despite significant discomfort [6,7]. Indeed, tear proteins and lipids are immediately deposited on the surface of the lens when a contact lens is put into the eye. Tear proteins are also easily accumulated on the lens and may cause immune reactions if lenses are not being cleaned completely [8,9].

Ortho-k lenses can be reused for at least one year; thus, lens care is a more important and critical compared with soft contact lenses that are made as disposable daily. It has been shown that cleaning rigid contact lenses with lens care solutions without finger rubbing was not an effective method for removing stubborn materials (such as mascara and hand cream) from the lens [10]. Rigid contact lens multipurpose care solutions, hydrogen peroxide, and povidone–iodine are all advised for cleaning ortho-k lenses, but the related studies only focused on disinfecting microorganisms [7]. The studies about removing tear components from ortho-k lenses have not yet been investigated intensively. In addition, it is also possible that an accumulation of tear components may affect the reverse geometry of ortho-k lens, resulting in ineffectiveness in flattering the cornea. The relationship between tear components accumulation and the optical characteristics of ortho-k lenses is still unclear.

In this study, we first investigated protein deposition in the absence or presence of tear lipids. Two tear proteins were analyzed here: the lysozyme and albumin. Lysozyme is the most abundant tear protein, while the concentration of albumin increases when the eye is closed or when wearing ortho-k lenses [11,12]. Protein adsorption amounts on ortho-k lenses were analyzed by cleaning with or without finger rubbing. Both short-term and long-term protein deposition analyses were conducted, and the accumulated protein amounts were quantified daily. In addition, the optical characteristics of ortho-k lens after a long-term protein deposition procedure were also investigated.

2. Materials and Methods

2.1. Orthokeratology Lenses, Contact Lens Care Solution, and Artificial Tear solution

The material of ortho-k lenses used in the study was Boston XO^{TM}, and the material generic name was Hexafocon A (Brighten Optix Co., Taipei, Taiwan). The contact lens care solution used for cleaning and rinsing was Menicon Care Plus multipurpose solution for all rigid gas permeable lenses (Menicon, Nagoya, Japan). The preparation of artificial tear solution has been published previously [13]. In general, a complex of salt solution was made according to the concentration listed in Table 1 [13]. The pH value of a complex of salt solution was adjusted to 7.4 and was stored at room temperature for 3 or more days. The 2000 times lipid stock solution was made in a solution of 1 hexane:1 ether, and the stock concentration was listed in Table 1. Then, 250 μL of 2000 times lipid stock solution was added into a complex of salt solution, and the mixed solution was placed into an ultra-sonic bath at 37 °C. The mixed solution was sonicated at 90 W and purged with nitrogen gas until the lipid stock solution was fully incorporated, and the odor of hexane and ether was cleared out. Then, either lysozyme or albumin was added into the mixed solution containing salts and lipids for the further experiments. All the components of salt, lipid, and protein were purchased from Sigma-Aldeich (St. Louis, MO, USA).

2.2. Short-Term Protein Deposition Analysis

The ortho-k lens was treated by an oxygen plasma system (Force State OP300, PFS Co., Ltd., Taipei, Taiwan) at 100 mTorr, 80 W, 10 standard cubic centimeter per minute (Sccm) for 120 s before the experiment, in order to improve the hydrophobicity. The orthokeratology lens was placed in 2 mL of solution 1, which was artificial tear solution containing either 2.0 mg/mL lysozyme or 0.2 mg/mL albumin, and incubated at 37 °C for 8 h (Step 1 in Figure 1). Then, the immersed lens was placed in 2 mL of care solution at 37 °C for 16 h (Step 2 in Figure 1). Finally, the ortho-k lens was not cleaned (no rubbing) by care solution and was placed into a new artificial tear solution. The other group was cleaned (rubbing), rinsed with fingers in gloves by 50 μL of care solution, and placed into a new artificial tear solution (Step 3 in Figure 1). A completed cycle (step 1 to 3) was repeated 5 times (5 days), and the protein concentrations in each solution were analyzed.

Table 1. The concentration of each component in artificial tear solution.

Category	Component	Stock Concentration (mg/mL)	Final Concentration in Artificial Tear Solution (mg/mL)
	Sodium chloride		5.26
	Potassium chloride		1.19
	Sodium citrate		0.44
	Glucose		0.036
	Urea		0.072
Complex of salt solution	Calcium chloride	N.A.	0.07
	Sodium carbonate		1.27
	Potassium hydrogen carbonate		0.30
	Sodium phosphate dibasic		3.41
	Hydrochloric acid		0.94
	ProClin 300		200 μL/liter of solution
	Oleic acid	3.6	0.0018
	Oleic acid methyl ester	24.0	0.012
Lipid stock solution	Triolein	32.0	0.016
	Cholesterol	3.6	0.0018
	Cholesteryl oleate	48.0	0.024
	Phosphatidylcholine	1.0	0.0005
Protein	Lysozyme	N.A.	2.0
	Albumin		0.2

N.A.: Non applicable.

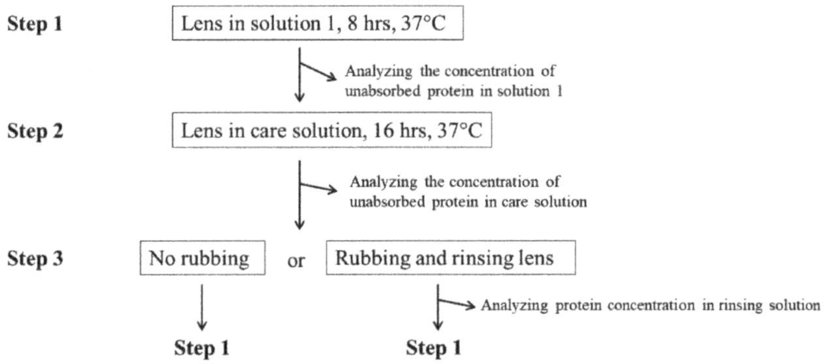

Figure 1. The procedure of protein deposition analysis. One completed cycle is from step 1 to step 3.

The Bio-Rad DC protein assay (Bio-Rad, Hercules, CA, USA) was used for measuring the amount of lysozyme or albumin in each solution [14]. The optical density (OD) value was obtained by an Enzyme-Linked Immunosorbent Assay (ELISA) reader with a wavelength of 280 nm. The deposited protein concentration on the orthokeratology lens after 3 steps on each was calculated as follows: (the original protein concentration)–(protein concentration in solution 1)–(protein concentration in care solution) for the no rubbing group. For the rubbing group, the deposited protein concentration was calculated as follows: (the original protein concentration)–(protein concentration in solution 1)–(protein concentration in care solution)–(protein concentration in rinsing solution). Five independent lenses were tested for each condition.

2.3. Long-Term Lysosomal Deposition Assay

In addition to a short-term protein deposition analysis, a long-term lysosomal deposition assay was also investigated. Ortho-k lenses were placed in artificial tear solution containing 2.0 mg/mL of lysozyme, and the procedure was same as shown in Figure 1. Thirty cycles (30 days) were conducted for a long-term analysis.

2.4. Optical Characteristics of Orthokeratology Lens

Light microscope VMS3020 (Shanghai Jingmi, Shanghai, China) was used for observing the surface of ortho-k lenses after protein deposition analysis. The pictures were taken with 10× objective and 10× ocular lens magnification. The base curve, central thickness, power and transmission of vision light (VIS), ultraviolet A (UVA), and ultraviolet B (UVB) light of ortho-k lenses were measured by CG Auto II (Neitz Instruments Co., Ltd., Tokyo, Japan), Contest plus (Rotlex, Omer, Israel), and UV/VIS Spectrophotometer (Kingtech Scientific Co., Ltd., Taipei, Taiwan). The water contact angle of lenses was measured by a MagicDroplet Contact Angle Meter Model 100SB (Sindatek Instruments Co., Ltd., Taipei, Taiwan). According to the standard ISO (International Standardization Organization) 18369-2 [15], the difference of base curve should be ±0.02 mm, central thickness should be ±0.02 mm, and power should be ±0.25 degree after any treatments. Otherwise, the measured value was considered as out of tolerance.

2.5. Statistical Analysis

The 2-tailed t-test was assessed in order to compare differences in lysozyme or albumin deposition amounts between two different conditions, such as comparison of protein deposition concentration between no rubbing and rubbing on day 1. A value of $p < 0.05$ was considered significant.

3. Results

3.1. Proteins Are Absorbed Increasingly in the Presence of Lipids

In order to mimic the condition of wearing ortho-k lenses, the lens was placed in artificial tear solution containing salts, lipids, and proteins. In addition, ortho-k lenses were placed in solution containing only salts and proteins to compare the amounts of protein deposition. The result showed that in the presence of lipids, the amounts of lysozyme or albumin were dramatically increased compared with the amounts in the absence of lipids (Figure 2).

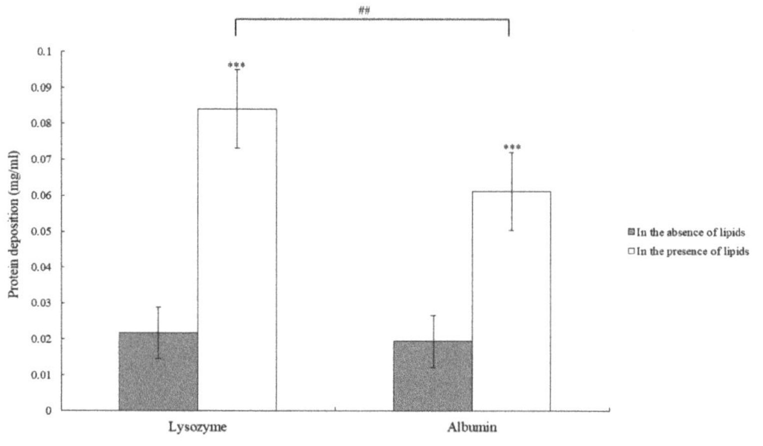

Figure 2. The concentration of protein deposition on the ortho-K lens in the absence of lipids (gray bars) or in the presence of lipids (white bars). *** $p < 0.001$ when comparing protein deposition amount in the absence of lipids versus in the presence of lipids. ## $p < 0.01$ when comparing the deposition amount of lysozyme versus albumin. Error bars represented standard deviation.

3.2. Rubbing the Lens Effectively Removes Absorbed Proteins from the Lens

Ortho-k lens wearers are advised to store lenses into care solution after wearing and then rub lenses to clean before putting back into the eye (Figure 1). However, many wearers may not rub the lenses to avoid breaking the lens. Then, the protein deposition on the lens with and without rubbing was investigated. The result demonstrated that protein deposition was increased daily regardless of no rubbing or rubbing (Figure 3). It was obvious that the amount of protein deposition on the lens without rubbing was more than the amount with rubbing. In addition, the amount of lysozyme deposition was significantly more than the amount of albumin when the lens was not rubbed to clean. The amount of lysozyme and albumin deposition was not similar when the lens was rubbed (Figure 3).

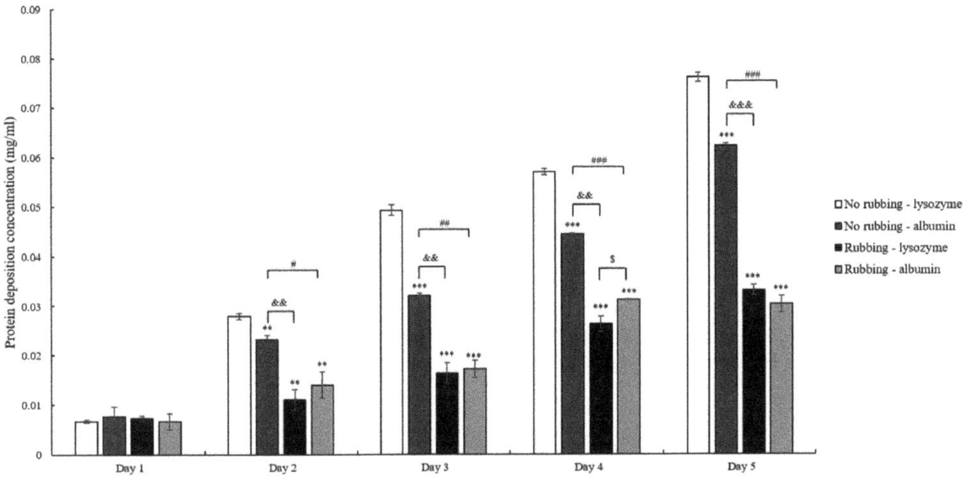

Figure 3. The concentration of protein deposition is accumulated when the lens is not rubbed (white or dark gray bars) or is rubbed (black or light gray bars) for cleaning. ** $p < 0.01$ and *** $p < 0.001$ when comparing protein deposition amount with lysozyme concentration on the lens without rubbing. && $p < 0.01$ and &&& $p < 0.001$ when comparing albumin deposition on no ribbing lens versus lysozyme deposition on rubbing lens. # $p < 0.05$, ## $p < 0.01$, and ### $p < 0.001$ when comparing albumin deposition on the lens without rubbing versus with rubbing. $ $p < 0.05$ when comparing lysozyme versus albumin deposition on the lens with rubbing. Error bars represented standard deviation.

3.3. Lysozyme Deposition on the Lens Tends to Be Stable after 14 Days

To understand the longer effect of cleaning methods on protein deposition, the procedure of protein deposition (Figure 1) was repeated for 30 days. The amount of lysozyme deposition was greatly reduced if the lens was rubbed compared with not rubbed (Figure 4). Lysozyme deposition was increased greatly during the first few days of the procedure no matter whether the lens was rubbed or not, which was similar with the observation when the procedure was repeated for 5 days (Figure 3). Although the concentration of lysozyme deposition was not increased dramatically after day 13, the current cleaning methods were also unable to remove lysozyme effectively once it was adsorbed onto the lens.

3.4. Optical Characteristics of Orthokeratology Lenses Changed after Long-Term of Lysozyme Deposition

Then, the optical characteristics of ortho-k lenses were investigated after 30 cycles of protein deposition procedure. There was contamination accumulated on the surface of the lens when the lens was not rubbed (Figure 5A) or rubbed (Figure 5B) with care solution. In addition, the power (PW) of each lens changed after 30 cycles of procedure (Table 2) as well as the transmission of VIS, UVA, and UVB (Table 3). The base curve of item 1 and the central thickness of item 3 in rubbing group were out of tolerance. The contact angle was also tested for each lens after 30 days, and the result showed that the contact angle was lower if the lens was not rubbed at the end of each cycle (Table 2).

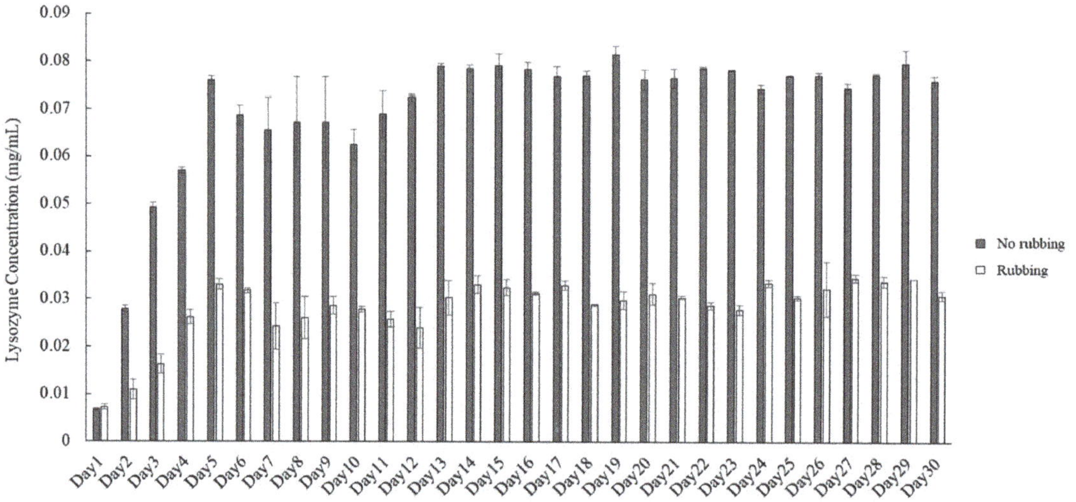

Figure 4. Deposited lysozyme concentrations are measured after the lens after one cycle of procedure. The lens is either not rubbed (gray bars) or rubbed (white bars) at the end of one cycle. The difference is statistically significant ($p < 0.001$) when comparing lysozyme deposition concentration on no rubbing versus rubbing lenses on the same day. Error bars represented standard deviation.

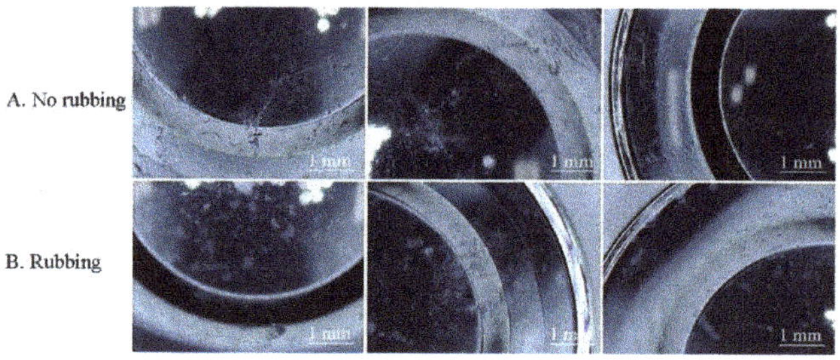

Figure 5. Pictures of lens surface after 30 cycles of protein deposition procedure when the lens was not rubbed (**A**) or rubbed (**B**) at the end of each cycle.

Table 2. Optical specifications of each tested lens before and after 30 cycles of protein deposition procedure.

Cleaning Method	Item	Before			After			
		BC (mm)	CT (mm)	PW (degree)	BC (mm)	CT (mm)	PW (degree)	Contact Angle (°)
No rubbing	1	8.60	0.23	+0.69	8.60	0.23	+0.66	15.09
	2	8.73	0.22	+0.77	8.72	0.22	+0.71	23.71
	3	9.11	0.23	+1.10	9.10	0.23	+1.11	13.02
Rubbing	1	9.01	0.24	+0.93	8.92 #	0.24	+0.74	80.29
	2	8.57	0.23	+0.76	8.57	0.24	+0.76	64.56
	3	8.71	0.21	−0.62	8.71	0.24 #	−0.48	52.32

BC: base curve; CT: central thickness; PW: power. # The measured data were out of tolerance.

Table 3. Optical transmission of each tested lens before and after 30 cycles of protein deposition procedure.

Cleaning Method	Item	Before			After		
		VIS	UVA	UVB	VIS	UVA	UVB
No Rubbing	1	83.85	12.63	0.734	85.18	12.86	0.779
	2	88.06	13.96	1.061	83.26	12.89	0.909
	3	82.98	12.24	0.677	76.69	11.52	0.785
Rubbing	1	87.86	13.55	0.831	78.19	10.74	0.523
	2	84.99	12.37	0.629	83.41	12.26	0.675
	3	84.12	13.44	0.987	83.73	13.23	1.014

VIS: vision light; UVA: ultraviolet A light; UVB: ultraviolet B light.

4. Discussion

We analyzed both short-term and long-term protein deposition on ortho-k lenses and the effect of protein deposition on optical characteristics of ortho-k lenses. We first investigated the effect of tear lipids on protein deposition, and the result demonstrated that the amounts of protein deposition were affected by the presence of lipids. Indeed, it has been shown that protein deposition increased dramatically in the presence of lipids on rigid gas-permeable contact lenses [16]. The previous study suggested that the hydrophobic nature of ortho-k lenses may attract the hydrophobic sites of lipids, resulting in the exposure of hydrophilic sites to attract protein binding [16]. Then, we next mimicked the possible cleaning methods that are used by ortho-k lens wearers. Although the wearers are advised to rub and rinse ortho-k lenses, many wearers start to skip rubbing because of being lazy or anxious about breaking expensive lenses [7,10]. The results showed that the amount of protein deposited on the lens was higher when the rubbing step was skipped, and the difference between rubbing and non-rubbing could be observed during the first few days (Figures 2 and 3). Therefore, rubbing the lens should continuously be advised to ortho-k lens wearers in order to remove deposited tear proteins.

A short-term protein deposition analysis showed that the deposition concentration of lysozyme and albumin was similar when the lens was rubbed to clean, whereas the concentration of lysozyme deposition was high when the rubbing step was skipped (Figure 2). The initial concentration of lysozyme was 10 times higher than albumin; thus, it was not surprising when lysozyme was adsorbed onto the lens more than albumin in the non-rubbing group. In addition, the surface of the ortho-k lenses is negatively charged [16]. The isoelectric point (pI) of albumin and lysozyme is 5.16 and 11.4, respectively [17,18]. Therefore, lysozyme is attracted and bound to the surface of the ortho-k lens more easily than albumin, resulting in more lysozyme deposition than albumin when the lens was not rubbed to clean. In contrast, lysozyme seemed to be removed more easily than albumin when the lens was rubbed to clean. Protein deposition onto the contact lens is not only affected by the charge of protein but other factors including the materials used for the contact lens, water content, pore size, protein size, protein structure, hydrophobicity, etc. can also play a vital role [17]. When the lens was rubbed, both lipids and proteins should be removed. We observed that the contact angle of the lens without rubbing was smaller than the lens with rubbing, suggesting that the lens with rubbing could maintain its hydrophobicity (Table 2). It has been shown that albumin was more easily denatured on the hydrophobic surface than on the hydrophilic surface [19], and it is possible that albumin was denatured after rubbing, resulting in it being difficult to be removed, and the final deposition concentration was similar to lysozyme. Whether albumin was more difficult to be removed from the ortho-k lens than lysozyme will require further investigation.

The result of a long-term protein deposition analysis demonstrated that the concentration of lysozyme deposition was saturated after 14 days whether the lens was rubbed to clean or not, suggesting that a balance between lysozyme adsorption and desorption was achieved. The assay we used for measuring protein concentration was an indirect method, because protein was not directly extracted from the lens. However, this indirect method allowed us to observe the daily accumulation of tear proteins, and the investigation could repeat for a long term in order to mimic the clinical observation. The result also suggested that the lens could not be completely cleaned by the current cleaning method for ortho-k lens wearers (Figure 5). Hydrogen peroxide and povidone–iodine can also be used for cleaning ortho-k lenses, especially for their effective anti-microbial activity [7]. Hydrogen peroxide has been shown that it can remove lipids or proteins on contact lenses when combining with surfactants or catalytic discs [20,21]. However, hydrogen peroxide cannot remove all the deposition on the lens, indicating that the cleaning ability of current commercial care solutions can still be improved.

In addition, lysozyme deposition changed the optical characteristics of ortho-k lenses, especially the power and the transmission of VIS, UVA, and UVB (Tables 2 and 3). The ortho-k lens utilizes the reverse geometry to provide hydraulic forces in post-lens tear film and causes stresses across the corneal epithelium, resulting in the reshaping of cornea and slowing the progression of myopia [22]. Therefore, the reduction of power and transmission of lights observed in the ortho-k lenses after a long-term lysosomal deposition might suggest that the reverse geometry design of the lens might be altered. We speculated that protein deposition on ortho-k lenses might not only increase the risk of infection but also reduce the effectiveness of myopia control. However, this possibility has not yet been observed clinically. The further clinical investigation should be analyzed to understand the relationship between tear protein deposition and myopia control of ortho-k lenses.

5. Conclusions

The current study demonstrated that tear proteins were more easily adsorbed on the surface of hydrophobic ortho-k lenses in the presence of tear lipids. Both short-term and long-term protein deposition analysis showed that proteins accumulated on the ortho-k lenses, and rubbing could remove significantly more adsorbed proteins than non-rubbing. Lysozyme deposition for a long term affected the optical characteristics of ortho-k lenses, and whether the changes of optical parameters affect the function of myopia control for ortho-k lenses will require clinical investigation. We mimicked clinical methods for cleaning ortho-k lenses, and our results provided in vitro evidence for tear protein accumulation on the lens that may increase risk for infection subsequently.

Author Contributions: Conceptualization, H.-W.F.; methodology, Y.-F.T., H.-F.H. and C.-C.L.; validation, W.-P.L., C.-H.H., Y.-F.T. and H.-F.H.; formal analysis, C.-Y.S. and L.-K.Y.; investigation, Y.-F.T., W.-P.L., C.-H.H. and C.-C.L.; data curation, C.-Y.S., L.-K.Y. and H.-W.F.; writing—original draft preparation, C.-Y.S.; writing—review and editing, L.-K.Y., W.-P.L., C.-H.H. and H.-W.F.; funding acquisition, L.-K.Y. and H.-W.F. All authors have read and agreed to the published version of the manuscript.

Funding: This research was supported by the Ministry of Science and Technology (MOST), Taiwan, under grant number 109-2622-E-027-019-CC1; National Taipei University of Technology and Chang Gung Memorial Hospital Joint Research Program (NTUT-CGMH-108-01); and Chang Gung Medical Research Project CORPG3K0121.

Institutional Review Board Statement: Not applicable.

Informed Consent Statement: Not applicable.

Data Availability Statement: The data presented in this study are available on request from the corresponding author.

Conflicts of Interest: The authors declare no conflict of interest.

References

1. Van Meter, W.S.; Musch, D.C.; Jacobs, D.S.; Kaufman, S.C.; Reinhart, W.J.; Udell, I.J. Safety of overnight orthokeratology for myopia: A report by the american academy of ophthalmology. *Ophthalmology* **2008**, *115*, 2301–2313 e2301. [CrossRef] [PubMed]
2. Bullimore, M.A.; Johnson, L.A. Overnight orthokeratology. *Cont. Lens Anterior Eye* **2020**, *43*, 322–332. [CrossRef] [PubMed]

3. Santodomingo-Rubido, J.; Villa-Collar, C.; Gilmartin, B.; Gutierrez-Ortega, R. Orthokeratology vs. Spectacles: Adverse events and discontinuations. *Optom. Vis. Sci.* **2012**, *89*, 1133–1139. [CrossRef] [PubMed]
4. Liu, Y.M.; Xie, P. The safety of orthokeratology–A systematic review. *Eye Contact Lens* **2016**, *42*, 35–42. [CrossRef] [PubMed]
5. Hsiao, C.H.; Lin, H.C.; Chen, Y.F.; Ma, D.H.; Yeh, L.K.; Tan, H.Y.; Huang, S.C.; Lin, K.K. Infectious keratitis related to overnight orthokeratology. *Cornea* **2005**, *24*, 783–788. [CrossRef] [PubMed]
6. Cope, J.R.; Collier, S.A.; Schein, O.D.; Brown, A.C.; Verani, J.R.; Gallen, R.; Beach, M.J.; Yoder, J.S. Acanthamoeba keratitis among rigid gas permeable contact lens wearers in the united states, 2005 through 2011. *Ophthalmology* **2016**, *123*, 1435–1441. [CrossRef] [PubMed]
7. Vincent, S.J.; Cho, P.; Chan, K.Y.; Fadel, D.; Ghorbani-Mojarrad, N.; Gonzalez-Meijome, J.M.; Johnson, L.; Kang, P.; Michaud, L.; Simard, P.; et al. Clear-orthokeratology. *Cont. Lens Anterior Eye* **2021**, *44*, 240–269. [CrossRef] [PubMed]
8. Allansmith, M.R.; Korb, D.R.; Greiner, J.V.; Henriquez, A.S.; Simon, M.A.; Finnemore, V.M. Giant papillary conjunctivitis in contact lens wearers. *Am. J. Ophthalmol.* **1977**, *83*, 697–708. [CrossRef]
9. Skotnitsky, C.; Sankaridurg, P.R.; Sweeney, D.F.; Holden, B.A. General and local contact lens induced papillary conjunctivitis (clpc). *Clin. Exp. Optom.* **2002**, *85*, 193–197. [CrossRef] [PubMed]
10. Cho, P.; Poon, H.Y.; Chen, C.C.; Yuon, L.T. To rub or not to rub?-effective rigid contact lens cleaning. *Ophthalmic Physiol. Opt.* **2020**, *40*, 17–23. [CrossRef] [PubMed]
11. Choy, C.K.; Cho, P.; Benzie, I.F.; Ng, V. Effect of one overnight wear of orthokeratology lenses on tear composition. *Optom. Vis. Sci.* **2004**, *81*, 414–420. [CrossRef] [PubMed]
12. Sack, R.A.; Tan, K.O.; Tan, A. Diurnal tear cycle: Evidence for a nocturnal inflammatory constitutive tear fluid. *Invest. Ophthalmol. Vis. Sci.* **1992**, *33*, 626–640. [PubMed]
13. Omali, N.B.; Subbaraman, L.N.; Heynen, M.; Ng, A.; Coles-Brennan, C.; Fadli, Z.; Jones, L. Surface versus bulk activity of lysozyme deposited on hydrogel contact lens materials in vitro. *Cont. Lens Anterior Eye* **2018**, *41*, 329–334. [CrossRef] [PubMed]
14. Su, C.Y.; Lai, C.C.; Yeh, L.K.; Li, K.Y.; Shih, B.W.; Tseng, C.L.; Fang, H.W. The characteristics of a preservative-free contact lens care solution on lysozyme adsorption and interfacial friction behavior. *Colloids Surf. B Biointerfaces* **2018**, *171*, 538–543. [CrossRef] [PubMed]
15. ISO. *18369-2 Ophthalmic Optics—Contact Lenses—Part 2: Tolerances*; International Standarization Organization: Geneva, Switzerland, 2017.
16. Bontempo, A.R.; Rapp, J. Protein-lipid interaction on the surface of a rigid gas-permeable contact lens in vitro. *Curr. Eye Res.* **1997**, *16*, 1258–1262. [CrossRef] [PubMed]
17. Luensmann, D.; Jones, L. Albumin adsorption to contact lens materials: A review. *Cont. Lens Anterior Eye* **2008**, *31*, 179–187. [CrossRef] [PubMed]
18. Omali, N.B.; Subbaraman, L.N.; Coles-Brennan, C.; Fadli, Z.; Jones, L.W. Biological and clinical implications of lysozyme deposition on soft contact lenses. *Optom. Vis. Sci.* **2015**, *92*, 750–757. [CrossRef] [PubMed]
19. Garrett, Q.; Griesser, H.J.; Milthorpe, B.K.; Garrett, R.W. Irreversible adsorption of human serum albumin to hydrogel contact lenses: A study using electron spin resonance spectroscopy. *Biomaterials* **1999**, *20*, 1345–1356. [CrossRef]
20. Kiel, J.S. Protein removal from soft contact lens using disinfection/neutralization with hydrogen peroxide/catalytic disc. *Clin. Ther.* **1993**, *15*, 30–35. [PubMed]
21. Lorentz, H.; Heynen, M.; Tran, H.; Jones, L. Using an in vitro model of lipid deposition to assess the efficiency of hydrogen peroxide solutions to remove lipid from various contact lens materials. *Curr. Eye Res.* **2012**, *37*, 777–786. [CrossRef] [PubMed]
22. Mountford, J. *A Model of Forces Acting in Orthokeratology*; Butterworth-Heinemann: Edinburgh, UK, 2004.

polymers MDPI

Article

Coaxial Electrospun PLLA Fibers Modified with Water-Soluble Materials for Oligodendrocyte Myelination

Zhepeng Liu [1,*], Jing Wang [1], Haini Chen [1], Guanyu Zhang [2], Zhuman Lv [2], Yijun Li [1], Shoujin Zhao [1] and Wenlin Li [2,*]

[1] School of Medical Instrument and Food Engineering, University of Shanghai for Science and Technology, Shanghai 200093, China; 202562371@st.usst.edu.cn (J.W.); 193832383@st.usst.edu.cn (H.C.); 172702210@st.usst.edu.cn (Y.L.); 183852335@st.usst.edu.cn (S.Z.)

[2] Department of Cell Biology, Second Military Medical University, Shanghai 200433, China; zhangguanyu555@foxmail.com (G.Z.); lvzhuman@163.com (Z.L.)

* Correspondence: zpliu@usst.edu.cn (Z.L.); liwenlin@smmu.edu.cn (W.L.)

Abstract: Myelin sheaths are essential in maintaining the integrity of axons. Development of the platform for in vitro myelination would be especially useful for demyelinating disease modeling and drug screening. In this study, a fiber scaffold with a core–shell structure was prepared in one step by the coaxial electrospinning method. A high-molecular-weight polymer poly-L-lactic acid (PLLA) was used as the core, while the shell was a natural polymer material such as hyaluronic acid (HA), sodium alginate (SA), or chitosan (CS). The morphology, differential scanning calorimetry (DSC), Fourier transform infrared spectra (FTIR), contact angle, viability assay, and in vitro myelination by oligodendrocytes were characterized. The results showed that such fibers are bead-free and continuous, with an average size from 294 ± 53 to 390 ± 54 nm. The DSC and FTIR curves indicated no changes in the phase state of coaxial brackets. Hyaluronic acid/PLLA coaxial fibers had the minimum contact angle ($53.1° \pm 0.24°$). Myelin sheaths were wrapped around a coaxial electrospun scaffold modified with water-soluble materials after a 14-day incubation. All results suggest that such a scaffold prepared by coaxial electrospinning potentially provides a novel platform for oligodendrocyte myelination.

Keywords: coaxial electrospinning; extracellular matrix; myelination; oligodendrocyte; water-soluble materials

Citation: Liu, Z.; Wang, J.; Chen, H.; Zhang, G.; Lv, Z.; Li, Y.; Zhao, S.; Li, W. Coaxial Electrospun PLLA Fibers Modified with Water-Soluble Materials for Oligodendrocyte Myelination. *Polymers* **2021**, *13*, 3595. https://doi.org/10.3390/polym13203595

Academic Editors: Ick-Soo Kim, Bramasta Nugraha and Faisal Raza

Received: 2 September 2021
Accepted: 15 October 2021
Published: 19 October 2021

1. Introduction

The myelin sheath wraps around the axons of neurons to provide protection, nutrition, and electrical insulation for axons [1]. Demyelinating diseases comprise a variety of disorders resulting from damage to oligodendrocytes, the myelin-forming cells, and consequent loss of myelin [2]. Demyelination could lead to devastating neurological impairments such as multiple sclerosis and cerebral palsy [3,4]. There are currently few effective therapies to regenerate the myelin [5,6]. The development of a platform for in vitro myelination would be highly useful for demyelinating disease modeling and drug screening [7,8]. Most studies have used a primary neuron and oligodendrocyte coculture system for an in vitro myelinating assay, which was time consuming and irreproducible [9]. Biocompatible polymers such as poly-L-lactic acid (PLLA), poly (lactic-co-glycolic) acid (PLGA), and poly (ε-caprolactone) (PCL) have been widely used as culture scaffolds to support cell proliferation and differentiation [10–12]. As the initiation of oligodendrocyte myelination does not depend on axonal signals [13], it is practicable to develop an artificial nanofiber scaffold for oligodendrocyte myelination. Previous efforts have used electrospun polystyrene or PLLA nanofibers as an artificial scaffold for oligodendrocyte myelination [14,15]. However, these scaffolds need to be coated with poly(l-lysine) to support cell attachment. Natural extracellular matrix (ECM) composition can provide biochemical and structural support for cell adhesion and regulate cell behaviors [16]. Scar formation is the biggest obstacle in the process of nerve regeneration. Studies have shown that hyaluronic acid (HA) can inhibit the generation of inflammation and promote the regeneration of nerve cells [17,18]. The non-antigenic nature of sodium alginate (SA) is more conducive to the repair of nerve cells [19]. SA gel was formed on the surface of the scaffold by the cross-linking method, which enhanced the biocompatibility of the scaffold and facilitated the proliferation and spread of cells on the scaffold surface [20]. Hossein et al. mixed chitosan (CS) particles with a scaffold to form a fibrous gel for sciatic nerve repair, and the results showed no significant difference in the sciatic nerve index compared with autograft [21]. However, most natural materials have high cell affinity and poor mechanical properties as cell scaffolds alone [22]. We reasoned that a coaxial stent structure with a water-soluble natural extracellular matrix outer layer and manmade polymer core could support better oligodendrocyte myelination. Therefore, in the present study, we aimed to develop a PLLA-based fiber scaffold with sodium hyaluronate, sodium alginate, or chitosan in the outer layer and to test their capacity to support myelination.

Common stent preparation methods include self-assembly [23,24], electrostatic spinning [25,26], and 3D printing [27,28], among others. The self-assembly method is an earlier method of preparation, and the process is simple and easy to operate. However, the self-assembled scaffold has weak mechanical properties, and it is difficult to create a stable three-dimensional structure, which results in the scaffold being unable to provide a stable place for cell growth and differentiation for a long time [29,30]. Three-dimensional (3D) printing is sought after by various industries due to its versatility and precision. However, the biological field requires far more resolution than most industries, resulting in slow printing processes and expensive equipment [31,32]. Electrospinning was used in the textile industry in its early days, but it has gradually expanded to many fields. This method has a relatively stable operation process and can produce uniform and continuous micron or nanofibers [33,34]. Currently, compared to electrospinning, many other stent preparation methods are relatively complicated to produce a suitable structure [35,36].

We designed a coaxial electrospinning setup to prepare a coaxial stent intended to promote the myelination of oligodendrocyte. The stent contained sodium hyaluronate, sodium alginate, or chitosan in the outer layer and a PLLA core (as illustrated in Figure 1). These stent structures greatly enhanced oligodendrocyte myelination. As far as we know, this is the first report on a coaxial scaffold modified with natural water-soluble materials by electrospinning as preparation for the culture and myelination of human oligodendrocytes.

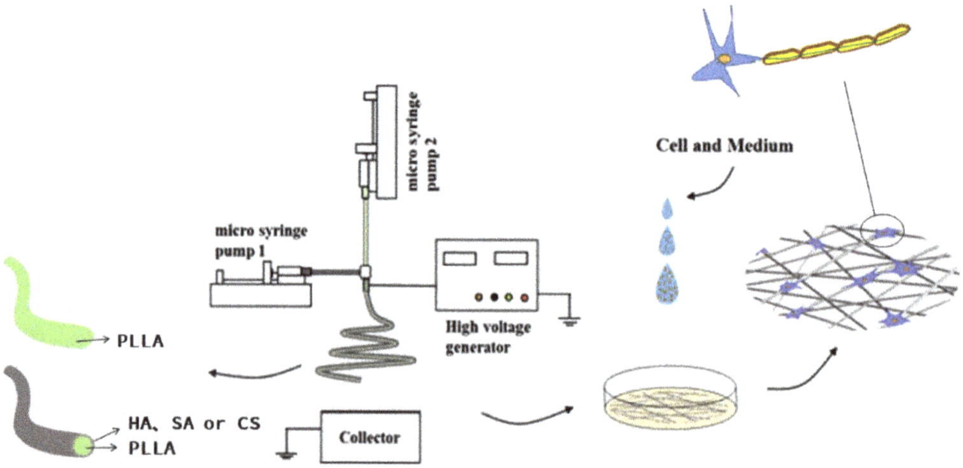

Figure 1. Coaxial electrospinning system.

2. Materials and Methods

2.1. Materials

Sodium hyaluronate (HA, Mw = 1800 kDa) was purchased from the Bloomage Freda Biopharma Co., Ltd. (Jinan, China). Poly(L-lactic acid) (PLLA, Mw = 30 Kda) was obtained from Jinan Daigang Biomaterial Co., Ltd. (Jinan, China). Sodium alginate (SA, Mw = 270 kDa) and chitosan (CS, Mw = 500,000, viscosity between 200 and 400 cP) were provided by Sinopharm Group Shanghai Chemical Reagent Company (Shanghai, China). Ethanol, dichloromethane (DCM), dimethyl sulfoxide (DMSO), and acetic acid were offered from Shanghai Vita Co., Ltd. (Shanghai, China).

MTT (4,5-dimethylthiazole-2))-2,5-diphenyltetrazolium bromide and 2-(4-amidinophenyl)-6-indole carbamidine dihydrochloride (DAPI) were purchased from Beyotime Biological Technology Co., Ltd. (Guangzhou, China). Rat adrenal pheochromocytoma cells (PC-12) were derived from the Cell Bank of the Type Culture Collection of the Chinese Academy of Sciences (Shanghai, China). Human embryonic stem cells (hESCs, H1 line) were obtained from WiCell (Madison, WI, USA).

2.2. Coaxial Electrospinning

The coaxial electrospinning platform used in this experiment was self-built, as shown in Figure 1. The inner and outer layers of spinning solution were controlled by two peristaltic pumps (KDS100, Scientific, Holliston, MA, USA), which were connected by homemade coaxial needles. The voltage controlled by the high-voltage generator (ZGF 60, Huatian Power Automation Co., Ltd., Wuhan, China) was applied to the needle through an alligator clip. An aluminum foil collector was used as a receiving device.

Firstly, the optimum parameters of the electrospinning (solution concentration/flow rate/voltage/needle–collector distance) were investigated, and subsequently, the coaxial fibers were prepared using the optimized conditions. Briefly, we added 3 g of PLLA to 50 mL (DCM: DMSO, 9:1/v:v) solution as the core solution. We configured three different shell spinning solutions: 0.1 g of HA was dissolved in 10 mL of a 30% ethanol aqueous solution, 0.1 g SA was dissolved in 10 mL of water, and 0.1 g of CS was added to 10 mL of 75% acetic acid aqueous solution. Pure PLLA spinning was obtained at a spinning solution flow rate of 0.8 mL/h, a voltage of 14 KV, and a distance needle to collector of 10 cm. The core layer and shell layer spinning solution flow velocity of coaxial electrospinning were 0.8 mL/h, the applied voltage was adjusted within the range of 14–16 KV, and the distance needle to collector was within 10–12 cm. All electrospinning processes were carried out under ambient conditions (22 ± 3 °C with a relative humidity of $50 \pm 5\%$).

2.3. Characterization

The fibers were characterized by size and appearance using an electron scanning microscope (SEM, Phenom ProX, Phenom, Eindhoven, The Netherlands). Before observing the fibers, the fibers were sprayed with gold. The diameter data of 100 random fibers in the photo were measured by ImageJ2x (Rawak Software Inc., Stuttgart, Germany), and the fiber diameter distribution was calculated to obtain the average fiber diameter. To visualize the core–sheath structure, transmission electron microscopy (Tecnai G^2 F20 S-TWIN, Hillsboro, OR, USA) at an accelerating voltage of 200 kV was employed. The chemical structure of the fiber was analyzed by the Fourier transform infrared spectrometer (FT-IR, Nicolet iS 5, Thermo Fisher, Waltham, MA, USA) to assess whether the chemical structure of the fiber was changed before preparation. All FTIR spectra were obtained in the spectral region of 500–2500cm^{-1}, with a resolution of 4 cm^{-1}, after 20 scans of each sample. A differential scanning calorimeter (DSC, DSC 204, NETZSCH, Selb, Germany) was used for thermal analysis of the fibers. Approximately 5 mg of the sample was placed in a clean crucible and heated from 25 to 300 °C (heating rate of 10 °C/min and a nitrogen purge of 10 mL/min). The hydrophilicity and hydrophobicity of the fiber were judged by the contact angle detection (DSA30, Kruss, Hamburg, Germany). During the measurement, 0.03 mL of deionized water were dropped on the spun fiber, and each sample was measured five times and averaged.

2.4. Cell Culture

Human oligodendrocytes were derived from hESCs as reported with modification [37]. Briefly, hESCs were maintained with E8 medium on a Matrigel coated surface. To induce neural differentiation, hESCs were treated with 2 μM TGFβ inhibitor SB43142 (Selleck, Houston, TX, USA), 1 μM BMP inhibitor DMH1 (Selleck, Houston, TX, USA), and 100 nM retinoic acid (Sigma-Aldrich, St. Louis, MO, USA) for 7 days in DMEM/F12 media supplemented with N2 and B27; then, it was treated with 100 nM SMO agonist SAG (Selleck, Houston, TX, USA) and 100 nM retinoic acid for an additional 7 days. The differentiated cells were dissociated with Accutase into single cells and plated into ultra-low attachment plates (Corning) for suspension culture supplemented with 10 ng/mL PDGF-AA, 5 ng/mL HGF, 10 ng/mL IGF1, and 10 ng/mL NT3 for 40 days. The cell aggregates were dissociated with Accumax into single cells (cells could be frozen for future experiments at this time point) and seeded on cover glasses with different fiber scaffolds at a density of 1.0×10^4 cells/cm^2. The cells were cultured with DMEM/F12 media with N2, B27, 60 ng/mL T3 (Sigma-Aldrich, St. Louis, MO, USA), 100 ng/mL biotin (Sigma-Aldrich, St. Louis, MO, USA), 1 μM cAMP (Sigma-Aldrich, St. Louis, MO, USA), and 60 μg/mL ascorbic acid-2-phosphate (Sigma-Aldrich, St. Louis, MO, USA) for an additional 14–21 days.

Rat adrenal pheochromocytoma cells (PC-12) were cultured in an incubator at 37 °C and 5% CO_2 concentration. The medium was a PC-12-defining medium (90% RPMI 1640 medium supplemented with 10% fetal bovine serum, 100 U/mL penicillin, and 100 μg/mL streptomycin). The medium was changed every two days. Prior to cell seeding, the four scaffolds prepared were placed in 24-well culture plates and UV-sterilized for 3 h. Cells were seeded on different scaffolds at a density of 1.0×10^4 cells cm^2.

All tissue culture products were obtained from Thermo Fisher Scientific except where otherwise specified.

2.5. Viability Assay

An MTT assay was used to evaluate the cytotoxicity of fiber scaffold to rat adrenal pheochromocytoma cells (PC-12). PC-12 were seeded onto different scaffolds at a density of 1.0×10^4 per well of 96-well plates. After 12 h, 24 h, 48 h, and 72 h, the old medium was discarded and washed three times with prewarmed PBS. A total of 360 μL of the prewarmed culture medium and 40 μL of 5 mg/mL MTT solution were added to each well, and the culture was incubated for 4 h. Then, the medium was discarded, and 400 μL of DMSO was added to each well. After shaking in the dark at 37 °C for 30 min, the DMSO solution was transferred to a 96-well plate. The absorbance was measured with a microplate reader (MODEL 680, Bio-Rad, Hercules, CA, USA) at a wavelength of 492 nm.

2.6. In Vitro Oligodendrocyte Myelination

In this experiment, the myelination of oligodendrocytes on the scaffolds in each group was observed by microscope and immunofluorescence staining. The scaffolds cocultured with oligodendrocytes for 14 days were fixed with 4% paraformaldehyde for 5 min and then permeabilized with PBS buffer containing 0.5% Triton X-100 (Sigma-Aldrich, St. Louis, MO, USA) and 5% donkey serum (Jackson ImmunoResearch, West Grove, PA, USA) for 30 min at room temperature. The cells were incubated with rat antimyelin basic protein (MBP, Abcam, Cambridge, UK) and mouse anti-rat O4 antibody (R&D system, Minneapolis, MN, USA) at 4 °C overnight. Next, the cells were washed with PBST and incubated with Alexa Fluor 488 conjugated donkey anti-mouse IgM and Alexa Fluor 555 conjugated donkey anti-rat IgG secondary antibodies (Invitrogen, 1000×) in PBST for one hour at room temperature. Nuclei were visualized by DAPI staining. Images were captured using a fluorescence microscope (Nikon ECLIPSE Ti2, Tokyo, Japan).

2.7. Statistical Analysis

All data are expressed as the mean value ± SD. Statistical analysis was performed with one-way analysis of variance (ANOVA) in Graph Pad Prism 7 software. A *p*-value of less than 0.05 was considered statistically significant.

3. Results and Discussion

3.1. Morphology and Microstructure of the Scaffolds

In order to compare the effects of different natural materials on the performance of fiber scaffolds, we prepared three different scaffolds. The shell materials were SA, HA, and CS. As shown in Figure 2a, all four fibers were bead-free and continuous. Lower magnitude SEM images are provided in Figure S1 (see Supplementary Materials). Among them, the pure PLLA spun was marked as A0, the spinning with SA as the shell was marked as A1, the outermost layer was HA spun as A2, and the outer layer of CS was labeled A3. It can be seen from Figure 2b that the diameter distribution of A0 fibers was relatively uniform, with an average diameter of 204 ± 44 nm. The diameter of the three types of coaxial electrospun fibers was basically larger than that of the A0. The smallest one was A1 with an average diameter of 294 ± 53 nm, and the largest was A3 with an average diameter of 390 ± 54 nm. This was due to the fact that the voltage and acceptance distance of A1 during the preparation process were larger than other groups. According to Maurya's research results, the increase in voltage or the distance needle to collector within a certain range can refine the fiber diameter [38]. The spinning condition of group A2 was similar to that of group A3, and the average fiber diameter was 334 ± 69 nm. The average fiber diameter of coaxial nanofibers is much bigger than that of neat PLLA nanofibers. The high viscosity and vapor pressure of the shell solution may be the reasons for the increasing of coaxial fiber diameter compared to single-component nanofiber. A similar trend was reported by Afshar et al. [39] on the fabrication of coaxial electrospun CS/PLA fibers, which had bigger average diameters than neat PLA fibers. In another work [40], it was also shown that the diameters of coaxial (PVP/PLA) and mono (PLA) electrospun scaffolds were 599.9 ± 112.0 nm and 136.8 ± 10 nm, respectively. TEM studies (Figure S2, Supplementary Materials) revealed a successful formation of the core–sheath structure.

3.2. DSC and FT-IR

Interaction between scaffold materials can be detected by FT-IR (Figure 2c). On the pure PLLA fiber spectra, two peaks caused by C=O and C-O-C stretching vibration appeared at 1760 cm^{-1} and 1170 cm^{-1}, which were consistent with the reports in the literature, and the absorption peaks at 1365 cm^{-1} and 1450 cm^{-1} were caused by CH_3 [41,42]. HA was formed by the polymerization of glucuronic acid and acetaminohexose, 1612 cm^{-1} and 1412 cm^{-1}, and the right corner of the valley was caused by the amide II [43,44]. The main functional groups in the SA molecule were carboxylate and glycosidic bonds, which corresponded to the characteristic peaks appearing at 1612 cm^{-1} and 1000–1150 cm^{-1} in the FT-IR spectrum [45]. Although CS is the product of deacetylation of chitin, the degree of deacetylation of CS used in the experiment was between 80% and 95%, so it still contained acyl groups. The absorption peaks at 1650 cm^{-1} and 1580 cm^{-1} in the spectrum were caused by acyl groups, while the glycosidic bonds were absorption peaks at 1100 cm^{-1} [44,46]. As expected, no new characteristic peaks appeared during the experiment, and the characteristic peaks of each component appeared in the spectrum of the coaxial bracket.

The DSC curves of different spun scaffolds are shown in Figure 2d. Compared with the other three materials, the pure PLLA showed an obvious endothermic peak at 178 °C. At the same time, this characteristic peak appeared in all coaxial bracket samples. The thermograms of SA and HA displayed an exothermic peak at about 236 °C and 240 °C, respectively, which were also observed in the coaxial fibers.

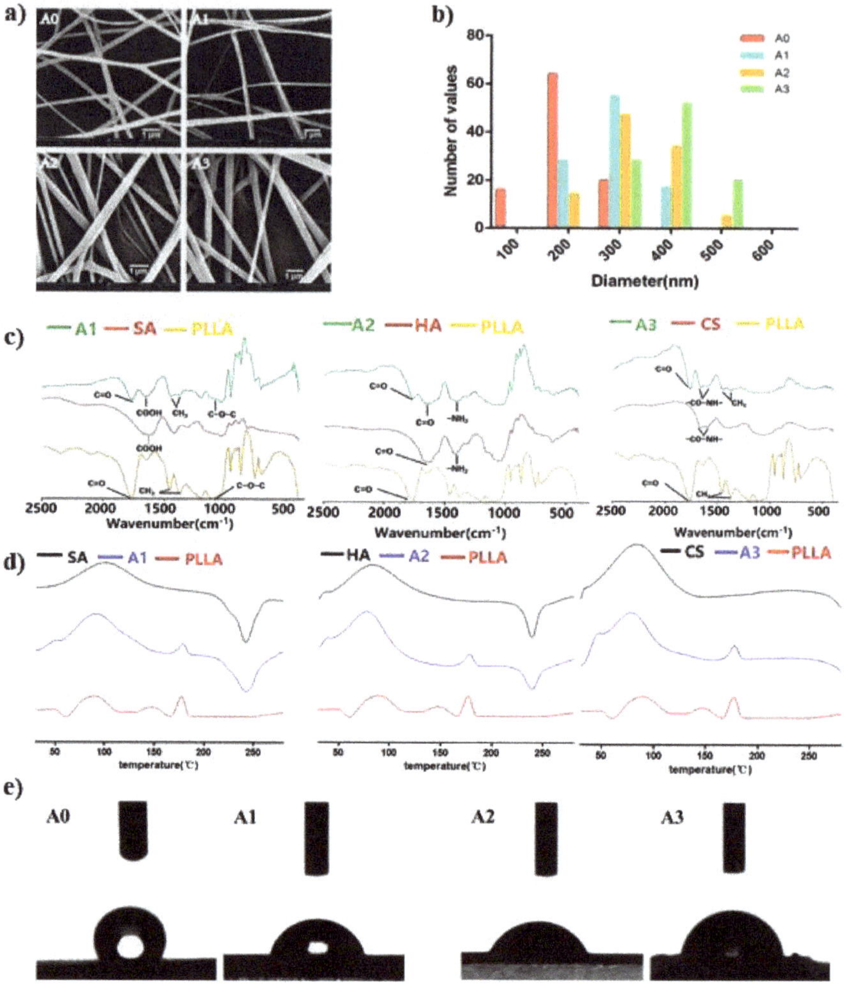

Figure 2. Physical and chemical properties investigation ((**a**,**b**) SEM of electrospinning fibers and diameter distribution; (**c**) Fourier transform infrared (FT-IR) of fiber scaffold; (**d**) DSC of fiber scaffold; (**e**) Experimental results of contact angles of spinning stent) (A0 6% PLLA; A1 1% sodium alginate (shell)—6% PLLA (core); A2 1% sodium hyaluronate (shell)—6% PLLA (core); A3 1% chitosan (shell)—6% PLLA (core)).

3.3. *Hydrophilicity of the Different Coaxial Scaffolds*

The contact angle of the liquid on the surface of the solid material is an important parameter to measure the wettability of the liquid on the surface of the material. As shown in Figure 2e, the contact angle of the pure PLLA fiber was 133° ± 0.45°, and the contact angles of the obviously coaxial electrospun scaffolds were 59.8° ± 0.36°, 53.1° ± 0.24°, and 77.3° ± 0.42°, among which the fibers of A2 had the smallest contact angle. This shows that the fiber surface is a natural material, which indirectly proves that the prepared spinning has a core–shell double-layer structure. Chang [47] et al. reported that the membranes prepared by hydrophilic materials reduced the contact angle and the membrane-containing HA had the smallest contact angle. In our study, A2 (HA) had the smallest contact angle.

3.4. *In Vitro Cytotoxicity of the Different Coaxial Scaffolds*

To evaluate the quality of cell scaffolds, the first consideration is the cytotoxicity of the scaffolds. Due to the postmitotic nature of oligodendrocytes, PC-12 was selected as the target cell for cytotoxic assay. Through the MTT cell viability experiments, as shown in Figure 3, all the scaffolds could sustain PC-12 cell proliferation. Specifically, the coaxial stents with an HA (A2) soluble extracellular matrix outer layer demonstrated even better cell proliferation after 24 and 48-h incubation ($p < 0.05$). It was attributed to the best hydrophilic effect of A2, which had the smallest contact angle. However, as the time went on, PC-12 proliferation on the coaxial stents showed no significant difference. These data suggested that the prepared scaffold was not cytotoxic.

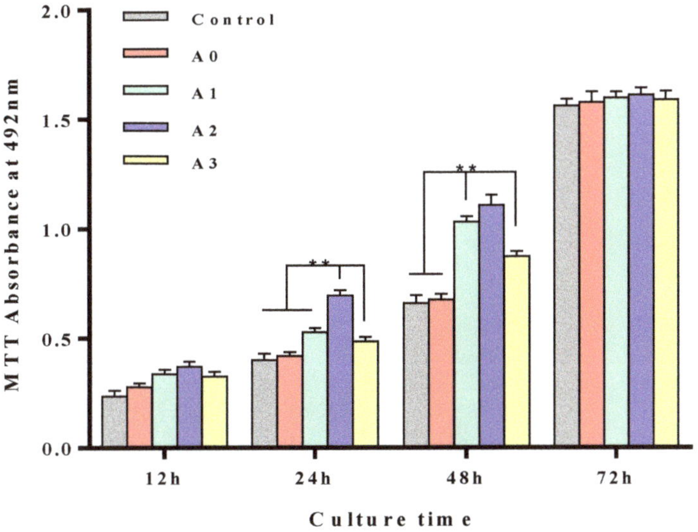

Figure 3. Cell viability of the different coaxial scaffolds. (Control) with no scaffold, (A0) 6% PLLA, (A1) 1% sodium alginate (shell)–6% PLLA (core), (A2) 1% sodium hyaluronate (shell)–6% PLLA (core), (A3) 1% chitosan (shell)–6% PLLA (core). * indicates $p < 0.05$, ** indicates $p < 0.01$.

3.5. *Oligodendrocytes Myelinate the Fiber Scaffolds*

After coculturing with different scaffolds for 14 days, the myelination of scaffolds by oligodendrocytes was analyzed by immunostaining. Oligodendrocytes formed MBP and O4 positive myelin sheaths along the fibers in all four tested scaffolds, which was consistent with the notion that oligodendrocytes can form myelin sheaths without the need of axonal signals. However, the MBP and O4 positive myelin sheaths were much longer in all three PLLA fibers modified with water-soluble materials than unmodified PLLA fibers, suggesting that the water-soluble matrixes used in this study, including sodium hyaluronate, sodium alginate, and chitosan, can enhance oligodendrocyte myelination (Figure 4). Makhijaa et al. reported that the stiffness, strain, topography, and spatial constraints of scaffolds play a key role in promoting the myelination of OPCs cells [48]. Hlavac et al. claimed that hydrogel scaffolds are suitable for nerve cell proliferation, differentiation, and repair [49]. In this study, PLLA scaffolds coated with hydrophilic material have played a very excellent role in promoting myelination.

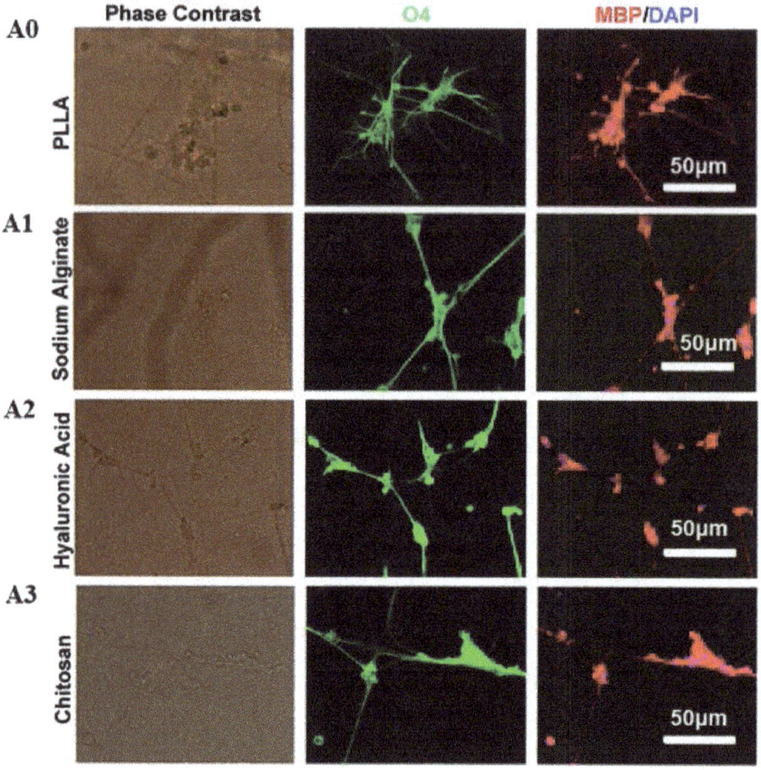

Figure 4. In vitro myelination of oligodendrocyte on different scaffolds after 14 days of cell seeding. Wrapped myelin positive for O4 and MBP was visualized by immunofluorescence staining. (A0) 6% PLLA, (A1) 1% sodium alginate (shell)–6% PLLA (core), (A2) 1% sodium hyaluronate (shell)–6% PLLA (core), (A3) 1% chitosan (shell)–6% PLLA (core).

4. Conclusions

In this experiment, the core–shell structured spinning scaffolds were prepared in one step by coaxial electrospinning technology for in vitro oligodendrocyte myelination. An MTT experiment showed that the scaffolds of each group were not cytotoxic. With 14 days of scaffold and oligodendrocyte coculturing, myelin sheaths were formed along the fibers. In particular, the fibers modified with water-soluble materials demonstrated longer myelin sheaths than unmodified PLLA fibers. These data suggested that these coaxial stents with a soluble natural extracellular matrix outer layer and synthetic polymer core could be better artificial scaffolds for oligodendrocyte myelination. This in vitro myelination culture system could be especially promising in screening candidates that can promote myelination for therapeutic purposes. However, although the initiation of myelination is an intrinsic property of oligodendrocytes, appropriate myelin compaction required an axon's instructive signaling that is still not fully understood. Previous studies demonstrated that myelin sheaths wrapped around artificial fibers were aberrantly organized, which could represent a disadvantage of using artificial fibers as surrogates for neuron axons. Therefore, it is important to further characterize the myelin structures wrapped around these coaxial stents in the future. Our study provided a strategy to modify nanofibers for better in vitro oligodendrocyte myelination.

Supplementary Materials: The following are available online at https://www.mdpi.com/article/10.3390/polym13203595/s1, Figure S1: SEM images of electrospinning fibers, Figure S2: TEM images of electrospinning fibers.

Author Contributions: Conceptualization, Z.L. (Zhepeng Liu) and W.L.; methodology, J.W.; software, H.C.; validation, G.Z. and Y.L.; formal analysis, Z.L. (Zhuman Lv); investigation, S.Z.; resources, H.C.; data curation, G.Z.; writing—original draft preparation, Z.L. (Zhepeng Liu); writing—review and editing, W.L.; visualization, Y.L.; supervision, Z.L. (Zhuman Lv); project administration, W.L.; funding acquisition, W.L. All authors have read and agreed to the published version of the manuscript.

Funding: This study received financial support from the National Natural Science Foundation of China (81571094).

Institutional Review Board Statement: Not applicable.

Informed Consent Statement: Not applicable.

Data Availability Statement: Not applicable.

Conflicts of Interest: The authors declare no conflict of interest.

References

1. Stadelmann, C.; Timmler, S.; Barrantes-Freer, A.; Simons, M. Myelin in the Central Nervous System: Structure, Function, and Pathology. *Physiol. Rev.* **2019**, *99*, 1381–1431.
2. Love, S. Demyelinating diseases. *Clin. Pathol.* **2006**, *59*, 1151–1159. [CrossRef]
3. Back, S.A.; Luo, N.L.; Borenstein, N.S.; Volpe, J.; Kinney, H. Arrested oligodendrocyte lineage progression during human cerebral white matter development: Dissociation between the timing of progenitor differentiation and myelinogenesis. *Neuropathol. Exp. Neurol.* **2002**, *61*, 197–211. [CrossRef]
4. Compston, A.; Coles, A. Multiple sclerosis. *Lancet* **2008**, *372*, 1502–1517. [CrossRef]
5. Qi, Z.P.; Zhang, T.H.; Kong, W.J.; Fu, C.; Chang, Y.X.; Li, H.R.; Yang, X.Y.; Pan, S. A dual-drug enhanced injectable hydrogel incorporated with neural stem cells for combination therapy in spinal cord injury. *Chem. Eng. J.* **2022**, *427*, 130906. [CrossRef]
6. Nemeth, C.L.; Fine, A.S.; Fatemi, A. Translational challenges in advancing regenerative therapy for treating neurological disorders using nanotechnology. *Adv. Drug Deliv. Rev.* **2019**, *148*, 60–67. [CrossRef]
7. Mozafari, S.; Evercooren, A.B.V. Human stem cell-derived oligodendrocytes: From humanized animal models to cell therapy in myelin diseases. *Semin. Cell Dev. Biol.* **2021**, *116*, 53–61. [CrossRef]
8. Catherine, L.; Bernard, Z.; Anna, W.; Christine, S.; Bruno, S. Remyelination in multiple sclerosis: From basic science to clinical translation. *Lancet Neurol.* **2020**, *19*, 678–688.
9. Rodrigues, G.; Gaj, T.; Adil, M.; Wahba, J.; Rao, A.T.; Lorbeer, F.K.; Kulkarni, R.U.; Diogo, M.M.; Cabral, J.; Miller, E.W.; et al. Defined and Scalable Differentiation of Human Oligodendrocyte Precursors from Pluripotent Stem Cells in a 3D Culture System. *Stem Cell Rep.* **2017**, *8*, 1770–1783. [CrossRef]
10. Parinaz, A.; Fatemeh, O.; Ahad, M. The triad of nanotechnology, cell signalling, and scaffold implantation for the successful repair of damaged organs: An overview on soft-tissue engineering. *J. Control. Release* **2021**, *332*, 460–492.
11. Luo, Y.Q.; Xue, F.; Liu, K.; Li, B.Q.; Fu, C.F.; Ding, J.X. Physical and biological engineering of polymer scaffolds to potentiate repair of spinal cord injury. *Mater. Des.* **2021**, *201*, 109484. [CrossRef]
12. Mneimneh, A.T.; Mehanna, M.M. Collagen-based scaffolds: An auspicious tool to support repair, recovery, and regeneration post spinal cord injury. *Int. J. Pharm.* **2021**, *601*, 120559. [CrossRef]
13. Rosenberg, S.S.; Kelland, E.E.; Tokar, E.; De la Torre, A.R.; Chan, J.R. The geometric and spatial constraints of the microenvironment induce oligodendrocyte differentiation. *Proc. Natl. Acad. Sci. USA* **2008**, *105*, 14662–14667. [CrossRef]
14. Nocita, E.; Giovane, D.A.; Tiberi, M.; Boccuni, L.; Fiorelli, D.; Sposato, C.; Romano, E.; Basoli, F.; Trombetta, M.; Rainer, A.; et al. EGFR/ErbB Inhibition Promotes OPC Maturation up to Axon Engagement by Co-Regulating PIP2 and MBP. *Cells* **2019**, *8*, 844. [CrossRef] [PubMed]
15. Nathalie, B.; Ana, M.; Sandra, V.; Abílio, A.; Maria, H.V.F.; Paula, M.V.; Odete, A.B.D.C. Electrically polarized PLLA nanofibers as neural tissue engineering scaffolds with improved neuritogenesis. *Colloids Surf. B Biointerfaces* **2018**, *167*, 93–103.
16. Marie, C.; Pierre, J.; Onnik, A.; Christophe, H. 3D models of dilated cardiomyopathy: Shaping the chemical, physical and topographical properties of biomaterials to mimic the cardiac extracellular matrix. *Bioact. Mater.* **2022**, *7*, 275–291.
17. Kumar, G.S.; Murugakoothan, P. Synthesis, spectral analysis, optical and thermal properties of new organic NLO crystal: N,N′-Diphenylguanidinium Nitrate (DPGN). *Spectrochim. Acta Part A Mol. Biomol. Spectrosc.* **2014**, *131*, 17–21. [CrossRef]
18. Wang, X.; He, J.; Wang, Y.; Cui, F.Z. Hyaluronic acid-based scaffold for central neural tissue engineering. *Interface Focus* **2012**, *2*, 278–291. [CrossRef]
19. Wu, Z.; Li, Q.; Xie, S.; Shan, X.; Cai, Z. In vitro and in vivo biocompatibility evaluation of a 3D bioprinted gelatin-sodium alginate/rat Schwann-cell scaffold. *Mater. Sci. Eng. C* **2020**, *109*, 1105–1130. [CrossRef] [PubMed]

20. Homaeigohar, S.; Tsai, T.Y.; Young, T.H.; Yang, H.J.; Ji, Y.R. An electroactive alginate hydrogel nanocomposite reinforced by functionalized graphite nanofilaments for neural tissue engineering. *Carbohydr. Polym.* **2019**, *224*, 112–115. [CrossRef] [PubMed]
21. Jahromi, H.K.; Farzin, A.; Hasanzadeh, E.; Barough, S.E.; Mahmoodi, N.; Najafabadi, M.R.Z.; Farahani, M.S.; Mansoor, K.; Shirian, S.; Ai, J. Enhanced sciatic nerve regeneration by poly-L-lactic acid/multi-wall carbon nanotube neural guidance conduit containing Schwann cells and curcumin encapsulated chitosan nanoparticles in rat. *Mater. Sci. Eng. C* **2020**, *109*, 2287–2299. [CrossRef]
22. Rajasekaran, R.; Seesala, V.S.; Sunka, K.C.; Ray, P.G.; Saha, B.; Banerjee, M.; Dhara, S. Role of nanofibers on MSCs fate: Influence of fiber morphologies, compositions and external stimuli. *Mater. Sci. Eng. C* **2020**, *107*, 110–218. [CrossRef]
23. Negah, S.S.; Oliazadeh, P.; Jahan-Abad, A.J.; Eshaghabadi, A.; Samini, F.; Ghasemi, S.; Asghari, A.; Gorji, A. Transplantation of human meningioma stem cells loaded on a self-assembling peptide nanoscaffold containing IKVAV improves traumatic brain injury in rats. *Acta Biomater.* **2019**, *92*, 132–144. [CrossRef]
24. Sarode, A.; Annapragada, A.; Guo, J.L.; Mitragotri, S. Layered self-assemblies for controlled drug delivery: A translational overview. *Biomaterials* **2020**, *242*, 119929. [CrossRef]
25. Wang, Z.; Wang, Y.C.; Yan, J.Q.; Zhang, K.S.; Lin, F.; Xiang, L.; Deng, L.F.; Guan, Z.P.; Cui, W.G.; Zhang, H.B. Pharmaceutical electrospinning and 3D printing scaffold design for bone regeneration. *Adv. Drug Deliv. Rev.* **2021**, *174*, 504–534. [CrossRef]
26. Mokhtari, F.; Azimi, B.; Salehi, M.; Hashemikia, S.; Danti, S. Recent advances of polymer-based piezoelectric composites for biomedical applications. *J. Mech. Behav. Biomed. Mater.* **2021**, *122*, 104669. [CrossRef] [PubMed]
27. Xu, W.H.; Jambhulkar, S.; Zhu, Y.X.; Ravichandran, D.; Kakarla, M.; Vernon, B.; Lott, D.G.; Cornella, J.L.; Shefi, O.; Miquelard-Garnier, G.; et al. 3D printing for polymer/particle-based processing: A review. *Compos. Part B Eng.* **2021**, *223*, 109102. [CrossRef]
28. Vijayavenkataraman, S.; Thaharah, S.; Zhang, S.; Lu, W.F.; Fuh, J.Y.H. Electrohydrodynamic jet 3D-printed PCL/PAA conductive scaffolds with tunable biodegradability as nerve guide conduits (NGCs) for peripheral nerve injury repair. *Mater. Des.* **2019**, *162*, 171–184. [CrossRef]
29. Stuart, K.; Amalia, A.; Eileen, L.; McPherson, M.J. Production of self-assembling biomaterials for tissue engineering. *Trends Biotechnol.* **2009**, *27*, 423–433.
30. Koss, K.M.; Unsworth, L.D. Neural tissue engineering: Bioresponsive nanoscaffolds using engineered self-assembling peptides. *Acta Biomater.* **2016**, *44*, 2–15. [CrossRef] [PubMed]
31. Ji, S.C.; Kang, H.-W.; Lee, I.H.; Ko, T.J.; Cho, D.-W. Development of micro-stereolithography technology using a UV lamp and optical fiber. *Int. J. Adv. Manuf. Technol.* **2009**, *41*, 281–286.
32. O'Brien, C.M.; Holmes, B.; Scott, F.; Zhang, L.J.G. Three-Dimensional Printing of Nanomaterial Scaffolds for Complex Tissue Regeneration. *Tissue Eng. Part B Rev.* **2015**, *21*, 103–104. [CrossRef] [PubMed]
33. Jain, R.; Shetty, S.S.; Yadav, K. Unfolding the electrospinning potential of biopolymers for preparation of nanofibers. *J. Drug Deliv. Sci. Technol.* **2020**, *57*, 1173–1185. [CrossRef]
34. Ghosal, K.; Agatemor, C.; Špitálsky, Z.; Thomas, S.; Kny, E. Electrospinning tissue engineering and wound dressing scaffolds from polymer-titanium dioxide nanocomposites. *Chem. Eng. J.* **2019**, *358*, 1262–1278. [CrossRef]
35. Ha, D.H.; Chae, S.H.; Lee, J.Y.; Kim, J.Y.; Yoon, J.B.; Sen, T.; Lee, S.W.; Kim, H.J.; Cho, J.H.; Cho, D.W. Therapeutic effect of decellularized extracellular matrix-based hydrogel for radiation esophagitis by 3D printed esophageal stent. *Biomaterials* **2021**, *266*, 120477. [CrossRef]
36. Kumar, R.; Aadil, K.R.; Ran, J.S.; Vijay, B.K. Advances in nanotechnology and nanomaterials based strategies for neural tissue engineering. *J. Drug Deliv. Sci. Technol.* **2020**, *57*, 1196–1205. [CrossRef]
37. Douvaras, P.; Fossati, V. Generation and isolation of oligodendrocyte progenitor cells from human pluripotent stem cells. *Nat. Protoc.* **2015**, *10*, 1143–1154. [CrossRef]
38. Maurya, A.K.; Narayana, P.L.; GeethaBhavani, A.; Hong, J.K.; Reddy, N.S. Modeling the relationship between electrospinning process parameters and ferrofluid/polyvinyl alcohol magnetic nanofiber diameter by artificial neural networks. *J. Electrost.* **2020**, *104*, 1416–1422. [CrossRef]
39. Afshar, S.; Rashedi, S.; Nazockdast, H.; Ghazaliand, M. Preparation and characterization of electrospun poly(lactic acid)-chitosan core-shell nanofibers with a new solvent system. *Int. J. Biol. Macromol.* **2019**, *138*, 1130–1137. [CrossRef]
40. Hajikhani, M.; Emam-Djomeh, Z.; Askari, G. Fabrication and characterization of mucoadhesive bioplastic patch via coaxial polylactic acid (PLA) based electrospun nanofibers with antimicrobial and wound healing application. *Int. J. Biol. Macromol.* **2021**, *172*, 143–153. [CrossRef]
41. Bonadies, I.; Longo, A.; Androsch, R.; Jehnichen, D.; Göbel, M.; Lorenzo, M.L.D. Biodegradable electrospun PLLA fibers containing the mosquito-repellent DEET. *Eur. Polym. J.* **2019**, *113*, 377–384. [CrossRef]
42. Liu, Z.X.; Yang, Y.; Zhang, K. Control of structure and morphology of highly aligned PLLA ultrafine fibers via linear-jet electrospinning. *Polymer* **2013**, *54*, 6045–6051. [CrossRef]
43. Safaei, M.; Taran, M. Optimal conditions for producing bactericidal sodium hyaluronate-TiO2 bionanocomposite and its characterization. *Int. J. Biol. Macromol.* **2017**, *104 Pt A*, 449–456. [CrossRef]
44. Coimbra, P.; Alves, P.; Valente, T.A.; Santos, R.; Correia, I.J.; Ferreira, P. Sodium hyaluronate/chitosan polyelectrolyte complex scaffolds for dental pulp regeneration: Synthesis and characterization. *Int. J. Biol. Macromol.* **2011**, *49*, 573–579. [CrossRef]

45. Salem, D.; Sallam, M.A.E.; Youssef, T. Synthesis of compounds having antimicrobial activity from alginate. *Bioorg. Chem.* **2019**, *87*, 103–111. [CrossRef] [PubMed]
46. Mauricio, A.; Salazar, R.; Luna-Bárcenas, G.; Mendoza-Galvan, A. FTIR spectroscopy studies on the spontaneous neutralization of chitosan acetate films by moisture conditioning. *Vib. Spectrosc.* **2018**, *94*, 1–6. [CrossRef]
47. Chang, P.H.; Chao, H.M.; Chern, E.; Hsu, S.H. Chitosan 3D cell culture system promotes naïve-like features of human induced pluripotent stem cells: A novel tool to sustain pluripotency and facilitate differentiation. *Biomaterials* **2021**, *268*, 120575. [CrossRef] [PubMed]
48. Makhijaa, E.P.; Espinosa-Hoyos, D.; Jagielska, A.; Van Vliet, K.J. Mechanical regulation of oligodendrocyte biology. *Neurosci. Lett.* **2020**, *717*, 134673. [CrossRef] [PubMed]
49. Hlavac, N.; Kasper, M.; Schmidt, C.E. Progress toward finding the perfect match: Hydrogels for treatment of central nervous system injury. *Mater. Today Adv.* **2020**, *6*, 100039. [CrossRef]

polymers MDPI

Article

Concentration Dependent Single Chain Properties of Poly(sodium 4-styrenesulfonate) Subjected to Aromatic Interactions with Chlorpheniramine Maleate Studied by Diafiltration and Synchrotron-SAXS

Felipe Orozco [1], Thomas Hoffmann [2], Mario E. Flores [2], Judit G. Lisoni [3], José Roberto Vega-Baudrit [1] and Ignacio Moreno-Villoslada [2,*]

[1] Laboratorio Nacional de Nanotecnología LANOTEC-CENAT, Centro Nacional de Alta Tecnología, Pavas, San José 1174-1200, Costa Rica; f.orozco.gutierrez@rug.nl (F.O.); jvegab@gmail.com (J.R.V.-B.)
[2] Laboratorio de Polímeros, Instituto de Ciencias Químicas, Facultad de Ciencias, Universidad Austral de Chile, Casilla 567, Valdivia 5090000, Chile; thomas.hoffmann@uach.cl (T.H.); mario.flores@uach.cl (M.E.F.)
[3] Facultad de Ciencias, Instituto de Ciencias Físicas y Matemáticas, Universidad Austral de Chile, Valdivia 5090000, Chile; judit.lisoni@uach.cl
* Correspondence: imorenovilloslada@uach.cl

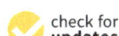

Citation: Orozco, F.; Hoffmann, T.; Flores, M.E.; Lisoni, J.G.; Vega-Baudrit, J.R.; Moreno-Villoslada, I. Concentration Dependent Single Chain Properties of Poly(sodium 4-styrenesulfonate) Subjected to Aromatic Interactions with Chlorpheniramine Maleate Studied by Diafiltration and Synchrotron-SAXS. *Polymers* **2021**, *13*, 3563. https://doi.org/10.3390/polym13203563

Academic Editor: Bramasta Nugraha

Received: 31 August 2021
Accepted: 1 October 2021
Published: 15 October 2021

Publisher's Note: MDPI stays neutral with regard to jurisdictional claims in published maps and institutional affiliations.

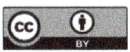

Abstract: The polyelectrolyte poly(sodium 4-styrenesulfonate) undergoes aromatic–aromatic interaction with the drug chlorpheniramine, which acts as an aromatic counterion. In this work, we show that an increase in the concentration in the dilute and semidilute regimes of a complex polyelectrolyte/drug 2:1 produces the increasing confinement of the drug in hydrophobic domains, with implications in single chain thermodynamic behavior. Diafiltration analysis at polymer concentrations between 0.5 and 2.5 mM show an increase in the fraction of the aromatic counterion irreversibly bound to the polyelectrolyte, as well as a decrease in the electrostatic reversible interaction forces with the remaining fraction of drug molecules as the total concentration of the system increases. Synchrotron-SAXS results performed in the semidilute regimes show a fractal chain conformation pattern with a fractal dimension of 1.7, similar to uncharged polymers. Interestingly, static and fractal correlation lengths increase with increasing complex concentration, due to the increase in the amount of the confined drug. Nanoprecipitates are found in the range of 30–40 mM, and macroprecipitates are found at a higher system concentration. A model of molecular complexation between the two species is proposed as the total concentration increases, which involves ion pair formation and aggregation, producing increasingly confined aromatic counterions in hydrophobic domains, as well as a decreasing number of charged polymer segments at the hydrophobic/hydrophilic interphase. All of these features are of pivotal importance to the general knowledge of polyelectrolytes, with implications both in fundamental knowledge and potential technological applications considering aromatic-aromatic binding between aromatic polyelectrolytes and aromatic counterions, such as in the production of pharmaceutical formulations.

Keywords: diafiltration; SAXS; aromatic interactions; poly(sodium 4-styrenesulfonate); chlorpheniramine; polyelectrolyte; aggregation

1. Introduction

During the last decades, we have studied the interactions between aromatic polyelectrolytes, such as poly(sodium 4-styrenesulfonate) (PSS), and low molecular-weight aromatic species (LMWS) acting as counterions, among which we can find xanthene dyes [1–7], redox-active tetrazolium salts [8–11], and different drugs [12–16]. Both complementary charged species bearing aromatic groups undergo secondary aromatic-aromatic interactions, additional to primary long-range electrostatic interactions, thus producing a reinforcement of the overall interaction. Contrary to the picture given by Manning's

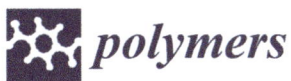

counterion condensation theory [17–21], in which the territorial binding of counterions to polyelectrolyte chains occurs, aromatic counterions and polymeric aromatic groups produce site-specific binding, losing water molecules from their respective hydration spheres, as deduced by 1D and 2D ^{1}H-NMR spectroscopies [3–6,8,13,16]. Verification of the nuclear Overhauser effect allowed for the demonstration that the interacting species approach each other by less than 5 Å. Another technique that allowed us to obtain information about the interaction between aromatic polyelectrolytes and low molecular-weight aromatic counterions was diafiltration (DF). This technique is a separation technique, which allowed the direct determination of the counterions bound to the polyelectrolyte in every instant, showing comparatively higher binding and resistance to the cleaving effect of added electrolytes in solution when contrasted with systems that do not undergo aromatic-aromatic interactions [6,12,13]. As a consequence of this interaction pattern, some properties of both the counterions and the polymers change, such as aggregation, acid-base, redox, and luminescent properties [2,4,10,13]. These interactions have also served to produce interesting higher order structures [11,22–25], and confer different properties to materials [26–31]. In particular, homogenously-dispersed photosensitizers and dyes with a controllable state of aggregation have been included in solid and semisolid materials by means of complexation with an aromatic polyelectrolyte [7,26,27]; nanoparticles of redox-active and acid-based reactive aromatic molecules have been produced in the presence of aromatic polyelectrolytes and included in solid and semisolid materials used as sensors [23,28,30].

Drug vehiculization and controlled release in matrices and nanoparticles based on aromatic-aromatic interactions have also been developed [15,16,23]. Importantly, outstanding drug loading of around 50% has been achieved, since the drug acts both as a bioactive molecule carried by the nanoparticle and as a main constituent of the carrier [15,16]. The mechanism for nanocarrier formation involving the dual function of the drug has been rationalized as the consequence of ion pair formation between the charged aromatic drug and the complementary charged polymeric aromatic residues through short-range aromatic-aromatic interactions. The occurrence of aromatic-aromatic interactions between the drug chlorpheniramine maleate (CPM) and the polyelectrolyte PSS has been reported in this context [12–14,16]. It was found that the extent of binding and the aggregation state of the complexes depend on the absolute and the relative concentration of the reactants. At a PSS concentration of 2 mM (in sulfonate groups per liter) DF showed drug binding of around 80% in a mixture of PSS/CPM at a sulfonate/drug stoichiometry 2:1 [12,14], forming clear solutions of non-aggregated complexes. On the contrary, at a PSS/CPM stoichiometry 2:3 and 5 mM of the polymer, higher binding, and the formation of nanoparticles were observed [16].

Ion pair formation between both charged aromatic species should imply drastic changes on chain properties in rigid polymers such as PSS. The rigidity of this polymer is due to both electrostatic repulsions between charged groups and the high volume of the aromatic rings, inducing an extended helical conformation of the polymer chain [32,33]. Chain properties of PSS have long been studied by SAXS and SANS in the presence of different salts and at several concentrations. Generally, a typical polyelectrolyte peak appears in scattering profiles, whose position depends on the concentration and nature of the counterions [34–38]. However, there are cases in which this typical peak does not appear, related with a high screening of electrostatic repulsions [37–40]. The effect of solvents or sulfonation degree on poly(styrene-co-styrenesulfonate) copolymers has also been studied by SANS and SAXS [41]. SANS and SAXS have been successfully used for the analysis of surfactants, colloids, powders, emulsions, nanocomposites, polymers, and macromolecules in general [42–46], and they offer complementary information to NMR, viscosimetry [47–49], conductimetry [50], and electron microscopies. It is worth mentioning the use of these techniques in complex electron-conductive system based on PSS and poly(3,4-ethylene dioxythiophene) (PEDOT), (PEDOT:PSS), whose chain properties and crystallinity are influenced by the solvent [51–53]. However, despite the different systems containing polymers, whose conformation properties in solution have been studied, there is no report in the literature, to the best of our knowledge, concerning the behavior of aromatic polyelectrolyte chains subjected to aromatic-aromatic interactions with aromatic low molecular-weight counterions as a function of the concentration.

In this work, we study the binding, aggregation, and chain properties in the system PSS/CPM at a sulfonate/drug stoichiometry 2:1 as a function of the system concentration in the dilute and semidilute regimes (crossover concentration between 10^{-3} and 10^{-2} M (in monomeric units) for PSS) [54,55]. DF results display novel and important features for this analytical tool for analyzing the binding of the drug to the polyelectrolyte. Synchrotron-SAXS and Dynamic Light Scattering (DLS) are used as complementary techniques to determine single correlation length chain parameters and the aggregation behavior of the system, respectively. Based on these results, we highlight a model picture for the binding and physicochemical behavior of these aromatic polyelectrolyte-aromatic counterion systems.

2. Theory

2.1. Diafiltration

Initially conceived as a separation technique for practical purposes [56–59], DF has served to calculate the thermodynamic and kinetic parameters of water-soluble polymers (WSP)/low molecular-weight species (LMWS) complexes after the development of a mathematical model to justify the DF profiles [2,3,5,8,12,60–62]. Thus, DF allowed the direct measurement of binding constants between WSP and LMWS, such as aromatic polyelectrolytes and aromatic counterions, providing the measurement of the stabilization effect associated to aromatic-aromatic interactions. A typical DF system is shown in Figure 1. The DF cell containing an aqueous solution of the WSP and the counterions of interest has, at the input, incoming water, and, at the output, a membrane only permeable to the LMWS. Therefore, as DF proceeds, the WSP is washed while the volume in the cell is kept constant. The filtered aqueous LMWS is collected in fractions, which are then quantified to obtain a DF profile as the plot of the natural logarithm of the concentration of the LMWS in the collected DF fractions ($ln\langle c_{LMWS}{}^{filtrate}\rangle$) versus the filtration factor (F), defined as the ratio between the accumulative filtrate volume and the constant volume in the DF cell.

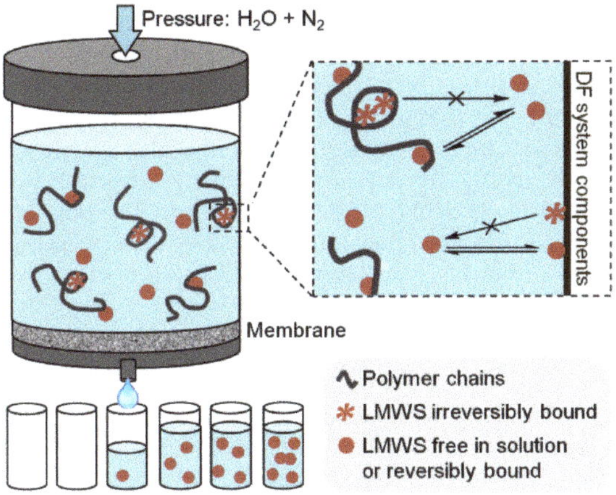

Figure 1. Scheme of a typical diafiltration system (**left**) and interaction model between low molecular-weight species, water-soluble polymers, and the diafiltration system components (**right**).

Several assumptions are made regarding the interactions between the LMWS and the WSP towards the disclosure of the information concealed in the DF profiles. (1) The total amount of LMWS is distributed in three different populations, namely free in solution, reversibly bound to the WSP (and/or to other components in the DF system), and irreversibly bound to the WSP (and/or to other components in the DF system) (see Figure 1). (2) Fast equilibrium is established between the reversibly bound fraction and the fraction free in the solution, so that the steady state approximation can be applied during filtration. (3) Interactions with the DF cell components, including the membrane, are additive to those with the WSP, so that experiments made in the absence of the WSP serve as control. Given these assumptions, a mathematical model fully described in the literature was applied to the DF profiles in order to obtain the information shown below [61–63].

The absolute value of the slope of the DF profile in the absence of the WSP (k^m) is related to the strength of the reversible interactions between the LMWS and the DF system components. Thus, an apparent dissociation constant between the LMWS and the DF system (${K_{diss}}^{LMWS/DS}$) can be defined and calculated as shown in Equations (1) and (2), respectively, where ${c_{LMWS}}^{free}$ is the concentration of LMWS free in solution, and ${c_{LMWS}}^{rev\text{-}bound\text{-}DF}$ the concentration of LMWS reversibly bound to the DF system components.

$$K_{diss}^{LMWS/DS} = \frac{C_{LMWS}^{free}}{C_{LMWS}^{rev-bound-DS}} \tag{1}$$

$$K_{diss}^{LMWS/DS} = \frac{k^m}{1-k^m} \tag{2}$$

Similarly, the absolute value of the slope in the presence of the WSP (j) is related with the strength of the reversible interactions between the LMWS and both the WSP and the DF system components. Thus, an apparent dissociation constant between the LMWS and the WSP (${K_{diss}}^{LMWS/WSP}$), defined in Equation (3), where ${c_{LMWS}}^{rev\text{-}bound\text{-}WSP}$ is the concentration of LMWS reversibly bound to the WSP, can be calculated by applying Equation (4) [62].

$$K_{diss}^{LMWS/WSP} = \frac{C_{LMWS}^{free}}{C_{LMWS}^{rev-bound-WSP}} \tag{3}$$

$$\frac{k^m j}{k^m - j} \le K_{diss}^{LMWS/DS} \le \frac{j}{k^m - j} \tag{4}$$

The values of k^m and j range between 0 and 1, lower values meaning stronger interaction. Theoretically $k^m \ge j$, so that ${K_{diss}}^{LMWS/WSP}$ ranges between 0 (j = 0) and infinite ($j = k^m$). Values of $j = k^m = 1$ indicate no interaction with both the DF system components and the WSP.

In Figure 1, the LMWS referred to as irreversibly bound are the molecules that present binding processes that may be reversible with an apparent dissociation constant that tend to zero at the conditions of the experiment or show much slower equilibrium kinetics than the DF process. The fraction of LMWS that is irreversibly bound at the beginning of the DF (i.e., when F tends to 0) (u) is determined from Equation (5), where b is the intercept of the DF profile; m, the absolute value of the slope (k^m or j); ${c_{LMWS}}^{cell\text{-}init}$, the total initial LMWS concentration; and ΔF, the difference in F value at which the filtered fractions are collected.

$$u = 1 - \frac{b\ \Delta F}{C_{LMWS}^{cell-init}(1 + e^{m\Delta F})} \tag{5}$$

By subtracting the u value of control experiments from that of the experiments made in the presence of the WSP, the initial fraction of LMWS irreversibly bound to the WSP is obtained. Likewise, the initial fraction of LMWS that is involved in association–dissociation processes (v) is determined from Equation (6).

$$v = 1 - u \tag{6}$$

2.2. SAXS

SAXS stands among the most important techniques used to analyze the conformation of polymers in solution. A simplified experimental setup is shown in Figure 2. A collimated X-ray beam impacts the sample, and the elastic component of the scattered beam is detected. The intensity pattern I is the fingerprint of the electron density of the sample and is a continuous function of the momentum transfer q, i.e., $I = I(q)$. From the analysis and modelling of $I(q)$, one can obtain the characteristic lengths, shape (including surface/volume ratio), assembling state (un/folding, aggregation, internal conformation), crystalline phases with large lattice parameters, and porosity, among other materials characteristics. In SAXS, the detection angle is far below 10°, and, depending on the wavelength of the X-ray beam, one can analyze characteristic dimensions that vary between 1 and 100 nm.

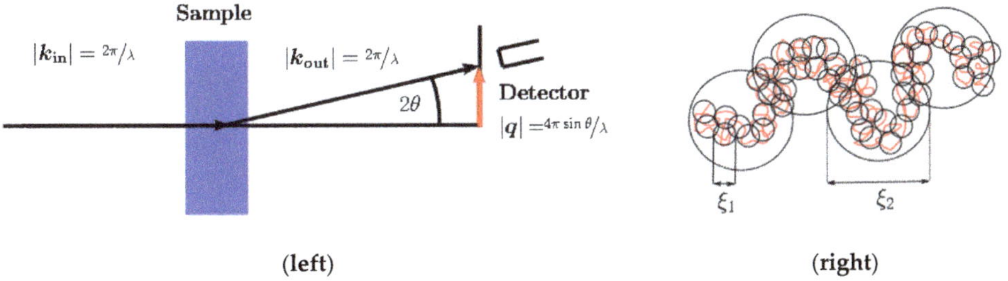

Figure 2. (**Left**) SAXS setting with incident and scattered wave vectors, $|k_{in}|$ and $|k_{out}|$, respectively, and momentum transfer $|q|$; (**right**): correlation length representing the static screening length, ξ_1, and fractal correlation length for larger domain size, ξ_2, as determined from Equations (8) and (9).

The theoretical aspects that describe $I(q)$ are reviewed in several papers and books and the reader is directed to them for more information [36,64–66]. In SAXS and SANS experiments, scattering profiles may be analyzed at the very low-q region ($q < 0.1$ nm^{-1}), where the scattering from solidlike density fluctuations is predominant, following the Guinier approximation for spherical particles:

$$I(q) \approx I_G(0) \exp[-(R_G{}^2 q^2)/3] \tag{7}$$

where $I_G(0)$ is the extrapolation of the intensity to $q \to 0$ from the observed q range, and R_G represents the radius of gyration of the polymeric chain, typically of some tenths of nm.

On the other hand, scattering from liquid-like or solution-like density fluctuations may be described by the Ornstein–Zernike scattering function applied in a q-range in both low- and high-q regions, where the intermolecular scattering function (the form factor) can be assumed constant [67,68], given by:

$$I(q) = I_{OZ}(0)/[1 + (q\xi_1)^2] \tag{8}$$

where $I_{OZ}(0)$ is the extrapolation of the intensity to $q \to 0$ from the observed q range, and ξ_1 is the correlation length representing the static screening length (see Figure 2), corresponding to the thermal blob size. The exponent 2 is typically obtained for linear polymers in semi-dilute θ-solutions, adopting a random walk conformation [66]. However, a fractal exponent 1.7 (equivalent to 5/3) has been also reported to properly describe $I(q)$ for larger domain size ξ_2 that corresponds to the arrangement of the smaller domains represented by ξ_1 to swallowed agglomerates (see also Figure 2) [66]. At these scale lengths, the chain conformation is a self-avoiding walk of thermal blobs. Thus, accordingly,

$$I(q) = I_{OZ}(0)/[1 + (q\xi_2)^{5/3}] \tag{9}$$

Plotting the inverse of $I(q)$, i.e., $I(q)^{-1}$, against q^2 and $q^{5/3}$ as described in Equations (10) and (11), respectively, will lead to straight lines, from which x_1 and x_2 can be extracted:

$$I(q)^{-1} = I_{OZ}(0)^{-1} + I_{OZ}(0)^{-1}\xi_1{}^2 q^2 \tag{10}$$

$$I(q)^{-1} = I_{OZ}(0)^{-1} + I_{OZ}(0)^{-1}\xi_2{}^{5/3} q^{5/3} \tag{11}$$

3. Experimental Section

3.1. Reagents

PSS (Aldrich; M_w 70,000 g/mol; 206.2 g/mol of sulfonate groups, CAS No. 25704-18-1) and PAA (received from Aldrich as poly(acrylic acid) and then neutralized in aqueous solutions by adjusting the pH value to 7.5 with NaOH; M_w 450,000 g/mol, 72.06 g/mol of acrylic units, CAS No. 9003-01-4) were purified by DF over a regenerated cellulose membrane of a nominal molecular weight limit (NMWL) of 10,000 Da (Millipore). After the polymer solutions were washed at least eight times their initial volume, the solvent was removed by freeze-drying. CPM (Sigma, racemic mixture), NaOH (Merck), and HCl (Merck) were used as received. For all experiments and purification procedures, deionized water was used. NaOH and HCl were used to adjust the pH. The structures of the polymers and CPM are shown in Figure 3.

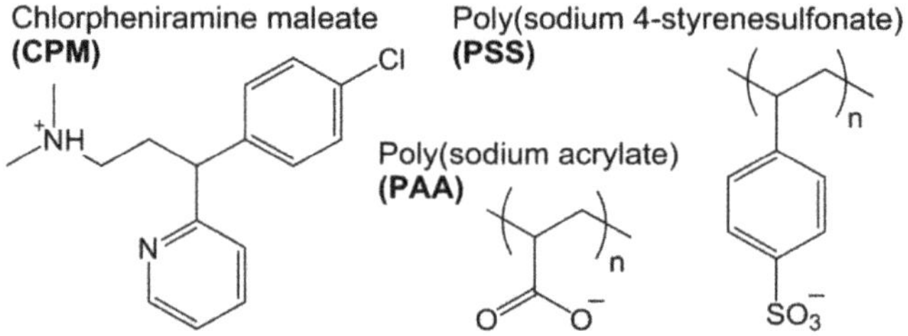

Figure 3. Molecular structure of CPM, PAA, and PSS.

3.2. Equipment

The pH was controlled with a Thermo Fisher Scientific pHmeter (Oakton pH700, Waltham, MA, USA). Dynamic light scattering (DLS) measurements were done in a Nano ZS zetasizer equipment (Malvern, Cambridge, UK) with backscatter detection (173°), controlled by the Dispersion Technology Software (DTS 6.2, Malvern, Cambridge, UK). DF cell Amicon 8010 (10 mL capacity) with a regenerated cellulose DF membrane (Millipore) of a 5000 Da NMWL was used for DF experiments. CPM concentration in the filtration fractions was quantified using HeλIos γ UV-vis spectrophotometer (Thermo Electron Corporation, Waltham, MA, USA). Synchrotron-SAXS experiments were done in the SAXS1 beamline of the Brazilian Synchrotron Light Laboratory (LNLS) in Campinas, Brazil (Full details of the SAXS line (6 October 2021) are found in https://www.lnls.cnpem.br/facilities/saxs1-en/ accessed on 31 August 2021.

3.3. Procedures

3.3.1. Sample Preparation

WSP/CPM aqueous solutions with 2:1 molar ratio ($WSP_n/CPM_{n/2}$, n being the polymer concentration in mmol of sulfonate groups per liter (mM)) were prepared at pH 7.5, and a different total system concentration, with n ranging from 0.25 to 60 mM. A set of turbid suspensions of $PSS_n/CPM_{n/2}$ complex obtained at PSS concentration of 35, 40, and 50 mM were analyzed by DLS at 25 °C in triplicate. The hydrodynamic diameter and zeta potential values of the formed particles were considered valid under the criteria of the DTS 6.2 software (Malvern, Cambridge, UK); correlograms of the analyses is shown below.

3.3.2. Diafiltration Measurements

A volume of $WSP_n/CPM_{n/2}$ aqueous mixtures (10 mL), with n ranging from 0.25 to 1.5 mM, were placed in a 10 mL DF cell bearing a 5000 Da NMWL membrane. The pH in the reservoir was also adjusted to 7.5. The experiments were performed at room temperature. During the experiment, the volume of the solution (10 mL) and pressure (3 bar) in the cell were kept constant. Fractions of 5 mL of the filtered solution were collected and the CPM concentration was quantified by UV-vis spectroscopy. DF control experiments were done in the absence of the WSP to analyze the interaction with the cell components. All experiments were carried out at least in duplicate. The results are expressed as a mean value, and their uncertainty as the standard deviation. The significance of the correlation of the independent variables u and j (and thus $K_{diss}^{CPM/WSP}$) was evaluated by the Pearson correlation coefficient method applied to the experimental data [69].

3.3.3. Synchrotron-SAXS Measurements

The above prepared $PSS_n/CPM_{n/2}$ aqueous mixtures were injected in the in-vacuum liquid cell available on the beamline, consisting of two mica windows enclosing the solution with 1 mm X-ray pathlength. The total sample volume was 500 μL and the measurements were carried out at room temperature. The beamline energy was set at 8 keV, the sample to detector distance was 3 m, resulting in a q range spanning from 0.04 to 1.2 nm^{-1}. The total acquisition time was 1000 s, transmission was corrected, and background was subtracted from all data. Data fitting was done using the free software Python Spyder3. The q domains that satisfy Equations (10) and (11) were searched in order to calculate ξ_1 and ξ_2.

4. Results and Discussion

4.1. Sample Preparation and DLS Characterization

Several samples were prepared with a stoichiometry $WSP_n/CPM_{n/2}$, and different values of n. Samples presenting PSS concentration in the range of 0.5–30 mM resulted in clear solutions. Samples presenting PSS concentration in the range of 40–60 mM precipitated. Between 30 and 40 mM nanoaggregates were found. This did not occur when PAA (pure or with CPM) or pure PSS was used. Figure 4 shows the correlograms of the DLS analyses of the samples PSS_{35}/CPM_{18}, PSS_{40}/CPM_{20}, and PSS_{50}/CPM_{25}. It can be seen that only the sample PSS_{35}/CPM_{18} shows a steady decay on the correlation function. A hydrodynamic diameter of 322 ± 11 nm was obtained, with polydispersity index of 0.275. The zeta potential of the particles took a value of −30.90 ± 2.25 mV, high enough in absolute value to ensure stability of the aggregate. On the contrary, large, polydisperse particles were visible by the naked eye in the samples PSS_{40}/CPM_{20} and PSS_{50}/CPM_{25}, which produced the shoulders and noisy correlograms at high correlation time values. For the PSS chain, entanglement is reported to occur beyond 100 mM for salt-free PSS ($M_w \sim$ 100,000 g/mol) solutions, without undergoing precipitation [44]. Thus, it can be concluded that the presence of CPM and the occurrence of aromatic-aromatic interactions between the drug and PSS enhances polymer aggregation and system collapse in this concentration regime.

4.2. Diafiltration Analysis

We performed DF experiments for $PSS_n/CPM_{n/2}$ and $PAA_n/CPM_{n/2}$ samples in the dilute regime, n between 0.5 and 2.5 mM. The corresponding DF profiles are shown in Figure 5, and the corresponding DF parameters are listed in Table 1. All the DF profiles show good linearity, with values of $R^2 \geq 0.98$. At first sight, it is evident that PSS present much stronger interactions with CPM than PAA. The strength of the reversible interaction is given by the slopes of the profiles, whereas the ordinate at the origin is related with the u value, i.e., with the initial fraction of molecules irreversibly bound to the polymer. The difference between the two polymers regarding the strength of the interaction with CPM stands on the ability of PSS to undergo aromatic-aromatic interactions with the LMWS.

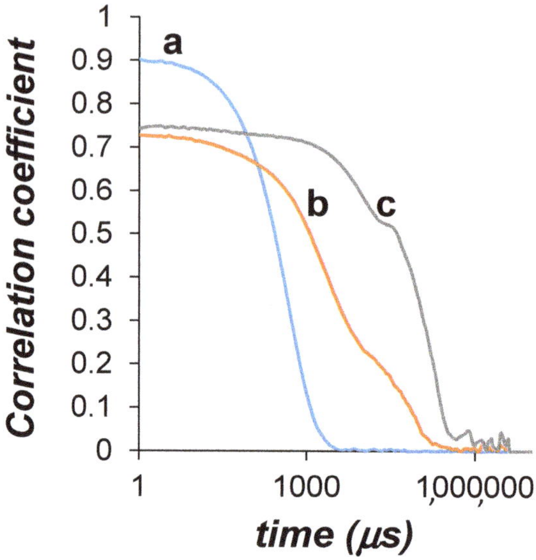

Figure 4. Correlograms obtained by DLS of samples PSS_{35}/CPM_{18} (a), PSS_{40}/CPM_{20} (b), and PSS_{50}/CPM_{25} (c).

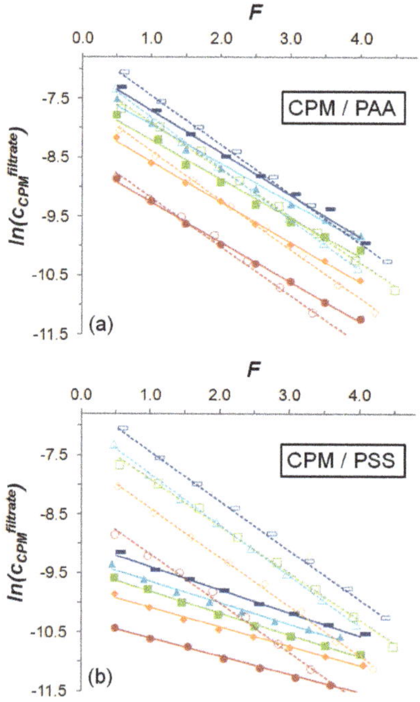

Figure 5. Diafiltration profiles of (**a**) $PAA_n/CPM_{n/2}$ and (**b**) $PSS_n/CPM_{n/2}$ systems at n = 0.50 (red circles), 1.0 (orange rhombuses), 1.5 (green squares), 2.0 (light blue triangles), and 2.5 (blue rectangles). Corresponding blank experiments made in the absence of polyelectrolytes are plotted as empty symbols.

Table 1. $WSP_n/CPM_{n/2}$ system formulations, the resulting DF parameters, and the linear adjustment of the DF profiles with the corresponding linear regression factors (R^2).

	$c_{CPM}{}^{total}$ mM	$c_{WSP}{}^{total}$ mM	v	u	j and (k^m)	$K_{diss}{}^{LMWS/WSP}$ and ($K_{diss}{}^{LMWS/DS}$)	Linear Adjustment	R^2
Blank	0.25	-	1.03	−0.03	(0.83)	(4.9)	y = −0.83x − 7.6	0.99
	0.50	-	0.97	0.03	(0.81)	(4.3)	y = −0.81x − 7.6	0.99
	0.75	-	0.94	0.06	(0.79)	(3.8)	y = −0.79x − 7.1	1.00
	1.00	-	0.94	0.06	(0.86)	(6.1)	y = −0.86x − 6.9	1.00
	1.25	-	1.03	0.03	(0.84)	(5.3)	y = −0.84x − 6.6	1.00
PAA	0.25	0.5	0.95 ± 0.02	0.05 ± 0.02	0.59 ± 0.13	2.8 ± 2.0	(−0.59 ± 0.13)x + (−8.7 ± 0.2)	1.00 ± 0.00
	0.50	1.0	0.89 ± 0.05	0.11 ± 0.05	0.63 ± 0.08	3.5 ± 1.9	(−0.63 ± 0.08)x + (−8.0 ± 0.2)	0.99 ± 0.01
	0.75	1.5	0.92 ± 0.02	0.08 ± 0.02	0.63 ± 0.04	3.7 ± 1.1	(−0.63 ± 0.04)x + (−7.6 ± 0.1)	0.98 ± 0.01
	1.00	2.0	0.88 ± 0.01	0.12 ± 0.01	0.62 ± 0.04	2.5 ± 0.6	(−0.62 ± 0.04)x + (−7.4 ± 0.1)	0.99 ± 0.00
	1.25	2.5	0.86 ± 0.01	0.14 ± 0.01	0.69 ± 0.04	4.5 ± 1.5	(−0.69 ± 0.04)x + (−7.0 ± 0.1)	0.99 ± 0.00
PSS	0.25	0.5	0.41 ± 0.00	0.59 ± 0.00	0.28 ± 0.03	0.48 ± 0.07	(−0.28 ± 0.03)x + (−10.4 ± 0.1)	0.98 ± 0.02
	0.50	1.0	0.39 ± 0.08	0.61 ± 0.08	0.30 ± 0.04	0.54 ± 0.11	(−0.30 ± 0.04)x + (−9.7 ± 0.1)	0.98 ± 0.01
	0.75	1.5	0.27 ± 0.01	0.73 ± 0.01	0.35 ± 0.02	0.70 ± 0.09	(−0.35 ± 0.02)x + (−9.5 ± 0.0)	0.99 ± 0.00
	1.00	2.0	0.27 ± 0.01	0.73 ± 0.01	0.37 ± 0.01	0.69 ± 0.03	(−0.37 ± 0.10)x + (−9.2 ± 0.1)	0.98 ± 0.00
	1.25	2.5	0.24 ± 0.02	0.76 ± 0.02	0.38 ± 0.00	0.78 ± 0.01	(−0.38 ± 0.00)x + (−9.0 ± 0.1)	0.99 ± 0.01

The DF parameters v, u, k^m, j, $K_{diss}{}^{LMWS/DS}$, and $K_{diss}{}^{LMWS/WSP}$ listed in Table 1 show, for blank experiments, u values very close to zero and k_m values in the range of 0.79–0.86, indicating that there is no CPM irreversibly bound to the cell components, and that weak reversible interactions occur with the system components, with apparent dissociation constants ($K_{diss}{}^{CPM/DS}$) higher than 3.8. In the case of $PAA_n/CPM_{n/2}$ mixtures, low u values are also found, ranging from 0.05 to 0.14, as well as relatively high j values, ranging between 0.59 and 0.69, also indicating weak interaction forces, with $K_{diss}{}^{CPM/PAA}$ higher than 2.5. On the contrary, for the $PSS_n/CPM_{n/2}$ mixtures, relatively high u values are found, ranging between 0.59 and 0.76, indicating that a significant initial fraction of the drug is irreversibly confined in the polymer domain. In addition, the fraction subjected to reversible binding presented $K_{diss}{}^{CPM/PSS}$ ranging between 0.48 and 0.78, related with j values ranging between 0.28 and 0.38, showing that the fraction of molecules in equilibrium that are bound to the polyelectrolyte is significantly higher than that of molecules free in solution.

It can be seen that, as the concentration of the $PSS_n/CPM_{n/2}$ system increases, u takes higher values (Figure 6a), indicating that a higher fraction of the total initial CPM molecules is irreversibly bound to the polymer at higher total concentration. A similar effect is found for the system $PAA_n/CPM_{n/2}$, in the low range of u values, presenting a smaller growth and higher relative standard deviations. The values of j, along with $K_{diss}{}^{CPM/WSP}$, also significantly increase as n increases, revealing that the fraction of reversible bound molecules, in addition to decreasing with respect to the irreversibly bound fraction, is less tightly bound to the polymer (Figure 6b,c). On the contrary, the data obtained for the $PAA_n/CPM_{n/2}$ system present considerable standard deviations, which prevent concluding a tendency for these two parameters.

These findings represent an interesting novelty in the development of DF as an analytical technique. The mathematical analysis of the DF profiles does not anticipate a direct physical correlation between j (or $K_{diss}{}^{LMWS/WSP}$) and u, i.e., between the strength of the reversible interactions and the fraction of molecules irreversibly bound to the polymer. However, a definite correlation between u and j (and $K_{diss}{}^{CPM/PSS}$) values for the $PSS_n/CPM_{n/2}$ system is found. Indeed, a linear dependency of j (and $K_{diss}{}^{CPM/PSS}$) with u is found with good linear regression factors in the range of concentration studied, as can be seen in Figure 6d. Pearson correlation coefficients of over 0.94 indicate a statistically significant linear positive correlation for both cases [69]. These results indicate that, for this system, the magnitudes represented by u and j, and thus $K_{diss}{}^{CPM/PSS}$, are physically linked, so that their values are directly correlated through the $PSS_n/CPM_{n/2}$ mixture's initial concentration.

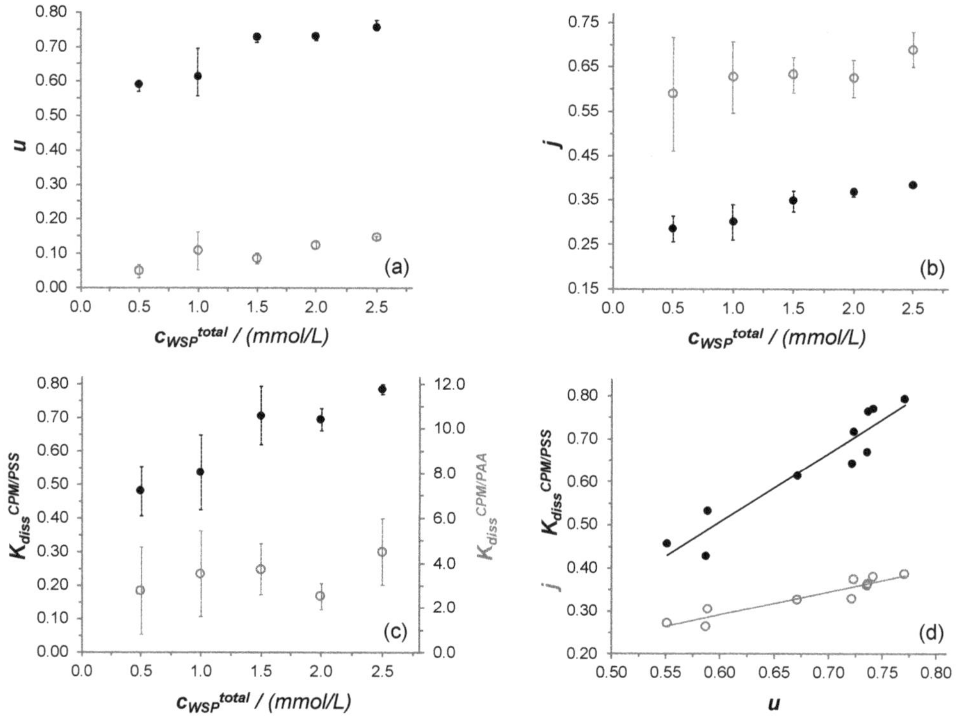

Figure 6. u values (**a**), j values (**b**), and $K_{diss}^{CPM/WSP}$ values (**c**), plotted against the initial polyelectrolyte concentration (c_{WSP}^{total}) for $PAA_n/CPM_{n/2}$ (grey empty circles) and $PSS_n/CPM_{n/2}$, systems (black circles). $K_{diss}^{CPM/PSS}$ (black circles) (y = 1.6x − 0.44; R^2 = 0.90) and j (grey empty circles) (y = 0.53x − 0.029; R^2 = 0.89) values plotted against u (plotting each individual experiment for all $PSS_n/CPM_{n/2}$ systems) (**d**).

4.3. SAXS Analysis

Figure 7A shows SAXS results of the experimental scattering intensity $I(q)$ as a function of the modulus of the momentum transfer vector q for five distinctive $PSS_n/CPM_{n/2}$ concentrations, with n ranging from 0.5 to 60 mM.

It can be seen in Figure 7A that the typical polyelectrolyte peak of PSS is not present in the $PSS_n/CPM_{n/2}$ complexes. The first two plots *a* and *b* correspond to low concentrated samples. The scattering of sample *c*, corresponding to $PSS_{10}/CPM_{5.0}$, yet in the typical concentration range at which many studies are reported in the literature [37,38], is significantly more intense. Sample *d*, PSS_{35}/CPM_{18}, shows in DLS a scattering pattern that is consistent with the formation of colloidal particles of nanometric size (around 300 nm, see Figure 4). These new conglomerates pop out in the SAXS profile as a small shoulder beginning at $q \sim 0.06$ nm^{-1}. The shoulder is more clearly observed in sample *e*, PSS_{60}/CPM_{30}, corresponding to a system concentration at which the polymeric complexes display macroprecipitation.

The total scattering function has a positive component related with intrachain interactions and a negative component related with repulsive interchain interactions [38]. The disappearance of the polyelectrolyte peak for PSS in the presence of a large excess of NaCl or other metal counterions is explained by an increase in the compressibility of the polymeric chains and fluctuations of the interparticle distances which rises the intensity in the low-q region, and the increase in the fluctuations of the intersegmental distance, increasing the scattering intensity in the high-q region [38,70]. These effects have also been observed in the presence of divalent metal counterions where electrostatic attraction is stronger and the screening more intense [34,37,71,72]. The screening of electrostatic repulsive forces producing polymeric systems of neutral-like behavior is invoked, then, to explain the polyelectrolyte peak disappearance [38,72,73]. An interesting theoretical study analyzing expected SAXS profiles for different systems as a function of the form factor and the Bjerrum length has been reported [74]. Scattering profiles similar to those reported here are shown for polyelectrolyte systems bearing relatively high Bjerrum length, corresponding to sausage single chain conformations, provided that interchain interactions are considered negligible. However, models considering attractive interchain interactions and clustering have also been reported to be consistent with fluctuating transient aggregates that could fit to the SAXS profiles reported in this work [34,35,37,73,75]. Similar scattering profiles can be also found for rigid polyelectrolytes such as DNA [72], chondroitin sulfate, hyaluronate, or poly(aspartate) [68], proteins [76], coacervate interpolymer complexes [40,77], and even nonionic micelles formed in water [78].

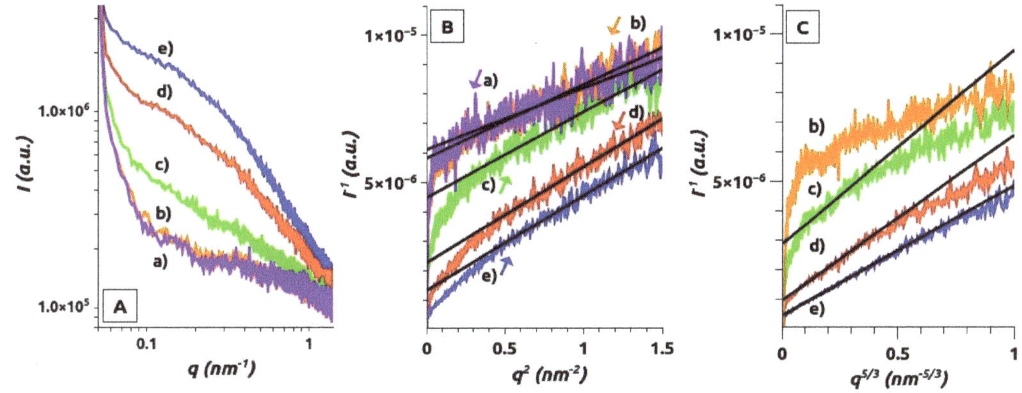

Figure 7. Synchrotron-SAXS results for selected $PSS_n/CPM_{n/2}$ concentration values: (**A**) $I(q)$ vs. q; (**B**) $I(q)^{-1}$ vs. q^2, and fitted curves obtained applying Equation (10) to a set of ($I(q)^{-1}$, q^2) values; (**C**) $I(q)^{-1}$ vs. $q^{5/3}$ and fitted curves obtained applying Equation (11) to a set of ($I(q)^{-1}$, $q^{5/3}$) values. (a) *$PSS_{0.5}/CPM_{0.25}$* (mauve), (b) *$PSS_{2.0}/CPM_{1.0}$* (orange), (c) *$PSS_{10}/CPM_{5.0}$* (green), (d) *PSS_{35}/CPM_{18}* (red), (e) *PSS_{60}/CPM_{30}* (blue).

Table 2 summarizes the ξ_1 and ξ_2 values obtained from curve fitting to Equations (10) and (11). The Ornstein-Zernike analysis shows good correlation of $I(q)^{-1}$ vs. q^2 for an extended range of data (see Figure 7B). The two more dilute samples seem to follow the signature of a Gaussian chain for a random walk conformation in a dilute environment. In addition, for samples where n is equal to or higher than 10, including those where nano- and macroprecipitates are observed, an also extended set of $I(q)^{-1}$ data correlates well with $q^{5/3}$ (Equation (11)), as observed in Figure 7C, showing a single polymer chain interacting equally well with itself and with the solvent producing self-avoiding walk conformations, characteristic of a fully swollen coil (Figure 2).

Table 2. ξ_1 and ξ_2 correlation lengths for different $PSS_n/CPM_{n/2}$ system formulations.

$PSS_n/CPM_{n/2}$ (mM/mM)	q Range for Equation (10) (nm^{-1})	R^2	$\xi_1 \pm \delta\xi_1$ (nm)	q Range for Equation (11) (nm^{-1})	R^2	$\xi_2 \pm \delta\xi_2$ (nm)
0.5/0.25	0.49–1.23	0.78	0.60 ± 0.01	-	-	-
2.0/1.0	0.53–1.27	0.90	0.70 ± 0.01	-	-	-
10/5.0	0.61–1.22	0.90	0.80 ± 0.01	0.20–0.52	0.924	1.70 ± 0.02
20/10	0.67–1.19	0.94	1.00 ± 0.01	0.22–0.53	0.978	2.30 ± 0.03
30/15	0.74–1.21	0.85	1.10 ± 0.02	0.20–0.54	0.976	2.70 ± 0.05
35/18	0.74–1.21	0.95	1.20 ± 0.02	0.20–0.55	0.989	2.90 ± 0.03
40/20	0.73–1.20	0.94	1.20 ± 0.02	0.20–0.55	0.992	3.00 ± 0.04
50/25	0.73–1.20	0.97	1.40 ± 0.02	0.20–0.55	0.993	3.40 ± 0.03
60/30	0.67–1.17	0.98	1.50 ± 0.02	0.18–0.53	0.995	4.0 ± 0.1

Figure 8 summarizes the correlation lengths obtained for the whole set of samples. The primary smaller thermal blobs showed static correlation lengths ξ_1 in the range of 0.5–1.5 nm, growing monotonously with the total concentration of the system. On the other hand, the secondary larger domains showed fractal correlation lengths ξ_2 in the range of 1.0–4.0 nm, also growing monotonously with the total concentration of the system, showing a larger rate, as compared to the primary blobs. This behavior is outstanding since the increase in the concentration of the system normally produces shrinking of the polymer chains and a decrease in the correlation lengths [68,70].

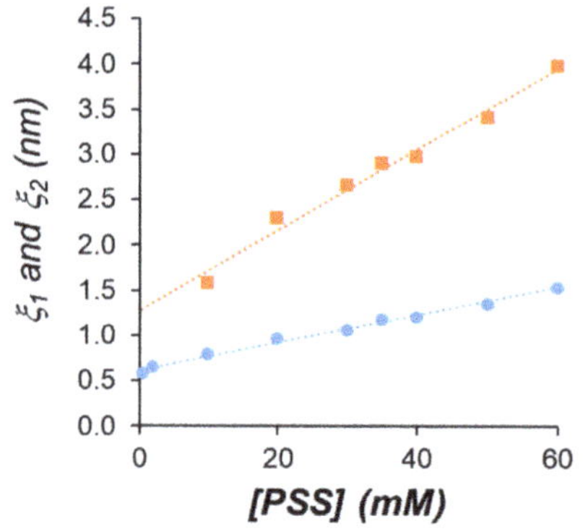

Figure 8. Correlation lengths ξ_1 (circles) and ξ_2 (squares) obtained from Equations (10) and (11), respectively. Linear regression functions are y = 0.0153 + 0.6238 (R^2 = 0.99) for ξ_1 vs. [PSS] and y = 0.0447 + 1.2751 (R^2 = 0.98) for ξ_2 vs. [PSS].

4.4. Aromatic WSP/Aromatic Counterion Complexation and Aggregation Model

At the concentration range of the experiments shown here for DF and synchrotron-SAXS, pure PSS does not form aggregates [44]. However, the occurrence of site-specific aromatic-aromatic interactions between CPM and the benzenesulfonate groups of PSS produces the decrease in the effective charge density of the polymer chains favoring intrachain attractive interactions and decreasing interchain repulsions, increasing the tendency of the macromolecule to fold. To explain the results shown in this paper, we should invoke the short-range character of aromatic-aromatic interactions. This involves the release of water from the hydration sphere of CPM and polymeric benzenesulfonate groups upon binding, producing ion pair formation. These ion pairs show a tendency to aggregate in hydrophobic domains. As depicted in Figure 9, these hydrophobic domains, composed of ion pairs and polymeric backbone folds and bundles, although transient, should contain the irreversibly bound fraction of CPM observed by DF and essentially determine the size of the thermal blobs related to the static screening length ξ_1. The remaining charged hydrated polymeric segments provide charge for the system stabilization in water and the reversible interaction with the remaining fraction of the LMWS.

The confinement of CPM in hydrophobic domains increases with the system concentration, which should enhance both the compressibility of the system and intersegmental interactions [79]. The correlation between u and j in DF experiments indicates that polymer chains fold and ion pairs aggregate in hydrophobic domains, confining a higher number of CPM molecules in polymeric blobs (increasing the value of the u parameter). As more benzenesulfonate/CPM ion pairs are confined in hydrophobic domains, the net charge of the polymeric particles decreases, decreasing the strength of the interaction with the non-confined fraction of the LMWS (increasing the value of the j parameter). Together with an increase in the system concentration, an arrangement of the polymeric chain containing the thermal blobs into swollen agglomerates represented by the characteristic length ξ_2 occurs. It is interesting to note that both ξ_1 and ξ_2 do increase with the total concentration. Short-range aromatic-aromatic interaction with the drug CPM should influence the size and mobility of the PSS segments. The thermal blobs, involving a higher number of unhydrated ion pairs stabilized in hydrophobic domains as the concentration increases, grow, and it is probable that they form clusters due to a certain tendency of CPM to self-aggregate [80]. These facts may be responsible for the increase in the thermal blob size, which further triggers an increase in the swollen fractal blobs size.

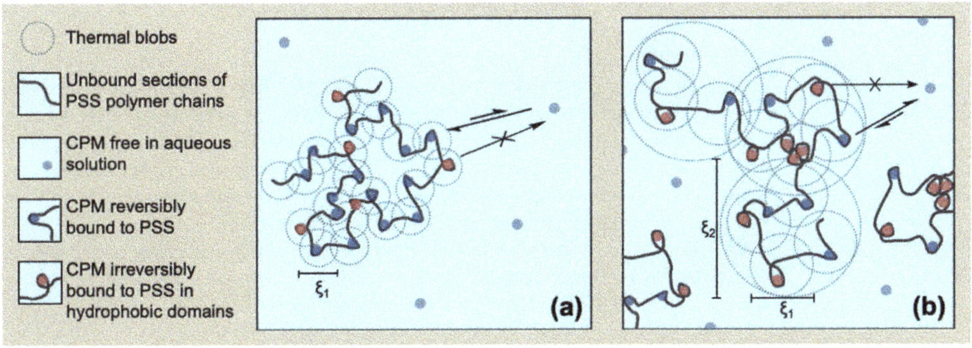

Figure 9. Molecular diagram of the $PSS_n/CPM_{n/2}$ system at different concentrations where ξ_1 and ξ_2, as well as the irreversibly bound fraction of CPM confined in folds and bundles of the polyelectrolyte chain increase at an increasing system concentration: (**a**) dilute regime; (**b**) semidilute regime.

Finally, when the net charge of the particles decreases below a certain value, interchain interactions become more favorable than chain-solvent interactions, the persistence length of the electrostatic interactions is favored over the entropic effect, and the $PSS_n/CPM_{n/2}$ complex precipitates [44,79].

4.5. Final Remarks

Here, we successfully showed a statistically significant linear correlation between j (and $K_{diss}{}^{CPM/PSS}$) and u for an aromatic WSP/aromatic LMWS system over a specific range of concentrations. In addition, we have shown the variation of the static and fractal correlation distances describing the behavior of the polymeric chains in the complex. Put together, the results shown here point at a binding and aggregation model that assumes the formation of hydrophobic domains upon the aggregation of polymeric hydrophobic segments and ion pairs formed through aromatic-aromatic interactions between the aromatic LMWS and the aromatic WSP. These separate domains, that may be considered to be two phases [35], consist of dynamic arrangements arising upon molecular interaction and aggregation: a discontinuous and transient inner hydrophobic phase, containing mainly the irreversibly bound fraction of LMWS confined in hydrophobic domains composed by ion pairs and polymeric backbone folds and bundles, and the hydrophilic phase, composed of the continuous aqueous phase. The interphase is composed by the remaining charged hydrated polymeric segments, which provides the system stabilization in water, and contains the reversibly bound counterions. Examples of two-phase aggregated systems have been described in the literature formed with PSS and cationic surfactants [39,81–83]. In addition to the study of polyelectrolyte/counterion interactions, DF has been shown to be a useful technique used to study interactions in nanophase-separated systems such nanodroplets of oily core stabilized by anionic and cationic surfactants interacting with the antibiotic oxytetracycline [63].

The binding model presented here, consistent with DLS, DF, and synchrotron-SAXS results, may be relevant for the interpretation of out-of-equilibrium processes in which the solvent is removed, so that the concentration of the complex increases, keeping the LMWS/WSP ratio constant. This may contribute to new knowledge involving material design and application, material properties, and functionality projection in fields such as agriculture, sensors, photocatalysts, environmental remediation, etc. Regarding drugs, the behavior of medicines based on aromatic polyelectrolytes/aromatic drug complexes interpreted under this binding model may contribute to the design of controlled drug delivery materials. In particular, it allows for the interpretation of the formation of pharmaceutical nanoformulations, in which outstanding high drug loading is achieved in nanocarriers (of around 50%), since the drug acts both as a bioactive molecule carried by the nanoparticle, and as a main constituent of the carrier [15].

5. Conclusions

As the concentration of the mixture PSS/CPM 2:1 in water increases in the dilute and semidilute regimes, a higher amount of CPM confines in the polymer domain. At polymer concentrations between 0.5 and 2.5 mM, the strength of the $PSS_n/CPM_{n/2}$ reversible interactions given by j (and thus $K_{diss}{}^{CPM/PSS}$) and the irreversibly bound fraction of CPM bound to PSS (u) are directly correlated, showing a linear tendency of positive slope (with Pearson correlation coefficients over 0.94), evidenced upon increasing the system total concentration. Thus, u, j, and $K_{diss}{}^{CPM/PSS}$ increase along with the system total concentration. Lower affinity is found for CPM and the non-aromatic polyelectrolyte PAA, thus j and $K_{diss}{}^{CPM/PAA}$ values showed high standard deviations, and correlations with u could not be found, highlighting the role of aromatic-aromatic interactions in the system behavior. Synchrotron-SAXS results display an outstanding increase in characteristic chain correlation lengths, static screening lengths ξ_1 in the range 0.5–1.5 nm, and correlation lengths ξ_2 in the range of 1–4 nm, following an aggregation pattern with a fractal dimension of 1.7. Nanoprecipitates of around 300 nm are found in the range of 30–40 mM, and macroprecipitates are found at a higher system concentration. A binding model has been proposed to interpret these results, so that, due to aromatic-aromatic interactions, the probability of ion pair formation between CPM and the benzene sulfonate groups of PSS increases with the total concentration of the system, as well as the probability of their aggregation. Therefore, hydrophobic domains are increasingly formed where a larger fraction of the CPM becomes irreversibly confined. Additionally, as the hydrophobic domains increase, less polyelectrolyte charged segments are available at the interface, so that the attraction of CPM molecules free in solution decreases, and the reversible interaction between the opposite charged species weakens. The increase in the drug confinement should be responsible for the increase in the static and fractal correlation lengths, observed in the increasing concentrations of the complex, and also weakens the interaction of the polymer chains with the solvent, producing precipitation at the highest concentrations evaluated. These findings contribute to the general knowledge of polyelectrolytes, with implications both in fundamental knowledge and potential technological applications considering aromatic-aromatic binding between aromatic polyelectrolytes and aromatic counterions, and, in particular, in the design of new pharmaceutical nanoformulations with outstanding high drug loading.

Author Contributions: Conceptualization, F.O. and I.M.-V.; methodology, F.O., T.H., M.E.F., J.G.L. and I.M.-V.; software, T.H., M.E.F. and J.G.L.; formal analysis, F.O., T.H., M.E.F., J.G.L. and I.M.-V.; investigation, F.O., T.H., M.E.F., J.G.L. and I.M.-V.; resources, J.R.V.-B., J.G.L., M.E.F. and I.M.-V.; data curation, F.O., T.H., M.E.F., J.G.L. and I.M.-V.; writing—original draft preparation, F.O., T.H. and I.M.-V.; writing—review and editing, F.O., T.H., M.E.F., J.G.L., J.R.V.-B. and I.M.-V.; validation, F.O., T.H., M.E.F., J.G.L. and I.M.-V.; visualization, F.O., J.G.L., T.H. and I.M.-V.; supervision, I.M.-V.; project administration, I.M.-V.; funding acquisition, J.R.V.-B., J.G.L., M.E.F. and I.M.-V. All authors have read and agreed to the published version of the manuscript.

Funding: This research was funded by Fondecyt Regular No. 1150899, 1181695, and 1210968, and Fondecyt Iniciación No. 11181029.

Institutional Review Board Statement: Not applicable.

Informed Consent Statement: Not applicable.

Acknowledgments: We thank Bernal Sibaja for helpful discussions regarding this work. J.L. and M.F. are grateful for the support of LNLS through project No. 20170181 and 20180276 that allowed accessing the Synchrotron-SAXS facilities in Campinas-Brazil. We particularly appreciate the technical support of Florian Meneau who helped in defining the SAXS experiments together with the correction to the technical aspects of the Synchrotron-SAXS experimental setup.

Conflicts of Interest: The authors declare no conflict of interest.

References

1. Moreno-Villoslada, I.; Flores, M.E.; Marambio, O.G.; Pizarro, G.d.C.; Nishide, H. Polyaromatic-Anion Behavior of Different Polyelectrolytes Containing Benzenecarboxylate Units. *J. Phys. Chem. B* **2010**, *114*, 7753–7759. [CrossRef]
2. Moreno-Villoslada, I.; González, F.; Arias, L.; Villatoro, J.M.; Ugarte, R.; Hess, S.; Nishide, H. Control of CI Basic Violet 10 aggregation in aqueous solution by the use of poly (sodium 4-styrenesulfonate). *Dye. Pigment.* **2009**, *82*, 401–408. [CrossRef]
3. Moreno-Villoslada, I.; González, R.; Hess, S.; Rivas, B.L.; Shibue, T.; Nishide, H. Complex formation between rhodamine B and poly (sodium 4-styrenesulfonate) studied by 1H-NMR. *J. Phys. Chem. B* **2006**, *110*, 21576–21581. [CrossRef] [PubMed]
4. Moreno-Villoslada, I.; Jofré, M.; Miranda, V.; Chandía, P.; González, R.; Hess, S.; Rivas, B.L.; Elvira, C.; San Román, J.; Shibue, T. π-Stacking of rhodamine B onto water-soluble polymers containing aromatic groups. *Polymer* **2006**, *47*, 6496–6500. [CrossRef]
5. Moreno-Villoslada, I.; Torres, C.; González, F.; Shibue, T.; Nishide, H. Binding of methylene blue to polyelectrolytes containing sulfonate groups. *Macromol. Chem. Phys.* **2009**, *210*, 1167–1175. [CrossRef]
6. Moreno-Villoslada, I.; Torres-Gallegos, C.s.; Araya-Hermosilla, R.; Nishide, H. Influence of the linear aromatic density on methylene blue aggregation around polyanions containing sulfonate groups. *J. Phys. Chem. B* **2010**, *114*, 4151–4158. [CrossRef] [PubMed]
7. Araya-Hermosilla, E.; Muñoz, D.; Orellana, S.; Yáñez, A.; Olea, A.F.; Oyarzun-Ampuero, F.; Moreno-Villoslada, I. Immobilization of rhodamine 6G in calcium alginate microcapsules based on aromatic-aromatic interactions with poly (sodium 4-styrenesulfonate). *React. Funct. Polym.* **2014**, *81*, 14–21. [CrossRef]
8. Moreno-Villoslada, I.; González, F.; Rivera, L.; Hess, S.; Rivas, B.L.; Shibue, T.; Nishide, H. Aromatic—Aromatic Interaction between 2, 3, 5-Triphenyl-2 H-tetrazolium Chloride and Poly (sodium 4-styrenesulfonate). *J. Phys. Chem. B* **2007**, *111*, 6146–6150. [CrossRef]
9. Moreno-Villoslada, I.; Soto, M.; González, F.; Montero-Silva, F.; Hess, S.; Takemura, I.; Oyaizu, K.; Nishide, H. Reduction of 2, 3, 5-Triphenyl-2 H-tetrazolium Chloride in the Presence of Polyelectrolytes Containing 4-Styrenesulfonate Moieties. *J. Phys. Chem. B* **2008**, *112*, 5350–5354. [CrossRef]
10. Moreno-Villoslada, I.; Torres, C.; González, F.; Soto, M.; Nishide, H. Stacking of 2, 3, 5-Triphenyl-2 H-tetrazolium Chloride onto Polyelectrolytes Containing 4-Styrenesulfonate Groups. *J. Phys. Chem. B* **2008**, *112*, 11244–11249. [CrossRef]
11. Flores, M.E.; Garcés-Jerez, P.; Fernández, D.; Aros-Perez, G.; González-Cabrera, D.; Álvarez, E.; Cañas, I.; Oyarzun-Ampuero, F.; Moreno-Villoslada, I. Facile Formation of Redox-Active Totally Organic Nanoparticles in Water by In Situ Reduction of Organic Precursors Stabilized through Aromatic—Aromatic Interactions by Aromatic Polyelectrolytes. *Macromol. Rapid Commun.* **2016**, *37*, 1729–1734. [CrossRef]
12. Moreno-Villoslada, I.; Oyarzún, F.; Miranda, V.; Hess, S.; Rivas, B.L. Comparison between the binding of chlorpheniramine maleate to poly (sodium 4-styrenesulfonate) and the binding to other polyelectrolytes. *Polymer* **2005**, *46*, 7240–7245. [CrossRef]
13. Moreno-Villoslada, I.; González, F.; Rivas, B.L.; Shibue, T.; Nishide, H. Tuning the pK a of the antihistaminic drug chlorpheniramine maleate by supramolecular interactions with water-soluble polymers. *Polymer* **2007**, *48*, 799–804. [CrossRef]
14. Orozco, F.; Redondo-Gómez, C.; Vega-Baudrit, J.R.; Moreno-Villoslada, I. On the comparison between diafiltration and isothermal titration calorimetry: Determination of the amount of analytes bound to water-soluble polymers. *Polym. Test.* **2019**, *76*, 443–447. [CrossRef]
15. Villamizar-Sarmiento, M.G.; Molina-Soto, E.F.; Guerrero, J.; Shibue, T.; Nishide, H.; Moreno-Villoslada, I.; Oyarzun-Ampuero, F.A. A New Methodology to Create Polymeric Nanocarriers Containing Hydrophilic Low Molecular-Weight Drugs: A Green Strategy Providing a Very High Drug Loading. *Mol. Pharm.* **2019**, *16*, 2892–2901. [CrossRef] [PubMed]
16. Villamizar-Sarmiento, M.G.; Guerrero, J.; Moreno-Villoslada, I.; Oyarzun-Ampuero, F.A. The key role of the drug self-aggregation ability to obtain optimal nanocarriers based on aromatic-aromatic drug-polymer interactions. *Eur. J. Pharm. Biopharm.* **2021**, *166*, 19–29. [CrossRef]
17. Manning, G.S. The molecular theory of polyelectrolyte solutions with applications to the electrostatic properties of polynucleotides. *Q. Rev. Biophys.* **1978**, *11*, 179–246. [CrossRef]
18. Manning, G.S. Limiting laws and counterion condensation in polyelectrolyte solutions. 8. Mixtures of counterions, species selectivity, and valence selectivity. *J. Phys. Chem.* **1984**, *88*, 6654–6661. [CrossRef]
19. Manning, G.S. Counterion condensation theory constructed from different models. *Phys. A Stat. Mech. Its Appl.* **1996**, *231*, 236–253. [CrossRef]
20. Nordmeier, E.; Dauwe, W. Studies of Polyelectrolyte Solutions I. Counterion Condensation by Poly (styrene sulfonate). *Polym. J.* **1991**, *23*, 1297–1305. [CrossRef]
21. Nordmeier, E. Advances in polyelectrolyte research: Counterion binding phenomena, dynamic processes, and the helix-coil transition of DNA. *Macromol. Chem. Phys.* **1995**, *196*, 1321–1374. [CrossRef]

22. Flores, M.E.; Sano, N.; Araya-Hermosilla, R.; Shibue, T.; Olea, A.F.; Nishide, H.; Moreno-Villoslada, I. Self-association of 5, 10, 15, 20-tetrakis-(4-sulfonatophenyl)-porphyrin tuned by poly (decylviologen) and sulfobutylether-β-cyclodextrin. *Dye. Pigment.* **2015**, *112*, 262–273. [CrossRef]
23. Araya-Hermosilla, E.; Orellana, S.L.; Toncelli, C.; Picchioni, F.; Moreno-Villoslada, I. Novel polyketones with pendant imidazolium groups as nanodispersants of hydrophobic antibiotics. *J. Appl. Polym. Sci.* **2015**, *132*. [CrossRef]
24. Araya-Hermosilla, E.; Roscam Abbing, M.; Catalán-Toledo, J.; Oyarzun-Ampuero, F.; Pucci, A.; Raffa, P.; Picchioni, F.; Moreno-Villoslada, I. Synthesis of tuneable amphiphilic-modified polyketone polymers, their complexes with 5,10,15,20-tetrakis-(4-sulfonatophenyl)-porphyrin, and their role in the photooxidation of 1,3,5-triphenylformazan confined in polymeric nanoparticles. *Polymer* **2019**, *167*, 215–223. [CrossRef]
25. Fuenzalida, J.P.; Flores, M.E.; Móniz, I.s.; Feijoo, M.; Goycoolea, F.; Nishide, H.; Moreno-Villoslada, I. Immobilization of hydrophilic low molecular-weight molecules in nanoparticles of chitosan/poly (sodium 4-styrenesulfonate) assisted by aromatic-aromatic interactions. *J. Phys. Chem. B* **2014**, *118*, 9782–9791. [CrossRef]
26. Coronel, A.; Catalán-Toledo, J.; Fernández-Jaramillo, H.; Godoy-Martínez, P.; Flores, M.E.; Moreno-Villoslada, I. Photodynamic action of methylene blue subjected to aromatic-aromatic interactions with poly (sodium 4-styrenesulfonate) in solution and supported in solid, highly porous alginate sponges. *Dye. Pigment.* **2017**, *147*, 455–464. [CrossRef]
27. Pino-Pinto, J.P.; Oyarzun-Ampuero, F.; Orellana, S.L.; Flores, M.E.; Nishide, H.; Moreno-Villoslada, I. Aerogels containing 5, 10, 15, 20-tetrakis-(4-sulfonatophenyl)-porphyrin with controlled state of aggregation. *Dye. Pigment.* **2017**, *139*, 193–200. [CrossRef]
28. Sanhueza, L.; Castro, J.; Urzúa, E.; Barrientos, L.; Oyarzun-Ampuero, F.; Pesenti, H.c.; Shibue, T.; Sugimura, N.; Tomita, W.; Nishide, H. Photochromic Solid Materials Based on Poly (decylviologen) Complexed with Alginate and Poly (sodium 4-styrenesulfonate). *J. Phys. Chem. B* **2015**, *119*, 13208–13217. [CrossRef]
29. Araya-Hermosilla, E.; Catalán-Toledo, J.; Muñoz-Suescun, F.; Oyarzun-Ampuero, F.; Raffa, P.; Polgar, L.M.; Picchioni, F.; Moreno-Villoslada, I. Totally Organic Redox-Active pH-Sensitive Nanoparticles Stabilized by Amphiphilic Aromatic Polyketones. *J. Phys. Chem. B* **2018**, *122*, 1747–1755. [CrossRef] [PubMed]
30. Catalán-Toledo, J.; Nenen, A.; Vallejos, G.A.; Oyarzun-Ampuero, F.; Shibue, T.; Nishide, H.; Moreno-Villoslada, I. A simple and green methodology to assemble poly (4-vinylpyridine) and a sulfonated azo-dye for obtaining stable polymeric nanoparticles. *Polymer* **2018**, *158*, 289–296. [CrossRef]
31. Araya-Hermosilla, R.; Araya-Hermosilla, E.; Torres-Gallegos, C.; Alarcón-Alarcón, C.; Moreno-Villoslada, I. Sensing Cu^{2+} by controlling the aggregation properties of the fluorescent dye rhodamine 6G with the aid of polyelectrolytes bearing different linear aromatic density. *React. Funct. Polym.* **2013**, *73*, 1455–1463. [CrossRef]
32. Carrillo, J.-M.Y.; Dobrynin, A.V. Detailed Molecular Dynamics Simulations of a Model NaPSS in Water. *J. Phys. Chem. B* **2010**, *114*, 9391–9399. [CrossRef]
33. Mantha, S.; Yethiraj, A. Conformational Properties of Sodium Polystyrenesulfonate in Water: Insights from a Coarse-Grained Model with Explicit Solvent. *J. Phys. Chem. B* **2015**, *119*, 11010–11018. [CrossRef]
34. Zhang, Y.; Douglas, J.F.; Ermi, B.D.; Amis, E.J. Influence of counterion valency on the scattering properties of highly charged polyelectrolyte solutions. *J. Chem. Phys.* **2001**, *114*, 3299–3313. [CrossRef]
35. Matsuoka, H.; Schwahn, D.; Ise, N. Observation of cluster formation in polyelectrolyte solutions by small-angle neutron scattering. 1. A steep upturn of the scattering curves from solutions of sodium poly (styrenesulfonate) at scattering vectors below 0.01.ANG.-1. *Macromolecules* **1991**, *24*, 4227–4228. [CrossRef]
36. Combet, J. Polyelectrolytes and small angle scattering. *EPJ Web Conf.* **2018**, *188*, 03001. [CrossRef]
37. Ise, N.; Okubo, T.; Kunugi, S.; Matsuoka, H.; Yamamoto, K.; Ishii, Y. "Ordered" structure in dilute solutions of sodium polystyrenesulfonates as studied by small-angle x-ray scattering. *J. Chem. Phys.* **1984**, *81*, 3294–3306. [CrossRef]
38. Nishida, K.; Kaji, K.; Kanaya, T.; Shibano, T. Added Salt Effect on the Intermolecular Correlation in Flexible Polyelectrolyte Solutions: Small-Angle Scattering Study. *Macromolecules* **2002**, *35*, 4084–4089. [CrossRef]
39. Nause, R.G.; Hoagland, D.A.; Strey, H.H. Structural Evolution of Complexes of Poly (styrenesulfonate) and Cetyltrimethylammonium Chloride. *Macromolecules* **2008**, *41*, 4012–4019. [CrossRef]
40. Fares, H.M.; Ghoussoub, Y.E.; Delgado, J.D.; Fu, J.; Urban, V.S.; Schlenoff, J.B. Scattering Neutrons along the Polyelectrolyte Complex/Coacervate Continuum. *Macromolecules* **2018**, *51*, 4945–4955. [CrossRef]
41. Essafi, W.; Spiteri, M.-N.; Williams, C.; Boue, F. Hydrophobic Polyelectrolytes in Better Polar Solvent. Structure and Chain Conformation as Seen by SAXS and SANS. *Macromolecules* **2009**, *42*, 9568–9580. [CrossRef]
42. Mertens, H.D.T.; Svergun, D.I. Structural characterization of proteins and complexes using small-angle X-ray solution scattering. *J. Struct. Biol.* **2010**, *172*, 128–141. [CrossRef] [PubMed]
43. Agbabiaka, A.; Wiltfong, M.; Park, C. Small Angle X-Ray Scattering Technique for the Particle Size Distribution of Nonporous Nanoparticles. *J. Nanopart.* **2013**, *2013*, 11. [CrossRef]
44. Dobrynin, A.V.; Colby, R.H.; Rubinstein, M. Scaling Theory of Polyelectrolyte Solutions. *Macromolecules* **1995**, *28*, 1859–1871. [CrossRef]
45. Terao, K.; Morihana, N.; Ichikawa, H. Solution SAXS measurements over a wide temperature range to determine the unperturbed chain dimensions of polystyrene and a cyclic amylose derivative. *Polym. J.* **2014**, *46*, 155–159. [CrossRef]
46. Jouault, N.; Dalmas, F.; Said, S.; Di Cola, E.; Schweins, R.; Jestin, J.; Boué, F. Direct Measurement of Polymer Chain Conformation in Well-Controlled Model Nanocomposites by Combining SANS and SAXS. *Macromolecules* **2010**, *43*, 9881–9891. [CrossRef]

47. De, R.; Das, B. Concentration, medium and salinity-induced shrinkage/expansion of Poly (sodium styrenesulfonate) in 2-ethoxyethanol-Water mixed solvent media as probed by viscosimetry. *J. Mol. Struct.* **2020**, *1199*, 126992. [CrossRef]
48. Han, A.; Colby, R.H. Rheology of Entangled Polyelectrolyte Solutions. *Macromolecules* **2021**, *54*, 1375–1387. [CrossRef]
49. De, R.; Das, B. Coiling/uncoiling behaviour of sodium polystyrenesulfonate in 2-ethoxyethanol-water mixed solvent media as probed using viscometry. *Polym. Int.* **2014**, *63*, 1959–1964. [CrossRef]
50. De, R.; Ray, D.; Das, B. Influence of temperature, added electrolyte, and polymer molecular weight on the counterion-condensation phenomenon in aqueous solution of sodium polystyrenesulfonate: A scaling theory approach. *RSC Adv.* **2015**, *5*, 54890–54898. [CrossRef]
51. Bagchi, D.; Menon, R. Conformational modification of conducting polymer chains by solvents: Small-angle X-ray scattering study. *Chem. Phys. Lett.* **2006**, *425*, 114–117. [CrossRef]
52. Takano, T.; Masunaga, H.; Fujiwara, A.; Okuzaki, H.; Sasaki, T. PEDOT Nanocrystal in Highly Conductive PEDOT:PSS Polymer Films. *Macromolecules* **2012**, *45*, 3859–3865. [CrossRef]
53. Choudhury, P.K.; Bagchi, D.; Sangeeth, C.S.S.; Menon, R. Modified conformation and physical properties in conducting polymers due to varying conjugation and solvent interactions. *J. Mater. Chem.* **2011**, *21*, 1607–1614. [CrossRef]
54. Kaji, K.; Urakawa, H.; Kanaya, T.; Kitamaru, R. Phase diagram of polyelectrolyte solutions. *J. Phys.* **1988**, *49*, 993–1000. [CrossRef]
55. Nishida, K.; Kaji, K.; Kanaya, T. Improved phase diagram of polyelectrolyte solutions. *J. Chem. Phys.* **2001**, *115*, 8217–8220. [CrossRef]
56. Geckeler, K.E.; Bayer, E.; Spivakov, B.Y.; Shkinev, V.M.; Vorob'eva, G.A. Liquid-phase polymer-based retention, a new method for separation and preconcentration of elements. *Anal. Chim. Acta* **1986**, *189*, 285–292. [CrossRef]
57. Geckeler, K.E.; Volchek, K. Removal of Hazardous Substances from Water Using Ultrafiltration in Conjunction with Soluble Polymers. *Environ. Sci. Technol.* **1996**, *30*, 725–734. [CrossRef]
58. Palacio, D.A.; Rivas, B.L.; Urbano, B.F. Ultrafiltration membranes with three water-soluble polyelectrolyte copolymers to remove ciprofloxacin from aqueous systems. *Chem. Eng. J.* **2018**, *351*, 85–93. [CrossRef]
59. Stoner, M.R.; Fischer, N.; Nixon, L.; Buckel, S.; Benke, M.; Austin, F.; Randolph, T.W.; Kendrick, B.S. Protein–solute interactions affect the outcome of ultrafiltration/diafiltration operations. *J. Pharm. Sci.* **2004**, *93*, 2332–2342. [CrossRef]
60. Rivas, B.L.; Pereira, E.D.; Moreno-Villoslada, I. Water-soluble polymer-metal ion interactions. *Prog. Polym. Sci.* **2003**, *28*, 173–208. [CrossRef]
61. Moreno-Villoslada, I.; Miranda, V.; Gutiérrez, R.; Hess, S.; Muñoz, C.; Rivas, B.L. Interactions of 2, 3, 5-triphenyl-2H-tetrazolium chloride with poly (sodium 4-styrenesulfonate) studied by diafiltration and UV-vis spectroscopy. *J. Membr. Sci.* **2004**, *244*, 205–213. [CrossRef]
62. Moreno-Villoslada, I.; Miranda, V.; Jofré, M.; Chandía, P.; Villatoro, J.M.; Bulnes, J.L.; Cortés, M.; Hess, S.; Rivas, B.L. Simultaneous interactions between a low molecular-weight species and two high molecular-weight species studied by diafiltration. *J. Membr. Sci.* **2006**, *272*, 137–142. [CrossRef]
63. Orellana, S.L.; Torres-Gallegos, C.; Araya-Hermosilla, R.; Oyarzun-Ampuero, F.; Moreno-Villoslada, I. Association Efficiency of Three Ionic Forms of Oxytetracycline to Cationic and Anionic Oil-In-Water Nanoemulsions Analyzed by Diafiltration. *J. Pharm. Sci.* **2015**, *104*, 1141–1152. [CrossRef]
64. Barrat, J.-L.; Joanny, F. Theory of Polyelectrolyte Solutions. In *Advances in Chemical Physics*; Prigogine, I., Rice, S.A., Eds.; Wiley: Hoboken, NJ, USA, 1996; pp. 1–66.
65. Chalal, M.; Ehrburger-Dolle, F.; Morfin, I.; Bley, F.; Aguilar de Armas, M.-R.; López Donaire, M.-L.; San Roman, J.; Bölgen, N.; Pişkin, E.; Ziane, O.; et al. SAXS Investigation of the Effect of Temperature on the Multiscale Structure of a Macroporous Poly (N-isopropylacrylamide) Gel. *Macromolecules* **2010**, *43*, 2009–2017. [CrossRef]
66. Rubinstein, M.; Colby, R.H. *Polymer Physics*; Oxford University Press: Oxford, UK, 2003.
67. Hayashi, H.; Morita, T.; Nishikawa, K. Interpretation of correlation length by small-angle X-ray scattering experiments on fluids near critical point. *Chem. Phys. Lett.* **2009**, *471*, 249–252. [CrossRef]
68. Horkay, F.; Basser, P.J.; Hecht, A.-M.; Geissler, E. Ionic effects in semi-dilute biopolymer solutions: A small angle scattering study. *J. Chem. Phys.* **2018**, *149*, 163312. [CrossRef] [PubMed]
69. Levin, J.; Fox, J.A.; Forde, D.R. *Elementary Statistics in Social Research*; Pearson Allyn & Bacon: Boston, MA, USA, 2010.
70. Nishida, K.; Urakawa, H.; Kaji, K.; Gabrys, B.; Higgins, J.S. Electrostatic persistence length of NaPSS polyelectrolytes determined by a zero average contrast SANS technique. *Polymer* **1997**, *38*, 6083–6085. [CrossRef]
71. Combet, J.; Rawiso, M.; Rochas, C.; Hoffmann, S.; Boué, F. Structure of Polyelectrolytes with Mixed Monovalent and Divalent Counterions: SAXS Measurements and Poisson-Boltzmann Analysis. *Macromolecules* **2011**, *44*, 3039–3052. [CrossRef]
72. Borsali, R.; Nguyen, H.; Pecora, R. Small-Angle Neutron Scattering and Dynamic Light Scattering from a Polyelectrolyte Solution: DNA. *Macromolecules* **1998**, *31*, 1548–1555. [CrossRef]
73. Ise, N. Ordering of Ionic Solutes in Dilute Solutions through Attraction of Similarly Charged Solutes—A Change of Paradigm in Colloid and Polymer Chemistry. *Angew. Chem. Int. Ed. Engl.* **1986**, *25*, 323–334. [CrossRef]
74. Limbach, H.J.; Holm, C. Single-Chain Properties of Polyelectrolytes in Poor Solvent. *J. Phys. Chem. B* **2003**, *107*, 8041–8055. [CrossRef]
75. Wu, D.Q.; Chu, B.; Lundberg, R.D.; MacKnight, W.J. Small-angle x-ray scattering (SAXS) studies of sulfonated polystyrene ionomers. 2. Correlation function analysis. *Macromolecules* **1993**, *26*, 1000–1007. [CrossRef]

76. Balu, R.; Mata, J.P.; Knott, R.; Elvin, C.M.; Hill, A.J.; Choudhury, N.R.; Dutta, N.K. Effects of Crowding and Environment on the Evolution of Conformational Ensembles of the Multi-Stimuli-Responsive Intrinsically Disordered Protein, Rec1-Resilin: A Small-Angle Scattering Investigation. *J. Phys. Chem. B* **2016**, *120*, 6490–6503. [CrossRef]
77. Leisner, D.; Imae, T. Interpolyelectrolyte Complex and Coacervate Formation of Poly (glutamic acid) with a Dendrimer Studied by Light Scattering and SAXS. *J. Phys. Chem. B* **2003**, *107*, 8078–8087. [CrossRef]
78. Shrestha, L.K.; Sharma, S.C.; Sato, T.; Glatter, O.; Aramaki, K. Small-angle X-ray scattering (SAXS) study on nonionic fluorinated micelles in aqueous system. *J. Colloid Interface Sci.* **2007**, *316*, 815–824. [CrossRef]
79. Brilliantov, N.V.; Kuznetsov, D.V.; Klein, R. Chain Collapse and Counterion Condensation in Dilute Polyelectrolyte Solutions. *Phys. Rev. Lett.* **1998**, *81*, 1433–1436. [CrossRef]
80. Srivastava, A.; Qiao, W.; Ismail, K. Physicochemical Interactions of Chlorpheniramine Maleate with Sodium Deoxycholate in Aqueous Solution. *J. Surfactants Deterg.* **2018**, *21*, 879–887. [CrossRef]
81. Skerjanc, J.; Kogej, K.; Vesnaver, G. Polyelectrolyte-surfactant interactions: Enthalpy of binding of dodecyl- and cetylpyridinium cations to poly (styrenesulfonate) anion. *J. Phys. Chem.* **1988**, *92*, 6382–6385. [CrossRef]
82. Popov, A.; Zakharova, J.; Wasserman, A.; Motyakin, M.; Kasaikin, V. Macromolecular and Morphological Evolution of Poly (styrene sulfonate) Complexes with Tetradecyltrimethylammonium Bromide. *J. Phys. Chem. B* **2012**, *116*, 12332–12340. [CrossRef]
83. Sitar, S.; Goderis, B.; Hansson, P.; Kogej, K. Phase Diagram and Structures in Mixtures of Poly (styrenesulfonate anion) and Alkyltrimethylammonium Cations in Water: Significance of Specific Hydrophobic Interaction. *J. Phys. Chem. B* **2012**, *116*, 4634–4645. [CrossRef]

polymers

MDPI

Article

A Novel Green Preparation of Ag/RGO Nanocomposites with Highly Effective Anticancer Performance

Maqusood Ahamed [1,*], Mohd Javed Akhtar [1], M. A. Majeed Khan [1] and Hisham A. Alhadlaq [1,2]

1 King Abdullah Institute for Nanotechnology, King Saud University, Riyadh 11451, Saudi Arabia; mjakhtar@ksu.edu.sa (M.J.A.); mmkhan@ksu.edu.sa (M.A.M.K.); hhadlaq@ksu.edu.sa (H.A.A.)
2 Department of Physics and Astronomy, College of Science, King Saud University, Riyadh 11451, Saudi Arabia
* Correspondence: mahamed@ksu.edu.sa

Abstract: The efficacy of current cancer therapies is limited due to several factors, including drug resistance and non-specific toxic effects. Due to their tuneable properties, silver nanoparticles (Ag NPs) and graphene derivative-based nanomaterials are now providing new hope to treat cancer with minimum side effects. Here, we report a simple, inexpensive, and eco-friendly protocol for the preparation of silver-reduced graphene oxide nanocomposites (Ag/RGO NCs) using orange peel extract. This work was planned to curtail the use of toxic chemicals, and improve the anticancer performance and cytocompatibility of Ag/RGO NCs. Aqueous extract of orange peels is abundant in phytochemicals that act as reducing and stabilizing agents for the green synthesis of Ag NPs and Ag/RGO NCs from silver nitrate and graphene oxide (GO). Moreover, the flavonoid present in orange peel is a potent anticancer agent. Green-prepared Ag NPs and Ag/RGO NCs were characterized by UV-visible spectrophotometry, transmission electron microscopy (TEM), scanning electron microscopy (SEM), energy dispersive spectroscopy (EDS), X-ray diffraction (XRD), and dynamic light scattering (DLS). The results of the anticancer study demonstrated that the killing potential of Ag/RGO NCs against human breast cancer (MCF7) and lung cancer (A549) cells was two-fold that of pure Ag NPs. Moreover, the cytocompatibility of Ag/RGO NCs in human normal breast epithelial (MCF10A) cells and normal lung fibroblasts (IMR90) was higher than that of pure Ag NPs. This mechanistic study indicated that Ag/RGO NCs induce toxicity in cancer cells through pro-oxidant reactive oxygen species generation and antioxidant glutathione depletion and provided a novel green synthesis of Ag/RGO NCs with highly effective anticancer performance and better cytocompatibility.

Keywords: Ag/RGO nanocomposites; green preparation; anticancer performance; potential mechanism; oxidative stress

check for updates

Citation: Ahamed, M.; Akhtar, M.J.; Khan, M.A.M.; Alhadlaq, H.A. A Novel Green Preparation of Ag/RGO Nanocomposites with Highly Effective Anticancer Performance. *Polymers* **2021**, *13*, 3350. https://doi.org/10.3390/polym13193350

Academic Editors: Bramasta Nugraha and Faisal Raza

Received: 31 August 2021
Accepted: 26 September 2021
Published: 30 September 2021

1. Introduction

Silver nanoparticles (Ag NPs), as one of the noble metals, possess unique physicochemical properties, including high thermal and electrical conductivity, high catalytic activity, good chemical stability, and surface-enhanced plasmon resonance effects [1,2]. Ag NPs also display excellent biological activities, e.g., broad-spectrum antimicrobial, antiviral, anti-inflammatory, and anticancer activities [3–5]. Additionally, due to their great optical properties, Ag NPs have also been used in electronics, catalysis, and biosensors [6]. However, the toxic potential of Ag NPs in human and environmental health are major hurdles to their biomedical and industrial applications [7,8]. The toxicity of Ag NPs has been reported in several in vitro and in vivo (mammalian and non-mammalian animals) studies [9–11].

Graphene derivatives, such as graphene oxide (GO) and reduced graphene oxide (RGO), have received great attention in the fields of electronics, sensing, and biomedicine due to their incredible physical and chemical features. RGO and its nanocomplex have been studied for antimicrobial, wound healing, drug delivery, and anticancer applications [12,13]. RGO surfaces have a large number of oxygen functional groups and surface defects, which makes them favourable for the development of nanocomposites (NCs) of RGO and metal/metal oxide for biomedical applications [14]. Currently, investigators are devoting a large amount of attention to the development of RGO and metal/metal oxide-based NCs due to their inherently superior biological activities that cannot be achieved by single composition [15–17].

Currently, NPs/NCs are being synthesized through three main routes: physical, chemical, and green methods [18,19]. Researchers are now recommending that the green method of NPs/NC synthesis is the best method due to its facile processing, use of non-toxic chemicals, and low cost [20–22]. The reducing and capping agents play important roles in the preparation of NPs/NCs. Highly toxic chemicals/solvents used in physical and chemical methods of NPs/NCs synthesis are responsible for environmental hazards [23,24]. Additionally, the use of toxic chemicals and solvents limits the application of NPs/NCs in medical and clinical fields [22]. Green synthesis requires the use of extracts from fruits, vegetables, or plants as reducing and stabilizing agents [25]. Biologically developed capping and reducing agents for the green synthesis of NPs/NCs are not harmful to the environment. Hence, the green method eliminates the use of expensive chemicals, consumes less energy, and produces eco-friendly NPs/NCs and by-products. However, it is still challenging to develop a simple, rapid, and inexpensive green protocol for the synthesis of Ag/RGO NCs with highly effective anticancer performance.

The green synthesis of Ag/RGO NCs is gaining momentum [18,26,27]. It is advisable to prepare Ag/RGO NCs with highly effective anticancer performance and negligible side effects to humans and the environment. This study aimed to develop a simple, inexpensive, and environmentally friendly approach for the preparation of Ag/RGO NCs using orange (*Citrus sinensis*) peel extract. Oranges are among the most productive fruits worldwide, and orange peels, their main agricultural waste product, contain a large number of phytochemicals [28]. Orange peels contain polyphenols and polysaccharides that act as reducing agents, and carboxylic groups, amino acid and citric acid, which act as stabilizing agents [29]. The major active biological constituents in citrus fruits and peels are flavonoids [30]. The high concentrations of flavonoids present in orange peel extract have shown anticancer activity, as well as the prevention of infectious and degenerative diseases [31].

Orange peel extract was prepared by the maceration process [22,32]. A number of studies reported that the maceration process for the preparation of orange peel extract is an excellent method for the green synthesis of NPs [28,33,34]. Green-synthesized Ag NPs and Ag/RGO NCs were characterized by modern analytical techniques, such as transmission electron microscopy (TEM), scanning electron microscopy (SEM), energy dispersive X-ray spectroscopy (EDS), X-ray diffraction (XRD), and dynamic light scattering (DLS). The anticancer efficiency of Ag NPs and Ag/RGO NCs was examined in human breast cancer (MCF7) and human lung cancer (A549) cells. The cytocompatibility of prepared samples was assessed in human normal breast epithelial (MCF10A) cells and human normal lung fibroblasts (IMR90). Furthermore, the potential mechanisms of the anticancer activity of Ag/RGO NCs were delineated through the oxidative stress pathway.

2. Materials and Methods

2.1. Preparation of Orange Peels Extract

Orange peels were obtained from locally purchased fresh orange fruit. Peels were washed with deionized water and dried in a food drier (12–15 h). Dried peels were ground into a fine powder by a locally purchased grinder. Then, 5 g of orange peel powder was soaked in 250 mL deionized water and continuously stirred for 5 h. Afterwards, the mixture was placed in a water bath (Cole-Parmer, Vernon Hills, IL, USA) at 60 °C for 2 h. At last, the mixture was filtered with filter paper (pore size 0.2 μm), and the resulting extract was stored at 4 °C for further application.

2.2. Synthesis of Ag NPs and Ag/RGO NCs

Silver nitrate (AgNO3, Millipore-Sigma, St. Louis, MO, USA), graphene oxide (GO, Millipore-Sigma), and orange peel extract were utilized as precursors for the synthesis of Ag NPs and Ag/RGO NCs. Briefly, an aqueous solution of 1 mM silver nitrate (1 mM) was prepared. Then, 50 mg of GO was also suspended in 100 mL of deionized water and kept in a water bath sonicator. The reaction was started by adding 20 mL of orange peel extract and 20 mL of GO suspension into 160 mL of aqueous solution of silver nitrate (1 mM) under mild stirring. The reaction mixture was incubated for 12 h in a dark setting at room temperature to avoid photo-activation of silver nitrate. After the completion of the incubation period, samples were dried at 90 °C for 3 h, and then ground into a fine powder for characterization and application. Pure Ag NPs were also prepared using the same method, without the addition of GO suspension. A schematic diagram of Ag/RGO NCs synthesis is presented in Figure 1.

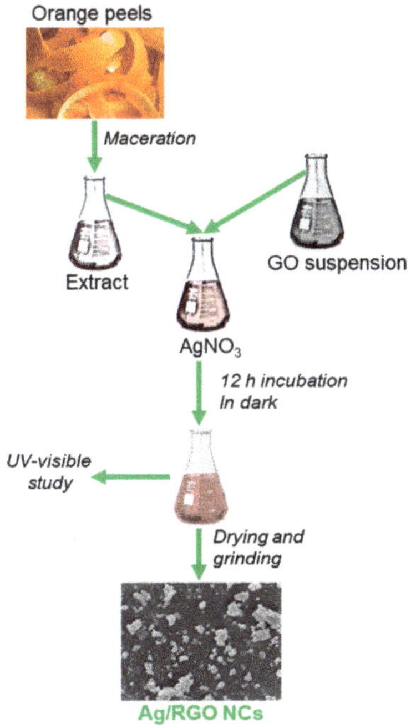

Figure 1. A schematic of green synthesis of Ag/RGO NCs using orange peel extract.

2.3. Characterization of Ag NPs and Ag/RGO NCs

UV-visible spectra of green-prepared Ag NPs and Ag/RGO NCs was evaluated between 250 and 750 nm using the Shimadzu UV-1800 spectrophotometer. X-ray diffraction (XRD) (Pan Analytic X'Pert Pro, Malvern Instruments, Malvern, WR14, 1XZ, UK) equipped with Cu-Kα radiation (λ = 0.15405 nm, at 45 kV and 40 mA) was used to assess the crystallinity and phase-purity of green-prepared Ag NPs and Ag/RGO NCs. Morphological analysis, elemental mapping, and other structural characterization were further carried out by field emission transmission electron microscopy (FETEM) (JEM-2100, JEOL, Inc., Tokyo, Japan) and field emission scanning electron microscopy (FESEM) (JSM-7600F, JEOL, Inc., Tokyo, Japan). The characterization of NPs/NCs in aqueous suspension (hydrodynamic size and zeta potential) was carried out by dynamic light scattering (DLS) (ZetaSizer, Nano-HT, Malvern Instruments).

2.4. Cell Culture

Human breast cancer cells (MCF7), human lung cancer cells (A549), human normal breast epithelial cells (MCF10A), and human lung fibroblasts (IMR90) were purchased from American Type Culture Collection (ATCC, Manassas, WV, USA). Cells were cultured in Dulbecco's Modified Eagle's Medium (DMEM) with the supplementation of 10% fetal bovine serum (FBS) and antibiotics (100 U/mL of penicillin and 100 µg/mL of streptomycin). Cells were grown at 37 °C in a humidified CO_2 incubator (Heracell 150i, Thermo Fisher Scientific, Waltham, MA, USA) with 5% CO_2 supply.

2.5. Exposure Procedure

The 1 mg/mL stock suspension of Ag NPs and Ag/RGO NCs was prepared in deionized water. Working concentrations (0.5–100 µg/mL) were diluted in culture medium. First, cells were exposed to different dosages (0.5–100 µg/mL) of Ag NPs and Ag/RGO NCs to examine their anticancer performance in a dose-dependent manner. Then, one moderate cytotoxic dosage (10 µg/mL) of each nanoscale material was chosen to explore potential mechanisms of anticancer activity through the oxidative stress pathway.

2.6. Anticancer Performance Assays

The anticancer activity of green-prepared NPs and NCs was examined by a tetrazolium dye 3-(4, 5-dimethylthiazol-2-yl)-2, 5-diphenyltetrazolium bromide (MTT) assay [35] with some specific modifications [36]. MTT assay is based on the principle that live cells are able to reduce yellow MTT salt into purple formazan crystals. These formazan crystals dissolved in acidified isopropanol, and absorbance was measured at 570 nm by a microplate reader (Synergy-HT, BioTek, Vinnoski, VT, USA). Potential mechanisms of anticancer activity of prepared samples were delineated by measuring the intracellular ROS and GSH levels. The ROS level was estimated using a cell-permeable probe 2′-7′-dichlorodihydrofluorescein diacetate (H_2DCFDA) (Millipore-Sigma) [37]. Upon reaction with ROS, the non-fluorescent H_2DCFDA was converted into highly fluorescent 2′-7′-dichlorofluorescein (DCF). The fluorescence intensity of DCF was measured at 485/520 nm (excitation/emission wavelength) using a microplate reader (Synergy-HT, BioTek). Ellman's protocol was used to estimate the intracellular glutathione level (GSH) [38]. The intracellular level of GSH was represented as nmol GSH/mg protein. Protein assay was performed using Bradford's method [39].

2.7. Statistical Analysis

One-way analysis of variance (ANOVA) followed by Dennett's multiple comparison tests was applied to analyse the biochemical data. The $p < 0.05$ was assigned as statistically significant. All the biochemical data are represented as the mean ± SD of three independent experiments ($n = 3$).

3. Results and Discussion

3.1. UV-Visible Spectrophotometer Study

The colour of orange peel extract changed from light orange to dark brown after incubation with $AgNO_3$ and GO for 12 h; the colour change reveals an indication of formation of Ag NPs and Ag/RGO NCs. The specific absorption peak of Ag NPs occurs in the range of 380–450 nm depending on shape, size, and agglomeration [40,41]. Hence, a UV-visible spectrophotometer was used to confirm the formation of Ag NPs and Ag/RGO NCs in the range of 250–750 nm. In the present study, Ag NPs and Ag/RGO NCs exhibited a strong plasma absorption band at ~395 nm (Figure 2). Our results were in agreement with those of other studies [42,43].

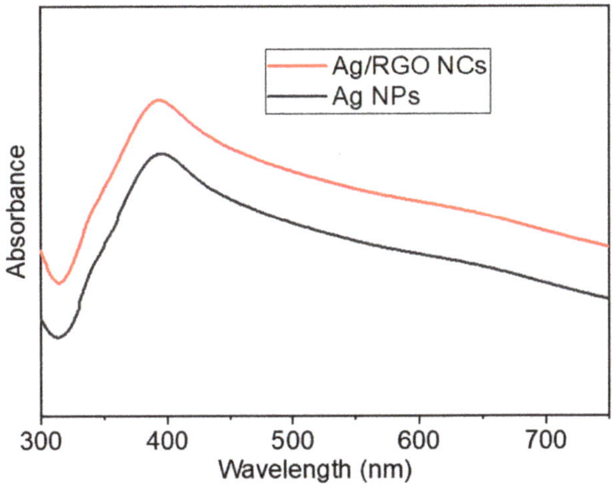

Figure 2. UV-visible spectra of Ag NPs and Ag/RGO NCs prepared from orange peel extract.

3.2. XRD Study

XRD spectra of green-prepared Ag NPs and Ag/RGO NCs are given in Figure 3A. The five distinct diffraction peaks at 2θ = 38.16, 44.32, 64.52, 77.45, and 81.59 correspond to the crystal planes (111), (200), (220), (311), and (222), respectively, for the Ag/RGO NCs, which occurs with the face-centred cubic structure of metallic Ag (JCPDS card no.04-0783) [44]. The incorporation of RGO did not alter the original structure of metallic Ag as all the peaks of Ag/RGO NCs were similar to those of pure Ag NPs [45]. The absence of diffraction peaks of RGO in Ag/RGO NCs suggests that the uniform integration of Ag NPs inhibited the restacking of RGO sheets [46], and indicates the successful synthesis of Ag/RGO NCs. No other peaks attributed to impurity were identified, which indicates the high purity of the prepared samples.

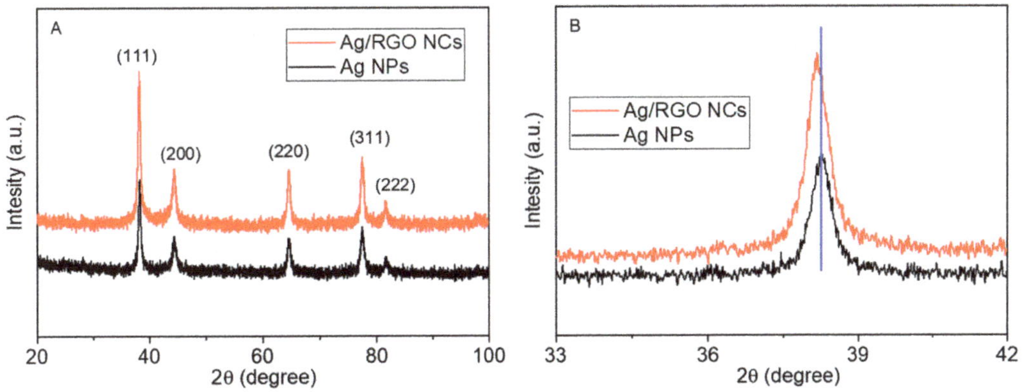

Figure 3. XRD characterization: (**A**) XRD spectra of Ag NPs and Ag/RGO NCs; (**B**) peak shifting.

Scherrer's formula [47] was applied to calculate the particle size of the prepared nanoscale materials corresponding to prominent peak (111). The average particle sizes of pure Ag NPs and Ag/RGO NCs were around 13 and 9 nm, respectively. We further observed that Ag/RGO NCs showed a slight shift of the XRD peak (111) towards a lower value in comparison to pure Ag NPs (Figure 3B). The shifting of the peak toward a lower value further supports the successful formation of Ag/RGO NCs.

3.3. TEM Study

The TEM characterization of pure Ag NPs and Ag/RGO NCs is presented in Figure 4. Pure Ag NPs were nearly spherical with some degree of agglomeration (Figure 4A). In Ag/RGO NCs, Ag NPs were almost uniformly anchored on RGO sheets (Figure 4B). The particle sizes calculated from TEM were approximately 12 and 8 nm for pure Ag NPs and Ag/RGO NCs, respectively, which agreed with the sizes calculated from XRD. Ag NPs on RGO sheets were less agglomerated than pure Ag NPs. Moreover, Ag NPs acted as spacers to avoid the restacking of RGO sheets, and enhanced the surface area of NCs. This could be a possible reason for the particle size reduction of Ag/RGO NCs. Decrements in the particle size of NPs after the incorporation of RGO were also reported in other studies [16,46,48]. Nanoscale materials with a smaller size and higher surface area exhibited higher biological activity [26]. High-resolution TEM images (Figure 4C,D) show the clear lattice fringes with measured interplanar distances of 0.233 and 0.229 nm for pure Ag NPs and Ag/RGO NCs, respectively, which corresponds to the (111) plane of the face-centred cubic structure of Ag [26]. Elemental analysis of Ag/RGO NCs by TEM-led EDS indicated the presence of Ag, C, and O elements with no impurities (Figure 5). The presence of Cu peaks was due to the utilization of a Cu-based grid.

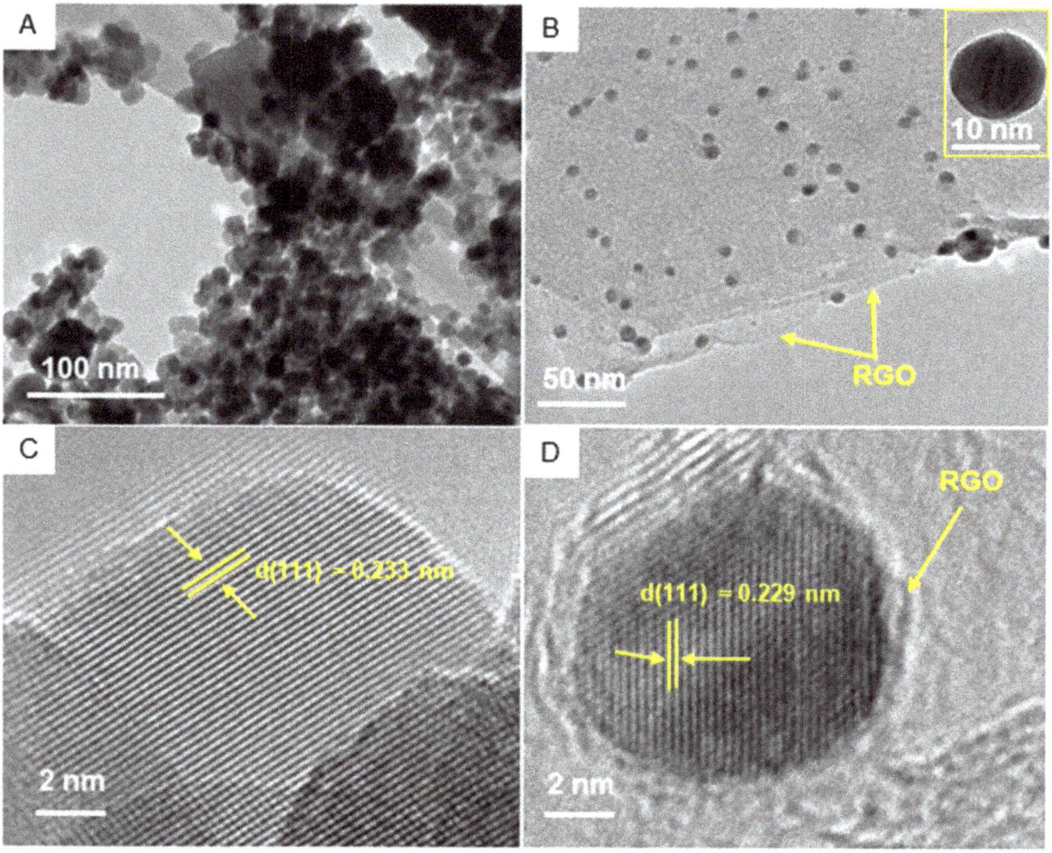

Figure 4. TEM characterization: (**A**) low-resolution TEM image of Ag NPs; (**B**) low-resolution TEM image of Ag/RGO NCs; (**C**) high-resolution TEM image of Ag NPs; (**D**) high-resolution TEM image of Ag/RGO NCs.

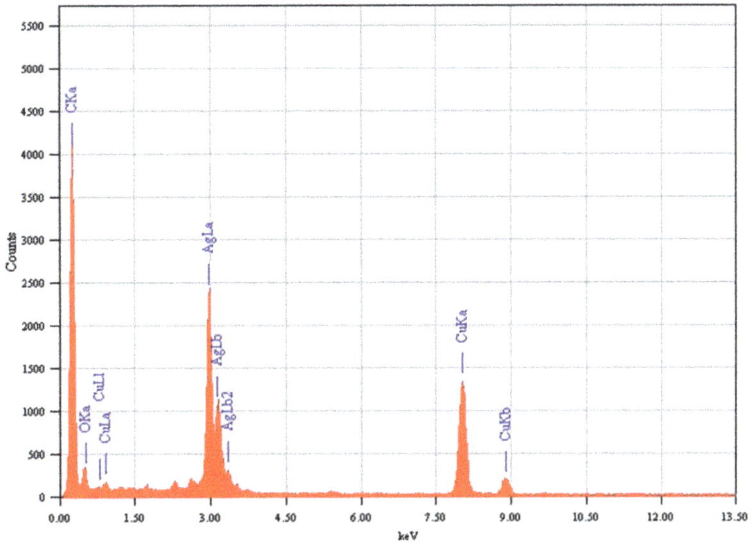

Figure 5. TEM-led EDS spectra of Ag/RGO NCs.

3.4. SEM Study

Figure 6 shows the surface morphology and elemental composition of green-prepared samples. SEM images suggested that the smooth morphology of Ag NPs (Figure 6A) and Ag NPs were well embedded on the surface of RGO sheets (Figure 6B), which is supported by TEM micrographs. The implanted Ag NPs on RGO sheets created a strong interaction between them, resulting in the effective migration of charge carriers (electrons and holes) from the inner part of NCs to the surface. Hence, charge carriers can participate in surface redox reactions [49]. This phenomenon could be helpful in photocatalysis and cancer therapy [50]. The quantitative elemental composition of Ag/RGO NCs is presented in Figure 6C. The presence of Ag, C, and O elements in Ag/RGO NCs was in agreement with TEM-led EDS data. Figure 7 shows the elemental mapping of Ag/RGO NCs, which further confirmed the homogenous distribution of Ag, C, and O in Ag/RGO NCs.

3.5. DLS Study

It is essential to examine the aqueous behaviour of nanomaterials (e.g., surface charge, particle distribution, and stability) before their biological activity assessments [51,52]. DLS is an important tool to assess the aqueous behaviour of nanoscale materials [53]. In this study, DLS data demonstrated that the hydrodynamic sizes of pure Ag NPs and Ag/RGO NCs in deionized water and culture medium were several times higher (43–65 nm) than particle sizes estimated from XRD and TEM (Table 1). This may be ascribed to the fact that DLS measures the Brownian motion, and the subsequent size distribution of a group of NPs/NCs in aqueous suspension provides an average hydrodynamic size. During the DLS study, there was a tendency of NPs/NCs to agglomerate in aqueous suspension, thereby showing the size of clumped NPs/NCs rather than individual NPs/NCs [53,54].

Zeta potential data suggested that colloidal suspensions of Ag NPs and Ag/RGO NCs in deionized water and culture medium were fairly stable, as these values ranged from 21 to 28 mV (Table 1). A higher value of zeta potential (either positive or negative) is directly proportional to the greater stability of colloidal suspension [55]. Additionally, positive surface charges (zeta potential value) of Ag NPs and Ag/RGO NCs offer encouraging conditions for their interaction with negatively charged cancer cells [56].

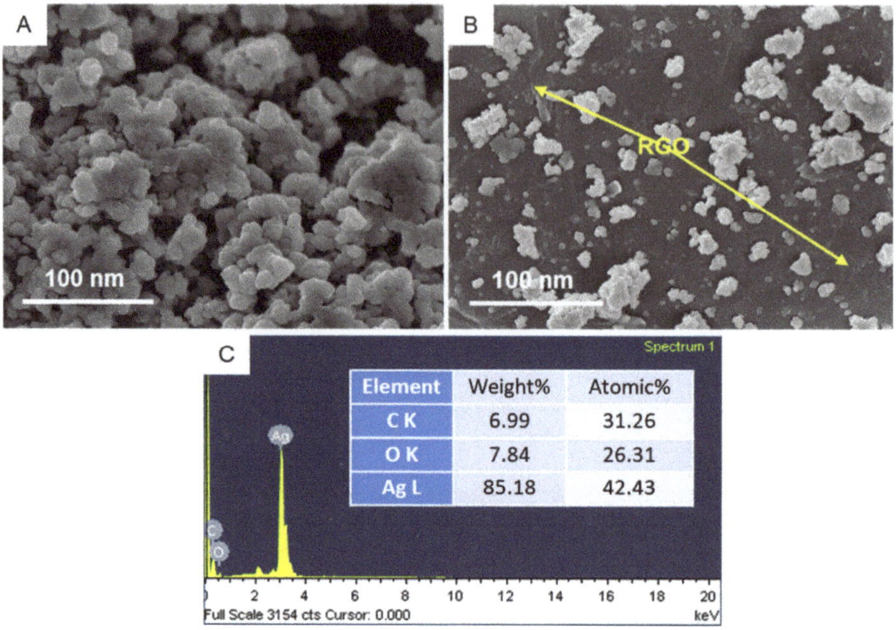

Figure 6. SEM characterization: (**A**) SEM image of Ag NPs; (**B**) SEM image of Ag/RGO NCs; (**C**) SEM-led EDS spectra of Ag/RGO NCs.

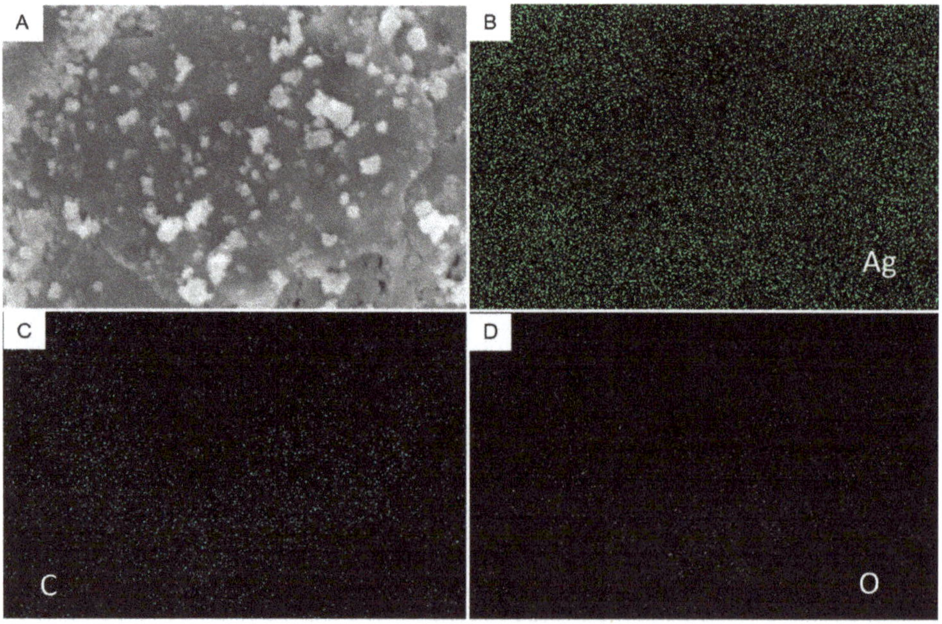

Figure 7. SEM elemental mapping of Ag/RGO NCs: (**A**) SEM micrograph; (**B**) Ag mapping; (**C**) C mapping; (**D**) O mapping.

Table 1. Dynamic light scattering (DLS) characterization of Ag NPs and Ag/RGO NCs.

NPs/NCs	Hydrodynamic Size (nm)		Zeta Potential (mV)	
	Deionized water	Culture medium	Deionized water	Culture medium
Ag NPs	59.8 ± 2.8	65.2 ± 3.3	25.7 ± 1.5	21.3 ± 1.3
Ag/RGO NCs	43.4 ± 1.6	46.7 ± 2.3	28.3 ± 0.9	23.7 ± 1.1

3.6. Anticancer Study

The anticancer performance of green-synthesized Ag NPs and Ag/RGO NCs was studied in two different types of cancer cells: human breast cancer (MCF7) and human lung cancer (A549) cells. Both types of cancer cells were treated with different concentrations of Ag NPs and Ag/RGO NCs, and anticancer performance was evaluated by MTT assay. Results showed that pure Ag NPs and Ag/RGO NCs kill both types of cancer cells in a dose-dependent manner (Figure 8A,B). Furthermore, the killing potential of Ag/RGO NCs against both cancer cells was twice that of pure Ag. The IC_{50} values of Ag/RGO NCs (10 μg/mL for MCF7 and 11 μg/mL for A549) were almost half of those of pure Ag NPs (19 μg/mL for MCF7 and 20 μg/mL for A549) (Table 2). The high anticancer efficacy of Ag/RGO NCs might be due to excellent green mediated (orange peel components) synergism between the two functional materials, Ag and RGO. Earlier reports suggested that bioactive flavonoid present in orange peel extract is a potent anticancer agent [31]. Therefore, orange peel extract-mediated green-synthesized Ag/RGO NCs have the potential to act as a chemotherapeutic drug. The high anticancer efficacy of Ag and graphene derivative-based NCs synthesized by different methods has also been reported by other studies. For example, Gurunathan and co-workers observed that chemically prepared RGO-Ag NCs showed higher cytotoxicity in ovarian cancer (A2780) than pure GO, RGO, and Ag NPs [27]. Another study also demonstrated that green-prepared (walnut husk) Ag-GO NCs exerted higher cytotoxicity to MCF7 cells in comparison to pure Ag NPs [57].

The application of anticancer drugs depends on their biocompatibility with normal cells/tissues. In this study, the cytotoxicity of Ag NPs and Ag/RGO NCs was examined in the normal counterparts of the above cancer cells: human normal breast epithelial (MCF10A) cells and human normal fibroblasts (IMR90). Results showed that green-synthesized pure Ag NPs and Ag/RGO NCs did not induce cytotoxicity to both types of normal cells (MCF10A and IMR90) (Figure 8C,D). Moreover, the cytocompatibility of Ag/RGO NCs in both normal cells was higher in comparison to pure Ag NPs. Overall, the anticancer study indicated that green-synthesized Ag/RGO NCs exhibited a higher potential of anticancer activity and better cytocompatibility than those of pure Ag NPs. Bioactive compounds present on green-prepared Ag NPs and Ag/RGO NCs might prevent their toxicity to normal cells.

3.7. Potential Mechanisms of Anticancer Activity

Oxidative stress has been suggested as a potential mechanism of the anticancer response of green-prepared Ag NPs. [46]. In the present study, the anticancer mechanism of green-prepared present nanoscale materials was delineated through assessing the oxidative stress pathway. Pro-oxidant ROS and antioxidant GSH were assessed in cancer and normal cells after exposure for 24 h to 10 μg/mL of pure Ag NPs and Ag/RGO NCs. Figure 9 demonstrates that pure Ag NPs and Ag/RGO NCs induced intracellular ROS generation and GSH depletion in both types of cancer cells (MCF7 and A549). However, Ag NPs and Ag/RGO NCs were not able to affect ROS and GSH levels in either of the normal cells (MCF10A and IMR90). Additionally, the oxidative stress-generating potential of Ag/RGO NCs was greater than pure Ag NPs, which supports the cytotoxicity data.

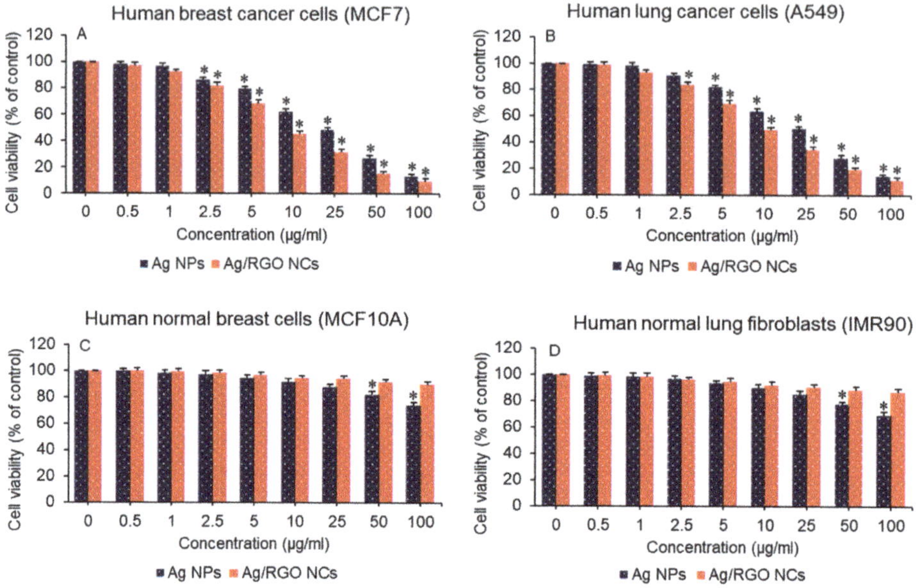

Figure 8. Anticancer performance of Ag NPs and Ag/RGO NCs in cancer cells. * $p < 0.05$ statistically different from control (0 concentration of NPs/NCs).

Table 2. IC_{50} values of pure Ag NPs and Ag/RGO NCs for human cancer cells.

NPs/NCs	Human Breast Cancer MCF7 Cells	Human Lung Cancer A549 Cells
Ag NPs	18.8 μg/mL	20.3 μg/mL
Ag/RGO NCs	9.7 μg/mL	10.9 μg/mL

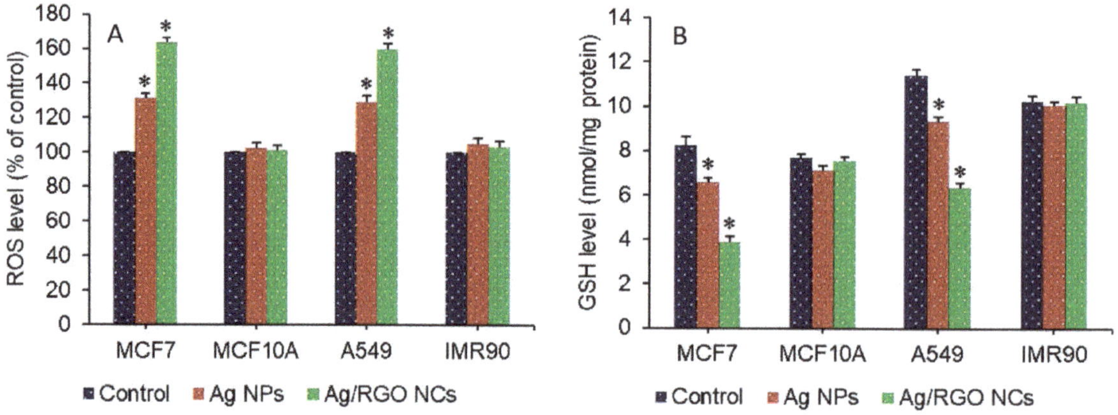

Figure 9. Oxidative stress response of cancer and normal cells against 10 μg/mL of Ag NPs and Ag/RGO NCs for 24 h: (**A**) ROS generation; (**B**) GSH depletion. * $p < 0.05$ statistically different from control.

The integration of RGO makes two crucial modifications in the physicochemical properties of Ag NPs, which play important roles in improving the anticancer performance of Ag/RGO NCs: (i) The firmly anchored Ag NPs on RGO sheets create a strong interaction between them that leads to an easy electron transfer process on the surface of NCs, resulting in highly effective anticancer performance through the intracellular generation of ROS [49]. (ii) The homogeneous anchoring of AG NPs on RGO sheets decreases the particle size and increases the surface of NCs. Smaller NPs generate greater intracellular ROS in comparison to higher NPs [58]. The oxidative stress-mediated anticancer activity of other nanoscale materials has also been proposed [50,59]. For example, our recent studies indicated that ZnO/RGO NCs and Zn-doped Bi_2O_3 NPs displayed anticancer activity through ROS generation [32,60,61]. The possible mechanism of anticancer performance in Ag/RGO NCs is depicted in Figure 10.

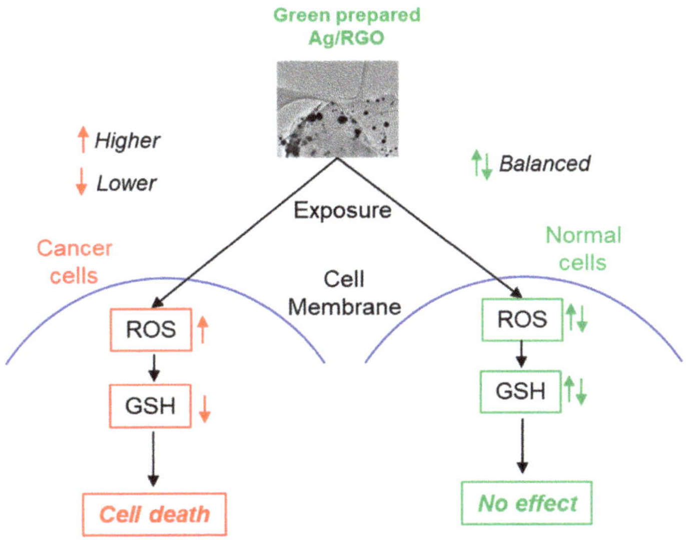

Figure 10. Possible mechanism of anticancer performance of Ag/RGO NCs.

4. Conclusions

A simple, cost-effective, and eco-friendly procedure was developed to prepare Ag NPs and Ag/RGO NCs. Green-synthesized Ag NPs and Ag/RGO NCs were characterized by UV-vis, XRD, TEM, SEM, EDS, and DLS techniques. XRD data confirm that the synthesis of face-centred cubic structures of metallic Ag and RGO implantation did not change the original crystal structure of Ag. A high-resolution TEM micrograph of Ag/RGO NCs indicated the presence of Ag and RGO with fine-quality lattice fringes without distortion. EDS elemental composition and mapping depicted the uniform presence of Ag, O, and C in Ag/RGO NCs. The DLS study demonstrated the outstanding colloidal stability of Ag NPs and Ag/RGO NCs. The anticancer study showed that the killing potential of Ag/RGO NCs against cancer (MCF7 and A549) was two-fold that of pure Ag NPs. Additionally, the cytocompatibility of Ag/RGO NCs in normal counterparts (MCF10A and IMR90) was higher than that of Ag NPs. Mechanistic data indicated that the anticancer activity of Ag NPs and Ag/RGO NCs was mediated through ROS generation and GSH depletion. Current work suggests a novel approach for highly effective cancer treatment through green-prepared Ag/RGO NCs. Further research on the antitumor efficacy of Ag/RGO NCs in animal models is warranted.

Author Contributions: Conceptualization, M.A.; investigation and methodology, M.A., M.J.A., M.A.M.K. and H.A.A.; writing—original draft preparation, M.A.; writing—review and editing, M.A. and M.J.A.; funding acquisition, M.A. All authors have read and agreed to the published version of the manuscript.

Funding: This work was supported by the National Plan for Science, Technology, and Innovation (MAARIFAH), King Abdulaziz City for Science and Technology, Kingdom of Saudi Arabia, under Award 13-NAN908-02.

Conflicts of Interest: The authors declare no conflict of interest.

References

1. Heo, S.; Lee, J.; Lee, G.H.; Heo, C.-J.; Kim, S.H.; Yun, D.-J.; Park, J.-B.; Kim, K.; Kim, Y.; Lee, D.; et al. Surface plasmon enhanced Organic color image sensor with Ag nanoparticles coated with silicon oxynitride. *Sci. Rep.* **2020**, *10*, 219. [CrossRef]
2. Sharma, R.K.; Yadav, S.; Dutta, S.; Kale, H.B.; Warkad, I.R.; Zbořil, R.; Varma, R.S.; Gawande, M.B. Silver nanomaterials: Synthesis and (electro/photo) catalytic applications. *Chem. Soc. Rev.* **2021**. [CrossRef]
3. Khorrami, S.; Zarrabi, A.; Khaleghi, M.; Danaei, M.; Mozafari, M.R. Selective cytotoxicity of green synthesized silver nanoparticles against the MCF-7 tumor cell line and their enhanced antioxidant and antimicrobial properties. *Int. J. Nanomed.* **2018**, *13*, 8013–8024. [CrossRef]
4. Sharmin, S.; Rahaman, M.; Sarkar, C.; Atolani, O.; Islam, M.T.; Adeyemi, O.S. Nanoparticles as antimicrobial and antiviral agents: A literature-based perspective study. *Heliyon* **2021**, *7*, e06456. [CrossRef] [PubMed]
5. Mane, P.C.; Sayyed, S.A.R.; Kadam, D.D.; Shinde, M.D.; Fatehmulla, A.; Aldhafiri, A.M.; Alghamdi, E.A.; Amalnerkar, D.P.; Chaudhari, R.D. Terrestrial snail-mucus mediated green synthesis of silver nanoparticles and in vitro investigations on their antimicrobial and anticancer activities. *Sci. Rep.* **2021**, *11*, 13068. [CrossRef] [PubMed]
6. Kästner, C.; Thünemann, A.F. Catalytic Reduction of 4-Nitrophenol Using Silver Nanoparticles with Adjustable Activity. *Langmuir* **2016**, *32*, 7383–7391. [CrossRef]
7. Stensberg, M.C.; Wei, Q.; McLamore, E.S.; Porterfield, D.M.; Wei, A.; Sepúlveda, M.S. Toxicological studies on silver nanoparticles: Challenges and opportunities in assessment, monitoring and imaging. *Nanomedicine* **2011**, *6*, 879–898. [CrossRef]
8. Burdușel, A.-C.; Gherasim, O.; Grumezescu, A.M.; Mogoantă, L.; Ficai, A.; Andronescu, E. Biomedical Applications of Silver Nanoparticles: An Up-to-Date Overview. *Nanomaterials* **2018**, *8*, 681. [CrossRef]
9. Leynen, N.; Van Belleghem, F.G.; Wouters, A.; Bove, H.; Ploem, J.-P.; Thijssen, E.; Langie, S.A.; Carleer, R.; Ameloot, M.; Artois, T.; et al. In vivo Toxicity Assessment of Silver Nanoparticles in Homeostatic versus Regenerating Planarians. *Nanotoxicology* **2019**, *13*, 476–491. [CrossRef]
10. Ferdous, Z.; Nemmar, A. Health Impact of Silver Nanoparticles: A Review of the Biodistribution and Toxicity Following Various Routes of Exposure. *Int. J. Mol. Sci.* **2020**, *21*, 2375. [CrossRef]
11. Ahamed, M.; AlSalhi, M.; Siddiqui, M. Silver nanoparticle applications and human health. *Clin. Chim. Acta* **2010**, *411*, 1841–1848. [CrossRef]
12. Anand, A.; Unnikrishnan, B.; Wei, S.-C.; Chou, C.P.; Zhang, L.-Z.; Huang, C.-C. Graphene oxide and carbon dots as broad-spectrum antimicrobial agents—A minireview. *Nanoscale Horiz.* **2018**, *4*, 117–137. [CrossRef] [PubMed]
13. Dash, B.; Jose, G.; Lu, Y.-J.; Chen, J.-P. Functionalized Reduced Graphene Oxide as a Versatile Tool for Cancer Therapy. *Int. J. Mol. Sci.* **2021**, *22*, 2989. [CrossRef] [PubMed]
14. McCallion, C.; Burthem, J.; Rees-Unwin, K.; Golovanov, A.; Pluen, A. Graphene in therapeutics delivery: Problems, solutions and future opportunities. *Eur. J. Pharm. Biopharm.* **2016**, *104*, 235–250. [CrossRef] [PubMed]
15. Rodwihok, C.; Wongratanaphisan, D.; Ngo, Y.L.T.; Khandelwal, M.; Hur, S.H.; Chung, J.S. Effect of GO Additive in ZnO/rGO Nanocomposites with Enhanced Photosensitivity and Photocatalytic Activity. *Nanomaterials* **2019**, *9*, 1441. [CrossRef] [PubMed]
16. Ahamed, M.; Akhtar, M.J.; Khan, M.A.M.; Alaizeri, Z.M.; Alhadlaq, H.A. Evaluation of the Cytotoxicity and Oxidative Stress Response of CeO2-RGO Nanocomposites in Human Lung Epithelial A549 Cells. *Nanomaterials* **2019**, *9*, 1709. [CrossRef] [PubMed]
17. Yang, K.; Feng, L.; Shi, X.; Liu, Z. Nano-graphene in biomedicine: Theranostic applications. *Chem. Soc. Rev.* **2013**, *42*, 530–547. [CrossRef] [PubMed]
18. Hemmati, S.; Heravi, M.M.; Karmakar, B.; Veisi, H. Green fabrication of reduced graphene oxide decorated with Ag nanoparticles (rGO/Ag NPs) nanocomposite: A reusable catalyst for the degradation of environmental pollutants in aqueous medium. *J. Mol. Liq.* **2020**, *319*, 114302. [CrossRef]
19. Divya, K.; Chandran, A.; Reethu, V.; Mathew, S. Enhanced photocatalytic performance of RGO/Ag nanocomposites produced via a facile microwave irradiation for the degradation of Rhodamine B in aqueous solution. *Appl. Surf. Sci.* **2018**, *444*, 811–818. [CrossRef]
20. Mescola, A.; Canale, C.; Fragouli, D.; Athanassiou, A. Controlled formation of gold nanostructures on biopolymer films upon electromagnetic radiation. *Nanotechnology* **2017**, *28*, 415601. [CrossRef]
21. Tan, N.P.B.; Lee, C.H.; Li, P. Green Synthesis of Smart Metal/Polymer Nanocomposite Particles and Their Tuneable Catalytic Activities. *Polymers* **2016**, *8*, 105. [CrossRef]
22. Castillo-Henriquez, L.; Alfaro-Aguilar, K.; Ugalde-Alvarez, J.; Vega-Fernandez, L.; Montes de Oca-Vasquez, G.; Vega-Baudrit, J.R. Green Synthesis of Gold and Silver Nanoparticles from Plant Extracts and Their Possible Applications as Antimicrobial Agents in the Agricultural Area. *Nanomaterials* **2020**, *10*, 1763. [CrossRef]
23. Jadoun, S.; Arif, R.; Jangid, N.K.; Meena, R.K. Green synthesis of nanoparticles using plant extracts: A review. *Environ. Chem. Lett.* **2021**, *19*, 355–374. [CrossRef]

24. Singh, J.; Dutta, T.; Kim, K.-H.; Rawat, M.; Samddar, P.; Kumar, P. 'Green' synthesis of metals and their oxide nanoparticles: Applications for environmental remediation. *J. Nanobiotechnol.* **2018**, *16*, 84. [CrossRef] [PubMed]
25. De Matteis, V.; Cascione, M.; Rizzello, L.; Liatsi-Douvitsa, E.; Apriceno, A.; Rinaldi, R. Green Synthesis of Nanoparticles and Their Application in Cancer Therapy. In *Green Synthesis of Nanoparticles: Applications and Prospects*; Springer Science and Business Media: New York, NY, USA, 2020; pp. 163–197.
26. Zhu, J.; Ni, H.; Hu, C.; Zhu, Y.; Cai, J.; Liu, S.; Gao, J.; Yang, H.; Liu, H. Rapid synthesis and characterization of silver-loaded graphene oxide nanomaterials and their antibacterial applications. *R. Soc. Open Sci.* **2021**, *8*, 201744. [CrossRef]
27. Gurunathan, S.; Han, J.W.; Park, J.-H.; Kim, E.S.; Choi, Y.-J.; Kwon, D.-N.; Kim, J.-H. Reduced graphene oxide–silver nanoparticle nanocomposite: A potential anticancer nanotherapy. *Int. J. Nanomed.* **2015**, *10*, 6257–6276. [CrossRef] [PubMed]
28. Thi, T.U.D.; Nguyen, T.T.; Thi, Y.D.; Thi, K.H.T.; Phan, B.T.; Pham, K.N. Green synthesis of ZnO nanoparticles using orange fruit peel extract for antibacterial activities. *RSC Adv.* **2020**, *10*, 23899–23907. [CrossRef]
29. Skiba, M.I.; Vorobyova, V.I. Synthesis of Silver Nanoparticles Using Orange Peel Extract Prepared by Plasmochemical Extraction Method and Degradation of Methylene Blue under Solar Irradiation. *Adv. Mater. Sci. Eng.* **2019**, *2019*, 8306015. [CrossRef]
30. Tajaldini, M.; Samadi, F.; Khosravi, A.; Ghasemnejad, A.; Asadi, J. Protective and anticancer effects of orange peel extract and naringin in doxorubicin treated esophageal cancer stem cell xenograft tumor mouse model. *Biomed. Pharmacother.* **2020**, *121*, 109594. [CrossRef] [PubMed]
31. Koolaji, N.; Shammugasamy, B.; Schindeler, A.; Dong, Q.; Dehghani, F.; Valtchev, P. Citrus Peel Flavonoids as Potential Cancer Prevention Agents. *Curr. Dev. Nutr.* **2020**, *4*, nzaa025. [CrossRef]
32. Ahamed, M.; Akhtar, M.J.; Khan, M.M.; Alhadlaq, H.A. Facile green synthesis of ZnO-RGO nanocomposites with enhanced anticancer efficacy. *Methods* **2021**, in press. [CrossRef] [PubMed]
33. Gao, Y.; Xu, D.; Ren, D.; Zeng, K.; Wu, X. Green synthesis of zinc oxide nanoparticles using Citrus sinensis peel extract and application to strawberry preservation: A comparison study. *LWT* **2020**, *126*, 109297. [CrossRef]
34. Niluxsshun, M.C.D.; Masilamani, K.; Mathiventhan, U. Green Synthesis of Silver Nanoparticles from the Extracts of Fruit Peel of Citrus tangerina, Citrus sinensis, and Citrus limon for Antibacterial Activities. *Bioinorg. Chem. Appl.* **2021**, *2021*, 6695734. [CrossRef]
35. Mosmann, T. Rapid colorimetric assay for cellular growth and survival: Application to proliferation and cytotoxicity assays. *J. Immunol. Methods* **1983**, *65*, 55–63. [CrossRef]
36. Ahamed, M.; Akhtar, M.; Siddiqui, M.A.; Ahmad, J.; Musarrat, J.; Al-Khedhairy, A.A.; AlSalhi, M.; Alrokayan, S.A. Oxidative stress mediated apoptosis induced by nickel ferrite nanoparticles in cultured A549 cells. *Toxicology* **2011**, *283*, 101–108. [CrossRef]
37. Siddiqui, M.; Alhadlaq, H.; Ahmad, J.; Al-Khedhairy, A.; Musarrat, J.; Ahamed, M. Copper Oxide Nanoparticles Induced Mitochondria Mediated Apoptosis in Human Hepatocarcinoma Cells. *PLoS ONE* **2013**, *8*, e69534. [CrossRef]
38. Ellman, G.L. Tissue sulfhydryl groups. *Arch. Biochem. Biophys.* **1959**, *82*, 70–77. [CrossRef]
39. Bradford, M.M. A rapid and sensitive method for the quantitation of microgram quantities of protein utilizing the principle of protein-dye binding. *Anal. Biochem.* **1976**, *72*, 248–254. [CrossRef]
40. Fernandes, I.J.; Aroche, A.F.; Schuck, A.; Lamberty, P.; Peter, C.R.; Hasenkamp, W.; Rocha, T. Silver nanoparticle conductive inks: Synthesis, characterization, and fabrication of inkjet-printed flexible electrodes. *Sci. Rep.* **2020**, *10*, 8878. [CrossRef]
41. Lotfy, W.A.; Alkersh, B.M.; Sabry, S.A.; Ghozlan, H.A. Biosynthesis of Silver Nanoparticles by Aspergillus terreus: Characterization, Optimization, and Biological Activities. *Front. Bioeng. Biotechnol.* **2021**, *9*, 265. [CrossRef]
42. Wu, T.; Liu, S.; Luo, Y.; Lu, W.; Wang, L.; Sun, X. Surface plasmon resonance-induced visible light photocatalytic reduction of graphene oxide: Using Ag nanoparticles as a plasmonic photocatalyst. *Nanoscale* **2011**, *3*, 2142–2144. [CrossRef]
43. Ahmad, M.A.; Aslam, S.; Mustafa, F.; Arshad, U. Synergistic antibacterial activity of surfactant free Ag–GO nanocomposites. *Sci. Rep.* **2021**, *11*, 196. [CrossRef]
44. Corsino, D.C.; Balela, M.D.L. Room temperature sintering of printer silver nanoparticle conductive ink. *IOP Conf. Ser. Mater. Sci. Eng.* **2017**, *264*, 12020. [CrossRef]
45. Devi, A.P.; Padhi, D.K.; Mishra, P.M.; Behera, A.K. Bio-Surfactant assisted room temperature synthesis of cubic Ag/RGO nanocomposite for enhanced photoreduction of Cr (VI) and antibacterial activity. *J. Environ. Chem. Eng.* **2021**, *9*, 104778. [CrossRef]
46. Mariadoss, A.V.A.; Saravanakumar, K.; Sathiyaseelan, A.; Wang, M.-H. Preparation, characterization and anti-cancer activity of graphene oxide—Silver nanocomposite. *J. Photochem. Photobiol. B Biol.* **2020**, *210*, 111984. [CrossRef] [PubMed]
47. Khan, M.A.M.; Khan, W.; Ahamed, M.; Alhazaa, A.N. Microstructural properties and enhanced photocatalytic performance of Zn doped CeO2 nanocrystals. *Sci. Rep.* **2017**, *7*, 12560. [CrossRef] [PubMed]
48. Swapna, R.; Kumar, M.S. Growth and characterization of molybdenum doped ZnO thin films by spray pyrolysis. *J. Phys. Chem. Solids* **2013**, *74*, 418–425. [CrossRef]
49. Qi, J.; Chang, Y.; Sui, Y.; He, Y.; Meng, Q.; Wei, F.; Ren, Y.; Jin, Y. Facile Synthesis of Ag-Decorated Ni3 S2 Nanosheets with 3D Bush Structure Grown on rGO and Its Application as Positive Electrode Material in Asymmetric Supercapacitor. *Adv. Mater. Interfaces* **2018**, *5*, 1700985. [CrossRef]
50. Ciccarese, F.; Raimondi, V.; Sharova, E.; Silic-Benussi, M.; Ciminale, V. Nanoparticles as Tools to Target Redox Homeostasis in Cancer Cells. *Antioxidants* **2020**, *9*, 211. [CrossRef]

51. Carvalho, P.; Felício, M.R.; Santos, N.; Gonçalves, S.; Domingues, M. Application of Light Scattering Techniques to Nanoparticle Characterization and Development. *Front. Chem.* **2018**, *6*, 237. [CrossRef]
52. Alhadlaq, H.; Akhtar, M.; Ahamed, M. Different cytotoxic and apoptotic responses of MCF-7 and HT1080 cells to MnO2 nanoparticles are based on similar mode of action. *Toxicology* **2019**, *411*, 71–80. [CrossRef] [PubMed]
53. Malm, A.V.; Corbett, J.C.W. Improved Dynamic Light Scattering using an adaptive and statistically driven time resolved treatment of correlation data. *Sci. Rep.* **2019**, *9*, 13519. [CrossRef]
54. Caputo, F.; Clogston, J.; Calzolai, L.; Rösslein, M.; Prina-Mello, A. Measuring particle size distribution of nanoparticle enabled medicinal products, the joint view of EUNCL and NCI-NCL. A step by step approach combining orthogonal measurements with increasing complexity. *J. Control. Release* **2019**, *299*, 31–43. [CrossRef] [PubMed]
55. Jiang, J.; Oberdörster, G.; Biswas, P. Characterization of size, surface charge, and agglomeration state of nanoparticle dispersions for toxicological studies. *J. Nanoparticle Res.* **2009**, *11*, 77–89. [CrossRef]
56. Ouyang, L.; Shaik, R.; Xu, R.; Zhang, G.; Zhe, J. Mapping Surface Charge Distribution of Single-Cell via Charged Nanoparticle. *Cells* **2021**, *10*, 1519. [CrossRef]
57. Khorrami, S.; Abdollahi, Z.; Eshaghi, G.; Khosravi, A.; Bidram, E.; Zarrabi, A. An Improved Method for Fabrication of Ag-GO Nanocomposite with Controlled Anti-Cancer and Anti-bacterial Behavior; A Comparative Study. *Sci. Rep.* **2019**, *9*, 9167. [CrossRef]
58. Yu, Z.; Li, Q.; Wang, J.; Yu, Y.; Wang, Y.; Zhou, Q.; Li, P. Reactive Oxygen Species-Related Nanoparticle Toxicity in the Biomedical Field. *Nanoscale Res. Lett.* **2020**, *15*, 115. [CrossRef]
59. Li, Y.; Yang, J.; Sun, X. Reactive Oxygen Species-Based Nanomaterials for Cancer Therapy. *Front. Chem.* **2021**, *9*, 152. [CrossRef]
60. Ahamed, M.; Akhtar, M.J.; Khan, M.A.M.; Alaizeri, Z.M.; Alhadlaq, H. Facile Synthesis of Zn-Doped Bi2O3 Nanoparticles and Their Selective Cytotoxicity toward Cancer Cells. *ACS Omega* **2021**, *6*, 17353–17361. [CrossRef]
61. Ahamed, M.; Akhtar, M.J.; Khan, M.M.; Alhadlaq, H.A. SnO2-Doped ZnO/Reduced Graphene Oxide Nanocomposites: Synthesis, Characterization, and Improved Anticancer Activity via Oxidative Stress Pathway. *Int. J. Nanomed.* **2021**, *16*, 89–104. [CrossRef] [PubMed]

polymers

MDPI

Article

Poloxamer 407 Based Gel Formulations for Transungual Delivery of Hydrophobic Drugs: Selection and Optimization of Potential Additives

Kamran Hidayat Ullah [1], Faisal Raza [2], Syed Mohsin Munawar [1], Muhammad Sohail [3], Hajra Zafar [2], Mazhar Iqbal Zafar [4] and Tofeeq Ur-Rehman [1,*]

1 Department of Pharmacy, Quaid-i-Azam University, Islamabad 45320, Pakistan; kamran_893@yahoo.com (K.H.U.); syedmohsin013@yahoo.com (S.M.M.)
2 School of Pharmacy, Shanghai Jiao Tong University, 800 Dongchuan Road, Shanghai 200240, China; faisalraza@sjtu.edu.cn (F.R.); hajrazafar@sjtu.edu.cn (H.Z.)
3 School of Pharmacy, Yantai University, Shandong 264005, China; sohailshah11@yahoo.com
4 Department of Environmental Sciences, Quaid-i-Azam University, Islamabad 45320, Pakistan; mazhariqbal.zafar@gmail.com
* Correspondence: tofeeq.urrehman@qau.edu.pk

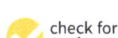

Citation: Ullah, K.H.; Raza, F.; Munawar, S.M.; Sohail, M.; Zafar, H.; Zafar, M.I.; Ur-Rehman, T. Poloxamer 407 Based Gel Formulations for Transungual Delivery of Hydrophobic Drugs: Selection and Optimization of Potential Additives. *Polymers* **2021**, *13*, 3376. https://doi.org/10.3390/polym13193376

Academic Editor: Constantinos Tsitsilianis

Received: 2 September 2021
Accepted: 24 September 2021
Published: 30 September 2021

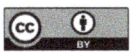

Abstract: The current study aimed to develop poloxamer 407 (P407) gel for transungual delivery of antifungal hydrophobic drugs with sufficient gel strength and drug loading. Gel strength and drug loading of P407 gel was improved by use of functional additives. Hydration enhancement effect was used to select optimum nail penetration enhancer. Face-centered central composite design (FCCCD) was used to observe the effect of the selected penetration enhancer (thioglycolic acid (TGA)) and cosolvent (ethanol) on gelation behavior to develop formulation with enough loading of hydrophobic drug, i.e., terbinafine HCl (TBN), and its permeation across the nail plate without compromising on gel strength. It was observed that increasing concentration of P407 and TGA significantly reduced gelation temperature and enhanced the gel strength of P407 gel and can be used to improve P407 gel strength. Under the scanning electron microscope, the significant effect of TGA as an ungual penetration enhancer was observed on the morphology of the nail plate. Optimized P407 gel prepared with modified cold method showed a gelation temperature of 8.7 ± 0.16 °C, gel strength of 122 ± 7.5 s and drug loading of 1.2% *w/w*, which was four times more than the drug loading in the gels prepared with conventional cold method. Rheological behavior was pseudoplastic with 47.75 ± 3.48% of gel erosion after 12 washings and 67.21 ± 2.16% of drug release after 12 h. A cumulative amount of TBN permeated from P407 gel with and without PE after 24 h was 27.30 ± 4.18 and 16.69 ± 2.31 μg/cm^2, respectively. Thioglycolic acid can be used as a nail penetration enhancer without the chemical modification or addition of extra additives while retaining the gel strength. Water miscible cosolvents with moderate evaporability such as ethanol, can be incorporated to P407 gel by minor modification in method of preparation to load the required dose of hydrophobic drugs. Developed P407 gel formulation with sufficient gel strength and drug loading will be a promising carrier for transungual delivery of hydrophobic antifungal agents.

Keywords: hydrogel; poloxamer 407 polymer; poloxamer 407 gel; transungual drug delivery; onychomycosis; ungual penetration enhancer; Terbinafine

1. Introduction

Onychomycosis accounts for 50% of nail diseases, which affect 10% of the general population with higher prevalence in people over 60 years of age. Oral systemic antifungal therapy is limited by its hepatotoxicity, drug interactions, a long duration of treatment, high cost of medication, increased microbial resistance and relapse of infection. Topical application of drug to nail is preferable because of its localized effects, minimum adverse effects and less drug interactions [1]. The major limitation of topical ungual drug delivery is low nail

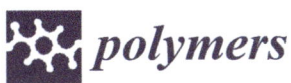

permeability due to the presence of highly stable disulfide and hydrogen bonds found in nail keratin [2]. Topical delivery of hydrophilic drugs may be facilitated through hydration of the nail plate and addition of nail penetration enhancers. However, the majority of recently approved drugs, including antifungals, are hydrophobic in nature and solubilization of the required dose is another challenge for transungual delivery of hydrophobic drugs. Nail permeation of drug molecules may be enhanced by the addition of reducing and oxidizing agents [3], keratolytic agents [4], keratinolytic enzymes [5] and surfactants [6].

Nail lacquer, a solution of drug and polymer in organic/vaporizing solvent, is one of the approaches where hydrophobic drugs and layer of the polymer deposits on the nail plate after evaporation of the organic solvent. Ciclopirox nail lacquer, approved by the FDA as topical treatment in onychomycosis, requires another organic solvent for removal which can damage barrier properties of the nail surface [7]. Unattended disposal of lacquers and organic solvents, just as nail polishes, may pose threat to the environment [8]. Moreover, rapid evaporation of organic solvent causes the formation of drug crystals, posing a barrier in its diffusion/permeation into the nail [9].

Polymer based platforms have been successfully used in various biomedical applications [10,11]. P407 gels, due to high water content, may hydrate the nail plate to facilitate permeation across the nail plate and can be a good alternate to nail lacquer for topical delivery of hydrophobic drugs such as terbinafine and efinaconazole [12]. P407 gels have an inherent tendency to improve the solubilization of hydrophobic drugs due to amphiphilic nature of polymer. Moreover, additives of different functionalities may be incorporated in gels without compromising their gelation ability [13,14]. Tanriverdi and Ozer reported the highest amount of drug accumulation in nail using poloxamer gel as compared to chitosan and carbopol gel [15]. However, P407 gels will be retained on the nail plate for a shorter period as compared to nail lacquer due to insufficient gel strength, weak stability and fast dissolution of the gels [16]. Drug loading capacity and gel strength of P407 gels may be improved either with the functional additives or by applying a chemical modification/conjugation approach [16–18]. Chemical modification and conjugation with crosslinker/polymers require costly and lengthy toxicity testing. The nail penetration enhancers and cosolvents are essential additives of P407 gels poised for transungual delivery of hydrophobic antifungal drugs and their impact on gel properties must be evaluated thoroughly.

In the present study, topical P407 gel formulation was developed with the aim to enhance the loading of hydrophobic drugs and to improve transungual permeation without compromising on thermogelation and washability of these gels. Nail permeation enhancers were screened based on the hydration enhancement factor [19]. TBN was selected as a model drug due to its strong antifungal activity against dermatophytes [20] and low aqueous solubility. Terbinafine is highly soluble in ethanol which is miscible with water and has a low vaporizing tendency as compared to ethyl acetate and acetone [21]. Optimized P407 gel was selected after assessing the effect of the selected PE (Thioglycolic acid), cosolvent (ethanol) and concentration of p407 on gel properties using face-centered central composite design (FCCCD).

2. Materials and Methods

2.1. Materials

Urea, tartaric acid, lactic acid, thiourea and oxalic acid were purchased through local supplier from BDH laboratories, Dorset, United Kingdom. Thioglycolic acid (TGA), chitosan, poloxamer P407 (Pluronic F127) and glycolic acid were purchased through local supplier from Sigma-Aldrich, Dorset, United Kingdom. Beta Cyclodextrin was purchased from Cydex Pharmaceuticals, Lenexa, Kansas, USA. Hydroxyl propyl cyclodextrin was supplied by Merck, United Kingdom. DMSO was purchased from Duksan Pure Chemicals, Ansan, Korea. Other chemicals used were of analytical grade.

2.2. Nail Clippings and Ethical Approval

This study was performed according to the principles of Declaration of Helsinki and ethical approval was obtained from the Bio-Ethical Committee (BEC) of Quaid-i-Azam University, Islamabad Pakistan (Protocol # BEC-FBS-QAU-2017-37). Human nail clippings were collected from healthy volunteers and informed consent was ensured in all cases.

2.3. Screening of Penetration Enhancers

PE were screened on the basis of hydration enhancement effect (HEF) [19]. Briefly, nail clippings, grouped on the basis of size and weight, were placed in 1 mL aqueous solution of each PE and control (deionized water) in a separate glass vial. The vials were sealed and stored at 25 ± 2 °C. After 24 h, nail clippings were removed from glass vials and dried with tissue paper to remove any residual solvent from the nail surface. The nail clippings were then weighed and HEF was calculated using following equation:

$$HEF = \frac{weight\ gain\ of\ nail\ clipping\ immersed\ in\ PE\ (\%)}{weight\ gain\ of\ nail\ clipping\ immersed\ in\ deionized\ water\ (\%)} \quad (1)$$

2.4. Topography of Nail

Effect of hydration and selected penetration enhancer on nail morphology was observed by scanning electron microscopy. Samples were sputtered with gold in sputter coater for 90 s at 30 mA. Images were taken by scanning electron microscope (SEM; Joel JSM-5910, Tokyo, Japan) available at the Central Resources Library (CRL), University of Peshawar, Pakistan. Morphology of untreated and treated nail clippings (3 mm central flat portion) was recorded. Treated nail clippings were either immersed in 5% *w*/*v* solution of thioglycolic acid or in deionized water for 72 h.

2.5. Preparation of P407 Gel

Previously reported "cold method" was used for preparation of poloxamer gels [22] and modified to accommodate high content of hydrophobic drug where required. Briefly, appropriate amount of TBN was dissolved in sufficient quantity of ethanol followed by addition of the calculated amount of P407. Whenever quantity of ethanol in final formulation was less than the quantity of ethanol required to dissolve TBN, excessive ethanol was used and allowed to evaporate up to required level (semisolid mass/thin film was formed on the walls and bottom of the container depending upon the amount of ethanol). Cold thioglycolic acid aqueous solution (having calculated TGA and water) was added to semisolid mass/thin film slowly and placed for 24 h in refrigerator or freezer whatever required. The final gel formulation had the required concentration of P407, TGA, ethanol and TBN.

2.6. Estimation of Drug Loading in Gels

The drug content of gels was increased slowly with increments of 1 mg/g until the precipitates of drug in the gel were visible with naked eye. The gel samples below and above the saturation point were examined under microscope (Olympus microscope, Model CX41RF, Tokyo, Japan). The effect of increase in P407 (20–30% *w*/*w*), ethanol (3–10% *w*/*w*) and modification in method on drug loading was investigated.

2.7. Experimental Design

Response surface method based on FCCCD was used to investigate relationship between independent variable on responses which involved full factorial along 6 replicates in the center. Response surface methodology (RSM) helps in identifying the significant variables, best process conditions and to study the interaction between key variables and responses with fewer experiments. The levels of the studied factors were selected so that they were within practical use and their relative difference was adequate to have a measurable effect on the response. A design consisting of 20 runs of experiments was generated using Design-Expert® 6.0.6 software (State Ease Inc., Minneapolis, MN, USA). Independent variables employed were concentration of P407 concentration (X1) with a constraint of 30% *w*/*w*, ethanol (X2) with a constraint of 10% *w*/*w* and thioglycolic acid (X3) with a constraint of 10% *w*/*w*. Constraint was identified based on preliminary experiment and literature. Below 20% *w*/*w*, P407 solution was in liquid form, and above 30% *w*/*w*, it was difficult to dissolve. Similarly, maximum ethanol concentration was kept at 10% *w*/*w* due to its undesirable effect on gel strength. TGA was kept in a concentration limit which is considered safe (below 15% for topical use). The dependent variables were gelation temperature (Y1) and gel strength (Y2).

2.8. Determination of Gelation Temperature

The sol-gel transition temperature of the P407 solutions was evaluated by visual tube inversion method as reported previously [23]. The glass tube containing 1 g of the sample was kept in sample cooler (Shimadzu Corporation, Kyoto, Japan). The temperature was gradually increased and the temperature at which no flow of solution occurred after tube inversion was noted as the gelation temperature (t_1). After raising the temperature well above the t_1 and maintaining for 15 min, the temperature was then lowered and the temperature, at which flow of the gel started, was noted (t_2). The mean ± SD of t_1 and t_2 is reported here as the gelation temperature.

2.9. Determination of Gel Strength

The strength of poloxamer gel formulations was determined to optimize gel consistency [24]. A glass tube assembly (25 g) which was hollow from inside was placed on surface of gel (1 g) in a glass tube at 32 °C. Gel strength was measured by recording the time (s) taken by the glass tube to penetrate 1 cm into the P407 gel.

2.10. Rheology

The gel formulation was subjected to rheological characterization using a Brookfield rheometer (DV3T, Middleboro, MA, USA). Spindle CPA-52Z was employed to determine the viscosity in centipoises at 32 ± 2 °C and the flow pattern was studied by constructing the graph. The graphs were presented as apparent viscosity (η) to the function of shear rate (s-1). The experiment was performed in triplicate and reported as mean ± SD.

2.11. Washability/Erosion Profile of P407 Gel

The erosion profile of prepared gel was measured by gravimetric method [25] with slight modification. Briefly, gel formulation (1 g) in small glass tube was placed in a beaker containing water at 32 °C. To the glass tube, 3 mL of phosphate buffer (PB) pH 5.5 maintained at 32 °C was added. At regular interval, the amount of eroded gel was determined by noting reduction in weight of gel after removing the dissolved liquid. One cycle of solvent addition and removal of dissolved material was taken as one washing and number of washings required to remove the percentage of gel from glass tube were noted.

2.12. In Vitro Drug Release

Dialysis membrane diffusion model was used to determine in vitro release profile of TBF from optimized P407 gel [15]. Briefly, gel formulation equivalent to 5 mg of TBN was added to cellulose membrane (molecular weight of 12–14 kDa). The membrane was placed in 50 mL of PB (pH 5.5): ethanol (9:1 ratio) in beaker at 32 °C and stirred at 50 rpm using magnetic stirrer. Samples were taken at regular intervals, replenished by the fresh medium to maintain the sink condition. The amount of TBN released was quantified using UV spectrophotometer at 283 nm as reported previously [26] after constructing the standard curve ($y = 0.0181x - 0.0015$, R^2: 0.998) using TBN solutions of 1.56 to 50 µg/mL. In vitro release study of drug suspension was performed in a similar manner. All experiments were performed in triplicate ($n = 3$) and results presented as mean ± SD.

2.13. Kinetic Modelling of Erosion Profile and In Vitro Drug Release

Gel erosion profile and in vitro drug release data was evaluated to predict release kinetics and mechanism of drug release by applying mathematical models, i.e., zero order, 1st order, Korsmeyer–Peppas, Higuchi and Hixson–Crowell model using DDSolver, a Microsoft Excel Add-In program. Most suitable model was selected based on the goodness of fit test (calculation of R2). n value obtained from Korsmeyer–Peppas model was used to find mechanism of drug release.

2.14. In Vitro Drug Permeation

Permeation of TBN across human nail clippings was performed using Franz diffusion cell [15]. Nail clipping of known thickness was mounted between donor and receiver compartment of Franz cell. Interface of donor and receiver compartment was occluded with parafilm. The system was kept at 32 °C. Receiver compartment was filled with PB (pH 5.5): ethanol (9:1) and checked for leakage. Gel formulation (0.1 g equivalent to 1 mg TBN) was placed on the nail surface and covered the donor compartment with parafilm. Sample was taken after every hour and quantified using UV spectrophotometer at 283 nm as mentioned in 2.12 above. Cumulative amount of the drug (μg) permeating per unit surface area of the nail (cm^2) was plotted against time (h).

3. Results

3.1. Screening of Penetration Enhancers Based on Hydration Enhancement Factor

Table 1 shows HEF values obtained after treatment with the aqueous solutions of various chemicals screened as nail penetration enhancers. Reducers of disulphide bonds, i.e., thioglycolic acid and mercaptoethanol, were observed as the best nail penetration enhancers with the highest HEF values of 2.73 ± 0.43 and 1.76 ± 0.47, respectively. Second best penetration enhancers were organic acids, i.e., tartaric acid, oxalic acid, glycolic acid and lactic acid, with HEF values of 1.44 ± 0.07, 1.42 ± 0.15, 1.42 ± 0.15 and 1.32 ± 0.10, respectively. Wetting agents/surfactant also showed slight penetration enhancement (HEF values of 1.23 ± 0.08 and 1.20 ± 0.05 for Tween 20 and P407, respectively). Concentration dependent effect of ethanol was observed, i.e., HEF of 5% (w/v) solution was 1.06 ± 0.12 while that of 20% solution was 1.24 ± 0.22. Another prominent nail penetration enhancer was resorcinol with a HEF value of 1.39 ± 0.16.

Table 1. Comparison of HEF values of screened chemicals as potential nail penetration enhancers.

S.No.	Penetration Enhancer	Concentration in the Nail Treatment Solution % *w/v*	Hydration Enhancement Factor (HEF) Mean ± SD
1.	Thiourea	5	1.19 ± 0.06
2.	Sodium lauryl sulphate	5	0.91 ± 0.13
3.	Tween 20	5	1.23 ± 0.08
4.	Tween 80	5	1.14 ± 0.21
5.	DMSO	5	1.18 ± 0.46
6.	Oxalic acid	5	1.42 ± 0.15
7.	Urea	5	1.04 ± 0.19
8.	Thioglycolic acid	5	2.73 ± 0.43
9.	Glycolic acid	5	1.42 ± 0.15
10.	Mercaptoethanol	5	1.76 ± 0.47
11.	Resorcinol	5	1.39 ± 0.16
12.	Alpha cyclodextrin	5	1.22 ± 0.18
13.	Hydroxy Propyl-β-Cyclodextrin	5	0.87 ± 0.08
14.	Chitosan	1	1.08 ± 0.28
15.	Chitosan	0.5	0.86 ± 0.05
16.	Thiolated chitosan	0.5	1.23 ± 0.17
17.	β-Cyclodextrin	5	1.09 ± 0.13
18.	Tartaric acid	5	1.44 ± 0.07
19.	Methionine	5	0.98 ± 0.12
20.	Lactic acid	5	1.32 ± 0.10
21.	Ethanol	5	1.06 ± 0.12
22.	Ethanol	20	1.24 ± 0.22
23.	Poloxamer 407	5	1.20 ± 0.06

3.2. *Effect of Penetration Enhancer on the Surface Morphology of Human Nail*

Figure 1 shows 1500X and 10,000X magnification scanning electron microscope images of the dorsal surface of nails. The untreated nail shows a relatively smooth surface and compact surface with minor ridges (Figure 1a,d). In the hydrated nail (immersed in deionized water for 72 h), the ridges are prominent (Figure 1b,e). The nail clipping hydrated with TGA solution shows disturbed integrity with the creation of some pore-like appearances (Figure 1c,f).

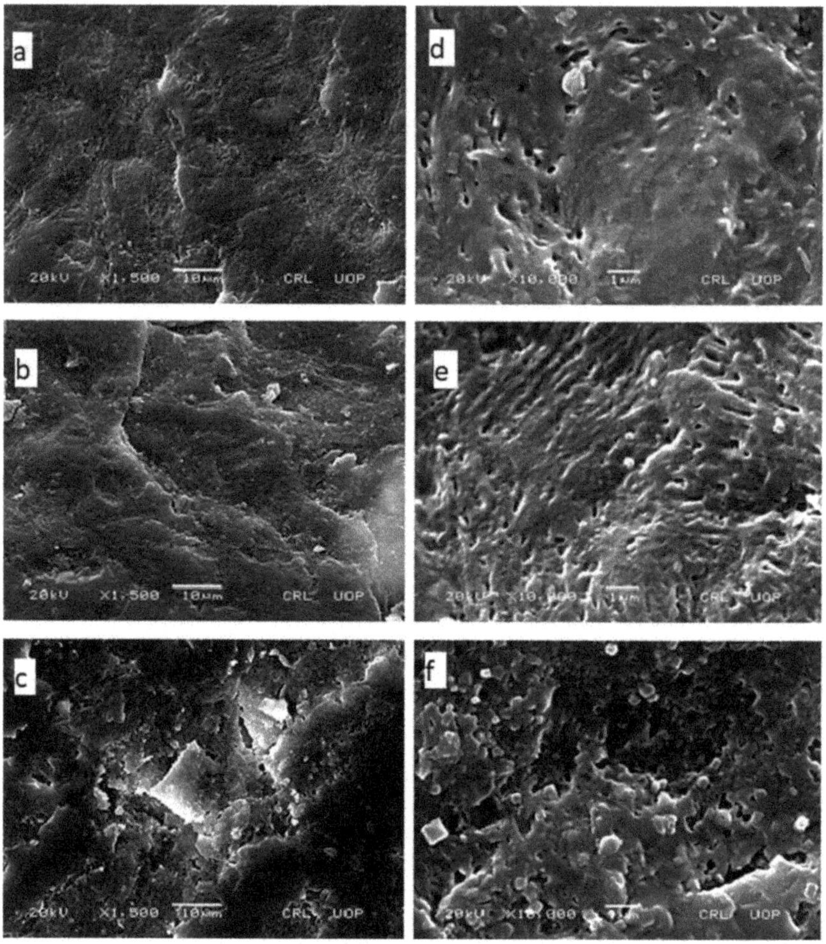

Figure 1. The impact of penetration enhancer on the surface morphology of nail observed under the electron microscope at low (1500×: left-side images) and high (10,000×: right-side images) magnification. Untreated nail (**a**,**d**), nail hydrated in water for 72 h (**b**,**e**) and nail hydrated in 5% TGA solution for 72 h (**c**,**f**).

3.3. *Effect of Independent Variables on Gelation Temperature of P407 Gel*

The formulated P407 gel containing TGA and ethanol was translucent and smooth. P407 gel with different formulation (20 runs as suggested by the Design Expert) showed varied gelation temperature ranging from 5.25 to 20.4 °C (Table 2). Analysis of variance (ANOVA) was carried out using Design Expert software to generate the polynomial equation of the responses. p value of less than 0.05 and F value of 164.16 showed that the quadratic model was significant to investigate the effect of dependent variables on gelation temperature. The "Predicted R-Squared" of 0.9488 is in reasonable agreement with the "Adj R-Squared" of 0.9872. This means, 94% variation in response will be explained by this model. Coefficient of variation for the suggested model was 3.58%.

Table 2. Different runs of face-centered central composite design and corresponding responses.

Code	P407 (% *w/w*)	Ethanol (% *w/w*)	TGA (% *w/w*)	Gelation Temp (°C)	Gel Strength (s)
F1	26	2	10	13.46 ± 0.28	92.66 ± 5.13
F2	28	6	5	8.43 ± 0.28	122.33 ± 8.50
F3	30	10	0	11.85 ± 0.25	124.66 ± 9.50
F4	26	6	5	15.46 ± 0.18	93.66 ± 6.02
F5	30	2	10	5.25 ± 0.16	156 ± 7.21
F6	28	6	10	6.53 ± 0.09	119 ± 8.54
F7	28	10	5	10.4 ± 0.32	111 ± 7.54
F8	26	10	0	20.43 ± 0.23	69 ± 7.54
F9	30	10	10	6.33 ± 0.09	149 ± 9.16
F10	30	6	5	5.93 ±0.23	142.33 ± 6.65
F11	30	2	0	7.38± 0.35	131 ± 7.54
F12	28	6	5	8.53 ± 0.14	122 ± 4.35
F13	28	6	5	8.66 ± 0.16	121.33 ± 9.29
F14	26	2	0	17.35 ± 0.25	82 ± 5.56
F15	28	6	5	8.61 ± 0.32	124.3 ± 7.02
F16	28	6	5	9.2 ± 0.23	126.33 ± 7.57
F17	28	6	0	12.7 ± 0.21	112.66 ± 5.50
F18	28	2	5	7.71 ± 0.21	131 ± 8.88
F19	28	6	5	8.38 ± 0.22	124.33 ± 4.93
F20	26	10	10	14.3 ± 0.32	84.33 ± 5.50

"Adequate Precision" measures the signal to noise ratio. Here, the ratio of 48.49 indicates adequate signal. The "Lack of Fit *F*-value" of 3.95 implied that the Lack of Fit is not significant. Supplementary Figure S1 shows that predicted and actual experimental results have an acceptable agreement which shows less residual and no significant error. Supplementary Figure S2 confirmed normal distribution of residuals in the plot of residuals versus the predicted response due to closeness of points to the straight line.

Values of "Prob > F" less than 0.05 indicate model terms are significant. In this case, A, B, C, C2 are significant model terms. The equation fitted to the data was:

$$Y_1 = 480.72 - 4.43A + 1.21B - 2.38C + 0.2AB + 0.3AC - 0.3BC + 2.04A^2 + 0.4B^2 + 0.96C^2 \quad (2)$$

where A, B and C is the concentration (% *w/w*) of P407, ethanol and TGA, respectively. A positive sign in front of the terms shows synergistic effects while the negative sign indicates the inverse relation between the factors. The polynomial equation for Y1 showed that concentration of polymer has the most significant effect (regression coefficient = −4.43, F value = 911) on gelation temperature followed by thioglycolic acid (regression coefficient = −2.38, F value = 264) and ethanol (regression coefficient = 1.21, F value = 68). A significant ($p < 0.05$) decrease in gelation temperature was observed with increase in quantity of both P407 and TGA (Table 2 and Figure 2). However, elevation of gelation temperature was observed when ethanol concentration was increased (Table 2 and Figure 2).

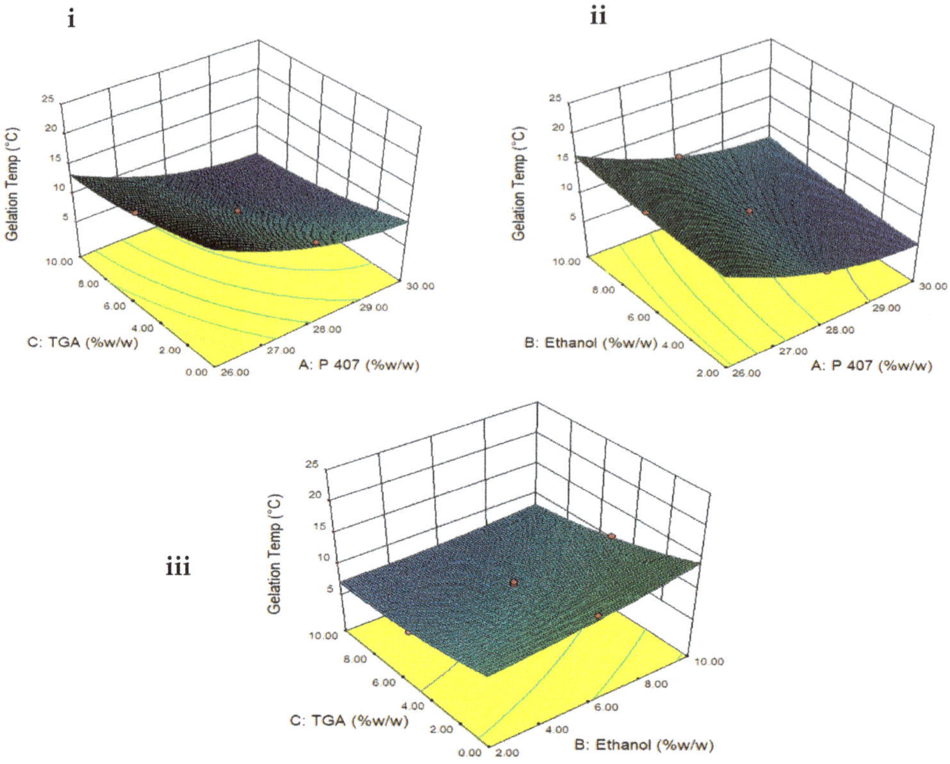

Figure 2. Three-dimensional surface plots showing effect of (**i**) TGA and P407 concentration on gelation temperature when ethanol is constant, (**ii**) ethanol and P407 concentration on gelation temperature when TGA is constant and (**iii**) TGA and ethanol concentration on gelation temperature when P407 is constant.

3.4. Effect of Independent Variables on Gel Strength

The gel strength of 20 different runs of P407 formulation was found in the range of 69 to 142 s. p value of 0.05 and F value of 60.26 showed that the quadratic model was significant to investigate the effect of dependent variables on gel strength and response optimization. The "Predicted R-Squared" of 0.8672 was in reasonable agreement with the "Adj R-Squared" of 0.9656. This means, 86% variation in response will be explained by this model. Coefficient of variation for suggested model was 3.58%.

"Adequate Precision" measures the signal to noise ratio. A ratio greater than four is desirable. Here, the ratio of 28.19 indicates adequate signal. The "Lack of Fit *F*-value" of 8.92 implied that the Lack of Fit is significant. This occurred due to noise. Supplementary Figure S3 showed that predicted values were close to the actual experimental value which shows less residual and no significant error. Supplementary Figure S4 confirmed normal distribution of residuals in the plot of residuals versus the predicted response due to closeness of points to the straight line.

Values of "Prob > F" less than 0.05 indicate model terms were significant. In this case, A, B, C, BC, A2, C2 were significant model terms.

Following polynomial equation was generated to investigate the effect of independent variables on gel strength.

$$Y_2 = 122.9 + 28.13A - 5.47B + 8.17C + 1.0AB + 2.92AC + 0.5BC - 4.3A^2 - 1.3B^2 - 6.47C^2 \quad (3)$$

where A, B and C is concentration (% *w*/*w*) of P407, ethanol and TGA, respectively. The polynomial equation for Y_2 showed that concentration of polymer (regression coefficient = +28.13, F value = 450) has the most significant effect on gel strength followed by thioglycolic acid (regression coefficient = +8.17, F value = 37.9) and ethanol (regression coefficient = −5.47, F value = 17.02). As depicted in Table 2 and Figure 3, gel strength was increased when quantity of both P407 and TGA was increased. *p* value of less than 0.05 showed that effect of both P407 and TGA was significant. Reduction in gel strength of P407 gel was observed with an increase in concentration of ethanol as depicted in Table 2 and Figure 3.

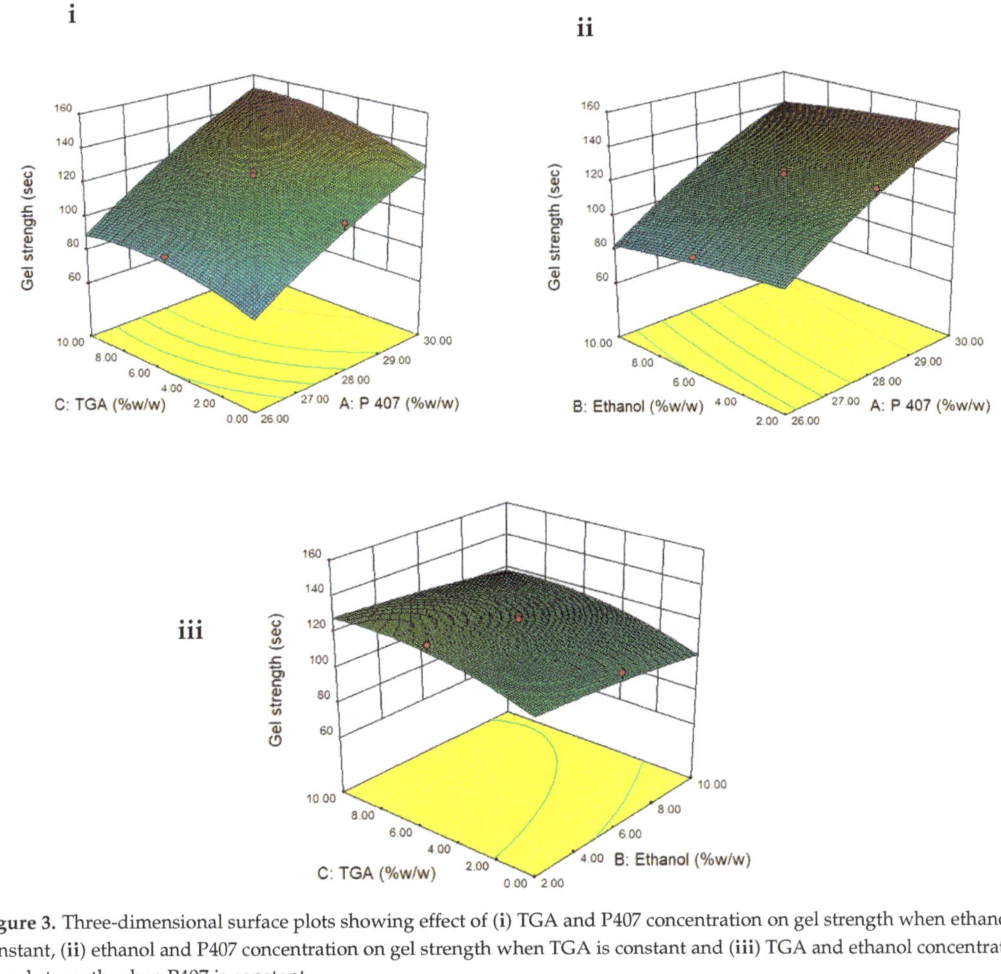

Figure 3. Three-dimensional surface plots showing effect of (**i**) TGA and P407 concentration on gel strength when ethanol is constant, (**ii**) ethanol and P407 concentration on gel strength when TGA is constant and (**iii**) TGA and ethanol concentration on gel strength when P407 is constant.

3.5. Response Optimization

Numerical optimization was performed to select formulation with gelation temperature below room temperature and enough gel strength. Constraints applied were to minimize gelation temperature and maximize gel strength. Optimum gel formulation with desirable properties (gelation temperature below room temperature and maximum strength) contains 27.32% P407, 3.18% ethanol and 4.72% TGA. Values of gelation temperature and gel strength predicted by quadratic model were 9.89 °C and 115 s, respectively. The model was validated by formulating optimum formulation and observing its response.

The actual gelation temperature and the gel strength of the optimized formulation were 8.68 °C and 122 s, respectively, which were close to the predicted values.

3.6. *Effect of Preparation Method on Loading of Drug*

Figure 4 shows the saturation limit of TBN loading in different formulations. For the gels prepared with cold method of preparation, the maximum loaded concentration of TBN in P407 gels (with no cosolvent and penetration enhancer) was 0.1, 0.2 and 0.4% *w/w* for gels containing 20% *w/w* (P20), 25% *w/w* (P25) and 30% *w/w* (P30) of P407, respectively. Similarly, maximum loaded concentration of TBN in gel containing 27% *w/w* of P407 having ethanol in concentration of 3% *w/w* (PE3), 6% *w/w* (PE6) and 10% *w/w* (PE10) was 0.3, 0.4 and 0.5% *w/w*, respectively. When the modified method was used, the maximum loaded drug in optimized gel was somewhere between 1.2 and 1.5% *w/w* (PE3F). No precipitate was observed until a concentration of 1.2 and at 1.5% *w/w* of TBN, precipitation of TBN was observed with naked eye. Microscopic images of optimized formulation with clear crystalline precipitates of insoluble TBN in P407 gel (with 1.5% of TBN) is shown in Figure 5.

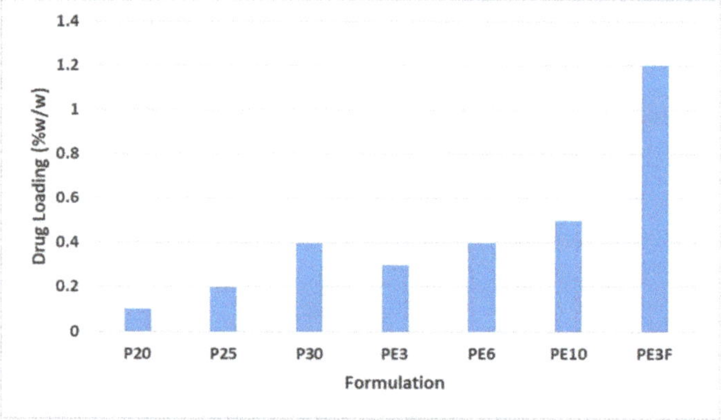

Figure 4. Saturation limit of terbinafine HCL loading in different formulations. P20, P25, P30 (simple P407 aqueous gels with increasing concentration of P407) and PE3, PE6, PE10 (gels containing 27% P407 with increasing concentration of ethanol) were prepared with simple cold method whereas PE3F is optimized formulation (27.32% of P407, 3.18% of ethanol and 4.76% of glycolic acid) prepared with film hydration method.

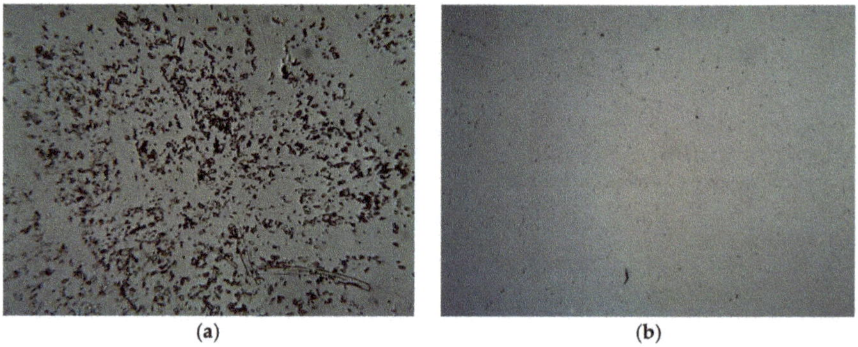

Figure 5. Images of optimized formulation under light microscope at 10X: (**a**) gel containing 1.5% *w/w* of TBN and (**b**) gel containing 1.2% *w/w* of TBN.

3.7. Rheology

The graph presented in Figure 6 shows apparent viscosity (η) of the gel to the function of applied shear rate (s^{-1}). It was observed that apparent viscosity of the gel decreased when applied shear rate was increased, which reflects that optimized gel will behave as non-Newtonian (pseudoplastic) type fluids.

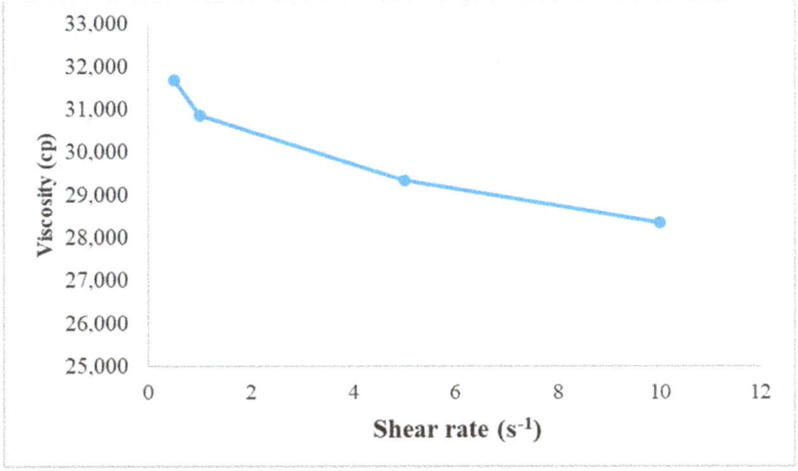

Figure 6. Apparent viscosity (η) vs. shear rate of P407 gel.

3.8. Washability/Gel Erosion

As shown in Figure 7, 76.46 ± 1.6% of the gel was retained after six washings while 23.54 ± 1.6% of P407 gel was eroded. After 12 washings, 52.25 ± 3.48% of the gel remained while 47.75 ± 3.48% of P407 gel was eroded after 12 washes, respectively.

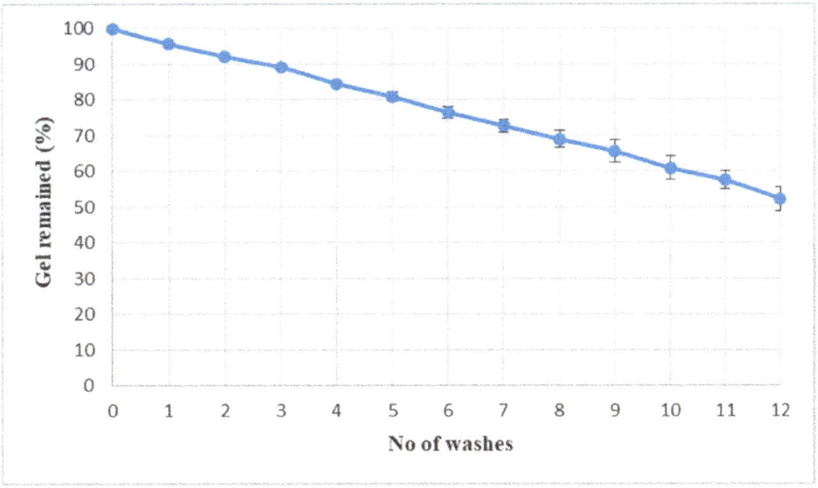

(**a**)

Figure 7. (**a**) Washability and (**b**) gel erosion pattern of P407 gel formulation in phosphate buffer.

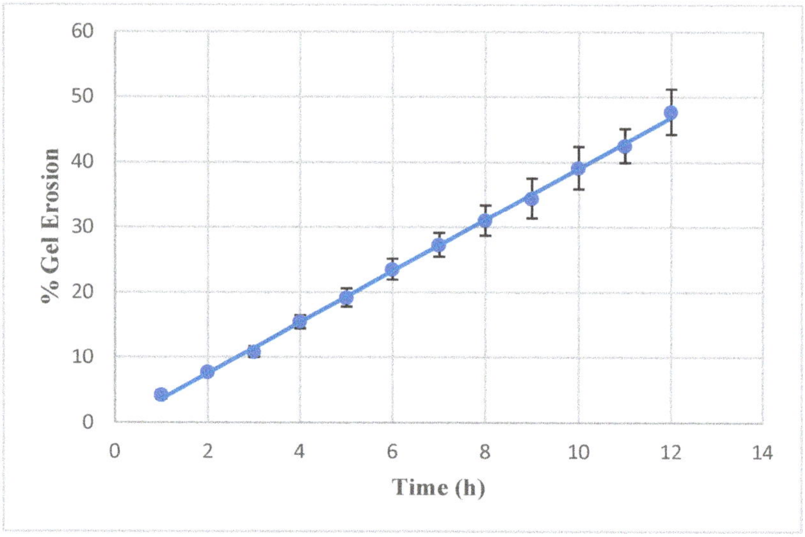

(**b**)

Figure 7. *Cont.*

3.9. In Vitro Release Profile

In vitro release profile of TBN loaded P407 gel showed that 44.23 ± 1.10 and 67.21 ± 2.16% of the drug was released after 6 and 12 h, respectively (Figure 8). The cumulative release was found to be >90% (94.36 ± 2.26%) in the case of drug suspension in just three hours.

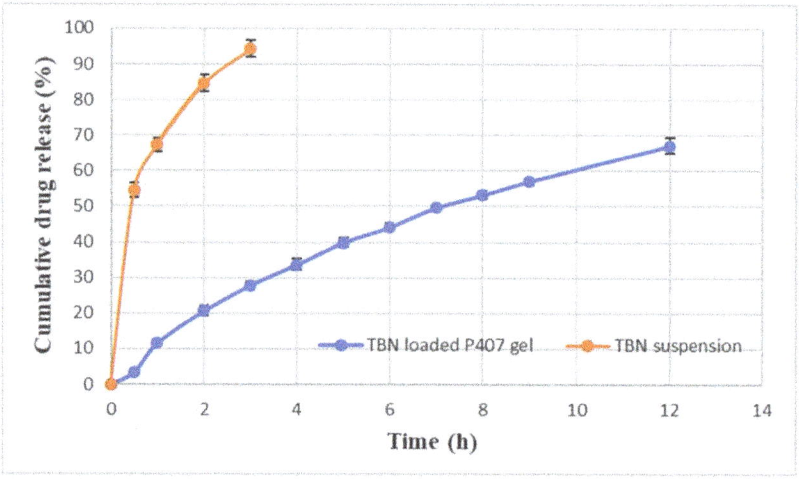

Figure 8. Comparison of in vitro release of terbinafine from optimized P407 gel formulation and TBN suspension.

3.10. Kinetic Modelling of Erosion Profile and Drug Release

Table 3 shows the kinetic parameters of erosion and drug release profile of optimized gel formulation. It appears that erosion of gel fits to zero order kinetics (R2 = 0.9989). The drug release data was fitted best to the first order kinetics (R2 = 0.9918) which showed that drug release was dependent on concentration of drug remaining in the formulation.

Anomalous behavior of drug release was observed as suggested by *n* value of 0.67 obtained from the Korsmeyer–Peppas model which suggests that release of drug from gel may be through both diffusion and erosion of gel.

Table 3. Kinetic modelling of erosion profile and in vitro drug release.

Model		For Gel Erosion	For Drug Release
Zero order	K	3.89	6.60
	R^2	0.9989	0.8894
First order	k1	0.048	0.098
	R^2	0.9814	0.9918
Higuchi	kH	11.01	18.14
	R^2	0.8142	0.9475
Korsmeyer–Peppas	kKP	3.72	12.99
	R^2	0.9990	0.9902
	n	1.02	0.67
Hixson–Crowell	kHC	0.015	0.02
	R^2	0.9898	0.9769

3.11. In Vitro Drug Permeation

The permeation of TBN obtained after placing optimized gel formulation with and without PE on the nail sample between donor and receiver compartment using Franz diffusion cell is shown in Figure 9. Concentration of TBN in receiver fluid was increased with the passage of time. The cumulative amount of TBN permeated from P407 gel with and without PE after 24 h was 27.30 ± 4.18 and 16.69 ± 2.31 μg/cm^2, respectively.

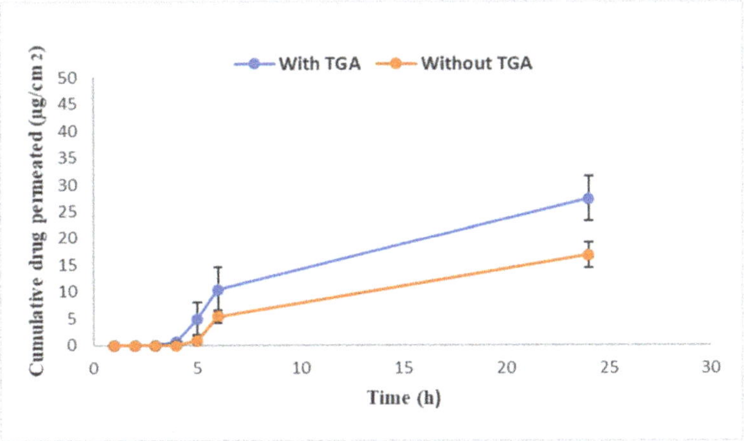

Figure 9. In vitro drug permeation across human nail.

4. Discussion

In the present study, permeation enhancers were screened based on HEF for their ability to enhance nail permeation. Weight of the human nail, when placed in water, increases due to ingress of water into the nail. Chemicals which cause any structural or physicochemical alteration in the nail will affect their ability to absorb water. Disulphide bonds in nail keratin are responsible for the nail barrier property so reducers of disulphide bonds will incorporate changes in nail keratin leading to the creation of pores in the nail which will increase the ability to hydrate the nail [27], as shown by the highest HEF for thioglycolic acid and mercaptoethanol. SEM analysis in our study confirms the formation of pores which create a pathway for permeant to penetrate intermediate and ventral layers of the nail plate. Tween 20 and P407 showed some penetration enhancing properties because they reduce surface tension in water-filled pores of the nail and enhance wetting [19]. Ethanol solution showed a concentration dependent increase in HEF; the higher the concentration of ethanol, the higher the HEF was. Khengar et al., 2007, observed that ethanol resulted in a very small amount of nail swelling which is in accordance with our finding [28].

Poloxamer polymer possesses surfactant properties [29] which is expected to help in nail penetration and solubilization of hydrophobic TBN. However, the solubilizing property of P407 aqueous solution was insufficient to hold the required dose of TBN (1% *w/w*). TBN was added to aqueous P407 solution, but this system was unable to solubilize the drug completely even at a concentration of 30% *w/w* P407, as shown in Figure 4. Ethanol was used as a cosolvent because of the higher solubility of TBN (up to 45 mg/mL) [30] and P407 polymer in ethanol [31]. However, P407 gel containing 10% *w/w* ethanol was also incapable of loading 1% w/w of TBN (Figure 4). As there was insignificant nail penetration enhancement by ethanol, our goal was to keep the quantity of ethanol as minimal as possible due to its undesirable effect on gel strength [31]. Film hydration method was employed as this method gave us the minimum amount of ethanol (3.18%) in the final formulation with enough drug loading (up to 1.2% *w/w*), as shown in Figure 4. Guiliano et al., 2020, incorporated the hydrophobic drug rutin to P407 gel prepared by cold method but was unable to load more than 0.1% *w/w* rutin, even in the presence of 2% *w/w* ethanol [32]. In a similar study to load hydrophobic drug doxorubicin, Xuan et al., 2011, prepared doxorubicin loaded P407 (15% *w/w*) and P188 (6% *w/w*). HCl (0.1% *w/w*) was used as a solubilizer of doxorubicin but it managed to load only 0.6% *w/w* of drug [33]. As poloxamer hydrogel has limitations of insufficient gel strength, weak stability and fast dissolution of the gels [34], both additives (TGA and ethanol) and P407 were investigated for their effect on gelation temperature and gel strength to overcome the soft gel properties with adequate loading of hydrophobic TBN. Thioglycolic was used in concentration of 4.72% *w/w* as this is claimed to be safe at a concentration of 15% and also sufficient to enhance permeation of TBN [35].

Design of experiments (DOE) is a widely employed organized method to determine the relationship between factors that influence outputs of a process. The DOE approach reduces the number of experiments and detects optimal response within the experimental space. Central composite design (CCD) is the most widely used response surface design. CCD design has advantages of less numbers of tests, high precision and good predictability. The FCCCD is recommended in many practical situations when the specified ranges of levels on the design variables are strict. In other words, the region of interest and the region of operability are the same [36].

The selected model (quadratic) for both responses showed a good fit with the experimental data, which was confirmed by high R^2 values and p value. Furthermore, "Adequate precision" is frequently used to assess signal to noise ratio (predicted response related to its associated error) and this ratio of greater than four is usually desirable. Gelation temperature and gel strength showed high signal to noise ratio, indicating the high adequacy of the selected model.

Supplementary Figures S1 and S3 show the predicted versus actual plots for gelation temperature and gel strength, which show closeness of the predicted value to the actual one. Each plot enables evaluation of the capability of the model for prediction. As the predicted values come closer to the actual ones, the points on the scatterplot fall closer to the line. If the points are all very close to the line, the model is expected to offer good predictability. Studentized residuals were distributed along a straight line with a slight deviation confirming low residual and non-significant error. In general, a coefficient of variation (CV) value of less than 10% normally signifies the reproducibility of the generated quadratic model. Relatively lower CV values recorded from the study (4.48% gelation temp, 3.58) confirm the reliability and accuracy of the model. If there is an inefficiency in the model in representing the data, this can be measured from the lack of fit value which was non-significant for gelation temperature but significant for gel strength, which could be due to noise. All these properties suggest that the quadratic model can be used to investigate the effect of P407, TGA and ethanol on gel properties.

The hydrophobic interaction of P407 copolymer chains is responsible for its thermogelation property. These copolymer chains exist in unimer form at concentration below critical micelle concentration (CMC) but start to self-assemble into a spherical micellar structure when its solution concentration exceeds the CMC or the solution temperature is increased above the critical micelle temperature (CMT) [31,37]. The formation of micelle occurs due to dehydration of the hydrophobic polypropylene oxide repeat units and defines the first step of gelation [38,39]. The core of micelles consist of a hydrophobic polypropylene oxide central core with their hydrophilic polyethylene oxide chains facing the external medium. When P407 concentration exceeds critical gel concentration, the micelle structures arrange into a lattice [40].

More the quantity of P407, more will be the physical entanglement which causes an increase in viscosity and lowering of the gelation temperature [38]. Ur-Rehman et al. observed that with an increasing concentration of P407, critical micellization temperature is reduced while intensity of micellization is increased [23]. Increasing poloxamer concentration increases the number of polymer chains per micelle up to a plateau value; above plateau value, increasing P407 concentration increases micelle concentration and reduces the average distance between micelles [40]. This results in strong entanglements of hydrophilic corona polyethylene oxide chains of micelles producing hard gels [41]. Addition of an external hydrophobic group reduces gelation temperature and enhances gel strength [42] which could be a possible explanation for the effect of TGA, as increasing its concentration replaces more polar hydroxyl group of water with the less polar thiol group. Further, replacing water with comparatively high molecular weight thioglycolic acid may also contribute to improved gel strength.

Addition of ethanol hinders the close packing of the block copolymer micelles which cause elevation of CMT and gelation temperature [23]. Further, weaker hydrogen bonding of ethanol as compared to deionized water resulted in gel strength reduction [24]. Although the presence of ethanol reduces the gel strength, this property may be exploited to prepare gel containing a very high concentration of P407, which otherwise is very difficult, time consuming and expensive. Initially, ethanol was used to solubilize TBN and P407 and then cold water was added slowly after the evaporation of ethanol. The finalized gel had a very minute amount of residual ethanol which would help in improving the flow of gel during application on nail.

Desirable behavior of gels for transungual applications is pseudoplastic (non-Newtonian) which corresponds to the decrease in apparent viscosity with an increase in shear rate [10]. This is important for easy application at the intended site. At the same time, the gel should be viscous enough in order to stay at the applied location for sufficient time [43].

P407 gel may erode from the nail surface when it comes in contact with water. This will have a two-way impact on topical gel formulation where i) the aqueous gel may not be retained on the nail for a longer period with exposure to accidental water contact and ii) it can be removed while washing with simple water. Our results demonstrate that two accidental washings may erode only 10% of the gel and more than 50% of the gel was available on the surface even after 12 possible accidental contacts of water. Goo et al., 2021, used hyaluronic acid (3.49% *w*/*w*) to enhance gel strength and reduce erosion of P407 gel (23.91% *w*/*w*). However, they observed 100% of gel erosion after seven washings despite the use of hyaluronic acid [44]. Cleansing of nails to remove nail polish or nail lacquer requires organic solvents which are not friendly to nails and the environment [45]. This study demonstrates that simple rinsing without rubbing may remove plenty of gel and erosion of gel is independent of the amount left on the nail. In the current study, erosion profile data were best fitted to zero order kinetics; however, drug release profile followed first order kinetics. This discrepancy might be due to the presence of ethanol in the release medium responsible for diffusion of drug, which is in accordance with the findings of Wang et al. [46]. The Korsmeyer–Peppas "n" value of 0.67 showed non-Fickian anomalous diffusion which suggests both diffusion and erosion were responsible for drug release [47]. It was observed that the presence of TGA enhances the permeation of TBN across the nail which may be due to breakage of nail disulphide bonds responsible for the nail barrier property [48]. Permeated drug concentration (7.6 μg/mL) was above minimum inhibitory concentrations (0.001–0.01 μg/mL) and minimal fungicidal concentrations (0.003–0.006 μg/mL) were against dermatophytes [49]. Gel formulation without TGA also showed permeation of TBN although less than that with TGA containing gel. It can be attributed to the nail uptake enhancing property of ethanol [48]. Rapid permeation of ethanol alters the solubility property of nail resulting in enhanced partitioning of drug into the nail. Optimized formulation with enough drug loading and gel strength.

5. Conclusions

Soft gel property and low drug loading of a water insoluble drug hinders the application of P407 gel in transungual delivery of hydrophobic drugs. TGA (up to 5%) can safely be added to P407 gels as a nail penetration enhancer. In addition, by applying a minor modification to the method of preparation, an evaporable cosolvent such as ethanol can be used to load the required dose of hydrophobic drugs which makes P407 gel a promising carrier for transungual delivery of hydrophobic antifungals in onychomycosis.

Supplementary Materials: The following are available online at https://www.mdpi.com/article/10.3390/polym13193376/s1, Figure S1: Design experts plot between predicted and actual values for gelation temperature; Figure S2: Normal plot of residuals for gelation temperature; Figure S3: Design experts plot between predicted and actual values for gel strength; Figure S4: Normal plot of residuals for gel strength.

Author Contributions: All authors uniformly contributed to the research work and the role of authors is as follows: conceptualization, T.U.-R., K.H.U. and M.I.Z.; design of methodology, T.U.-R., K.H.U. and S.M.M.; data acquisition, K.H.U. and S.M.M.; software (Design Expert and DDSolver), M.S. and H.Z.; data analysis and presentation, K.H.U. and F.R.; manuscript preparation, K.H.U. and F.R.; review and editing of MS, T.U.-R., H.Z., M.I.Z., S.M.M. and M.S.; project supervision, T.U.-R. All authors have read and agreed to the published version of the manuscript.

Funding: This study was supported with the funding from Higher Education Commission of Pakistan under Indigenous PhD fellowship program to KHU and National Research Program for Universities to TUR (Grant No: 9911/Federal/NRPU/R&D/HEC/2017).

Institutional Review Board Statement: The study was performed according to the guidelines of Declaration of Helsinki, and approved by the Bio-Ethical Committee (BEC) of Quaid-i-Azam University, Islamabad Pakistan (Protocol # BEC-FBS-QAU-2017-37).

Informed Consent Statement: Informed consent was obtained from all subjects involved in the study.

Data Availability Statement: Not applicable.

Acknowledgments: The authors are thankful to Higher Education Commission of Pakistan (for financial support), Central Resources Laboratory, University of Peshawar, Pakistan (for SEM analysis) and volunteers (for provision of nail clippings).

Conflicts of Interest: The authors declare no conflict of interest.

References

1. Barot, B.S.; Parejiya, P.B.; Patel, H.K.; Mehta, D.M.; Shelat, P.K. Microemulsion-Based Antifungal Gel Delivery to Nail for the Treatment of Onychomycosis: Formulation, Optimization, and Efficacy Studies. *Drug Deliv. Transl. Res.* **2012**, *2*, 463–476. [CrossRef]
2. Bseiso, E.A.; Nasr, M.; Sammour, O.A.; Abd El Gawad, N.A. Novel Nail Penetration Enhancer Containing Vesicles "NPEVs" for Treatment of Onychomycosis. *Drug Deliv.* **2016**, *23*, 2813–2819. [CrossRef]
3. Kobayashi, Y.; Miyamoto, M.; Sugibayashi, K.; Morimoto, Y. Enhancing Effect of N-Acetyl-L-Cysteine or 2-Mercaptoethanol on the in Vitro Permeation of 5-Fluorouracil or Tolnaftate through the Human Nail Plate. *Chem. Pharm. Bull.* **1998**, *46*, 1797–1802. [CrossRef] [PubMed]
4. Quintanar-Guerrero, D.; Ganem-Quintanar, A.; Tapia-Olguín, P.; Kalia, Y.N.; Buri, P. The Effect of Keratolytic Agents on the Permeability of Three Imidazole Antimycotic Drugs through the Human Nail. *Drug Dev. Ind. Pharm.* **1998**, *24*, 685–690. [CrossRef] [PubMed]
5. Mohorčič, M.; Torkar, A.; Friedrich, J.; Kristl, J.; Murdan, S. An Investigation into Keratinolytic Enzymes to Enhance Ungual Drug Delivery. *Int. J. Pharm.* **2007**, *332*, 196–201. [CrossRef] [PubMed]
6. Vejnovic, I.; Simmler, L.; Betz, G. Investigation of Different Formulations for Drug Delivery through the Nail Plate. *Int. J. Pharm.* **2010**, *386*, 185–194. [CrossRef] [PubMed]
7. Smith, K.A.; Hao, J.; Li, S.K. Effects of Organic Solvents on the Barrier Properties of Human Nail. *J. Pharm. Sci.* **2011**, *100*, 4244–4257. [CrossRef]
8. Felzenszwalb, I.; da Silva Fernandes, A.; Brito, L.B.; Oliveira, G.A.R.; Silva, P.A.S.; Arcanjo, M.E.; da Costa Marques, M.R.; Vicari, T.; Leme, D.M.; Cestari, M.M. Toxicological Evaluation of Nail Polish Waste Discarded in the Environment. *Environ. Sci. Pollut. Res.* **2019**, *26*, 27590–27603. [CrossRef]
9. Elsayed, M.M.A. Development of Topical Therapeutics for Management of Onychomycosis and Other Nail Disorders: A Pharmaceutical Perspective. *J. Control. Release* **2015**, *199*, 132–144. [CrossRef]
10. Ranch, K.M.; Maulvi, F.A.; Naik, M.J.; Koli, A.R.; Parikh, R.K.; Shah, D.O. Optimization of a Novel in Situ Gel for Sustained Ocular Drug Delivery Using Box-Behnken Design: In Vitro, Ex Vivo, in Vivo and Human Studies. *Int. J. Pharm.* **2019**, *554*, 264–275. [CrossRef]
11. Das, P.; Jana, N.R. Biomedical Applications of Functional Polyaspartamide-Based Materials. *ACS Appl. Polym. Mater.* **2021**. [CrossRef]
12. Hui, X.; Wester, R.C.; Barbadillo, S.; Lee, C.; Patel, B.; Wortzmman, M.; Gans, E.H.; Maibach, H.I. Ciclopirox Delivery into the Human Nail Plate. *J. Pharm. Sci.* **2004**, *93*, 2545–2548. [CrossRef] [PubMed]
13. Fuentes, S.; Dubo, J.; Barraza, N.; González, R.; Veloso, E. Hybrid Chitosan-Pluronic F-127 Films with BaTiO3:Co Nanoparticles: Synthesis and Properties. *J. Magn. Magn. Mater.* **2015**, *377*, 65–69. [CrossRef]
14. Jabarian, L.E.; Rouini, M.R.; Atyabi, F.; Foroumadi, A.; Nassiri, S.M.; Dinarvand, R. In Vitro and in Vivo Evaluation of an in Situ Gel Forming System for the Delivery of PEGylated Octreotide. *Eur. J. Pharm. Sci.* **2013**, *48*, 87–96. [CrossRef] [PubMed]
15. Tanriverdi, S.T.; Özer, Ö. Novel Topical Formulations of Terbinafine-HCl for Treatment of Onychomycosis. *Eur. J. Pharm. Sci.* **2013**, *48*, 628–636. [CrossRef] [PubMed]
16. Niu, G.; Du, F.; Song, L.; Zhang, H.; Yang, J.; Cao, H.; Zheng, Y.; Yang, Z.; Wang, G.; Yang, H.; et al. Synthesis and Characterization of Reactive Poloxamer 407s for Biomedical Applications. *J. Control. Release* **2009**, *138*, 49–56. [CrossRef]
17. Abou-Shamat, M.A.; Calvo-Castro, J.; Stair, J.L.; Cook, M.T. Modifying the Properties of Thermogelling Poloxamer 407 Solutions through Covalent Modification and the Use of Polymer Additives. *Macromol. Chem. Phys.* **2019**, *220*, 1900173. [CrossRef]
18. Ju, C.; Sun, J.; Zi, P.; Jin, X.; Zhang, C. Thermosensitive Micelles–Hydrogel Hybrid System Based on Poloxamer 407 for Localized Delivery of Paclitaxel. *J. Pharm. Sci.* **2013**, *102*, 2707–2717. [CrossRef]
19. Chouhan, P.; Saini, T.R. Hydration of Nail Plate: A Novel Screening Model for Transungual Drug Permeation Enhancers. *Int. J. Pharm.* **2012**, *436*, 179–182. [CrossRef]
20. Jessup, C.J.; Ghannoum, M.A.; Ryder, N.S. An Evaluation of the in Vitro Activity of Terbinafine. *Med. Mycol.* **2000**, *38*, 155–159. [CrossRef]
21. Tobiszewski, M.; Namieśnik, J.; Pena-Pereira, F. Environmental Risk-Based Ranking of Solvents Using the Combination of a Multimedia Model and Multi-Criteria Decision Analysis. *Green Chem.* **2017**, *19*, 1034–1042. [CrossRef]
22. Xuan, J.-J.; Balakrishnan, P.; Oh, D.H.; Yeo, W.H.; Park, S.M.; Yong, C.S.; Choi, H.-G. Rheological Characterization and in Vivo Evaluation of Thermosensitive Poloxamer-Based Hydrogel for Intramuscular Injection of Piroxicam. *Int. J. Pharm.* **2010**, *395*, 317–323. [CrossRef]
23. Ur-Rehman, T.; Tavelin, S.; Gröbner, G. Effect of DMSO on Micellization, Gelation and Drug Release Profile of Poloxamer 407. *Int. J. Pharm.* **2010**, *394*, 92–98. [CrossRef]
24. Choi, H.G.; Lee, M.K.; Kim, M.H.; Kim, C.K. Effect of Additives on the Physicochemical Properties of Liquid Suppository Bases. *Int. J. Pharm.* **1999**, *190*, 13–19. [CrossRef]
25. Ur-Rehman, T.; Tavelin, S.; Gröbner, G. Chitosan in Situ Gelation for Improved Drug Loading and Retention in Poloxamer 407 Gels. *Int. J. Pharm.* **2011**, *409*, 19–29. [CrossRef]
26. Vaghasiya, H.; Kumar, A.; Sawant, K. Development of Solid Lipid Nanoparticles Based Controlled Release System for Topical Delivery of Terbinafine Hydrochloride. *Eur. J. Pharm. Sci.* **2013**, *49*, 311–322. [CrossRef]

27. Murdan, S. Enhancing the Nail Permeability of Topically Applied Drugs. *Expert Opin. Drug Deliv.* **2008**, *5*, 1267–1282. [CrossRef]
28. Khengar, R.H.; Jones, S.A.; Turner, R.B.; Forbes, B.; Brown, M.B. Nail Swelling as a Pre-Formulation Screen for the Selection and Optimisation of Ungual Penetration Enhancers. *Pharm. Res.* **2007**, *24*, 2207–2212. [CrossRef]
29. Patel, H.R.; Patel, R.P.; Patel, M.M. Poloxamers: A Pharmaceutical Excipients with Therapeutic Behaviors. *Int. J. PharmTech Res.* **2009**, *1*, 299–303.
30. Meloun, M.; Bordovská, S.; Galla, L. The Thermodynamic Dissociation Constants of Clotrimazole, Terbinafine Hcl, Acetylsalicylic Acid, Salicylic Acid, and Galanthamine by the Nonlinear Regression of Multiwavelength Spectrophotometric Ph-Titration Data. *SRX Pharmacol.* **2010**. [CrossRef]
31. Kwon, K.-W.; Park, M.J.; Hwang, J.; Char, K. Effects of Alcohol Addition on Gelation in Aqueous Solution of PEO-PPO-PEO Triblock Copolymer. *Polym. J.* **2001**, *33*, 404–410. [CrossRef]
32. Giuliano, E.; Paolino, D.; Cristiano, M.C.; Fresta, M.; Cosco, D. Rutin-Loaded Poloxamer 407-Based Hydrogels for in Situ Administration: Stability Profiles and Rheological Properties. *Nanomaterials* **2020**, *10*, 1069. [CrossRef] [PubMed]
33. Xuan, J.-J.; Yan, Y.-D.; Oh, D.H.; Choi, Y.K.; Yong, C.S.; Choi, H.-G. Development of Thermo-Sensitive Injectable Hydrogel with Sustained Release of Doxorubicin: Rheological Characterization and in Vivo Evaluation in Rats. *Drug Deliv.* **2011**, *18*, 305–311. [CrossRef] [PubMed]
34. Fakhari, A.; Corcoran, M.; Schwarz, A. Thermogelling Properties of Purified Poloxamer 407. *Heliyon* **2017**, *3*, e00390. [CrossRef] [PubMed]
35. Burnett, C.L.; Bergfeld, W.F.; Belsito, D.V.; Klaassen, C.D.; Marks, J.G.; Shank, R.C.; Slaga, T.J.; Snyder, P.W.; Andersen, F.A. Final Amended Report on the Safety Assessment of Ammonium Thioglycolate, Butyl Thioglycolate, Calcium Thioglycolate, Ethanolamine Thioglycolate, Ethyl Thioglycolate, Glyceryl Thioglycolate, Isooctyl Thioglycolate, Isopropyl Thioglycolate, Magnesium Thiogl. *Int. J. Toxicol.* **2009**, *28* (Suppl. 4), 68–133. [CrossRef] [PubMed]
36. Elsayed, E.W.; El-Ashmawy, A.A.; Mursi, N.M.; Emara, L.H. Optimization of Gliclazide Loaded Alginate-Gelatin Beads Employing Central Composite Design. *Drug Dev. Ind. Pharm.* **2019**, *45*, 1959–1972. [CrossRef]
37. Giuliano, E.; Paolino, D.; Fresta, M.; Cosco, D. Drug-Loaded Biocompatible Nanocarriers Embedded in Poloxamer 407 Hydrogels as Therapeutic Formulations. *Medicines* **2019**, *6*, 7. [CrossRef]
38. Escobar-Chávez, J.J.; López-Cervantes, M.; Naïk, A.; Kalia, Y.N.; Quintanar-Guerrero, D.; Ganem-Quintanar, A. Applications of Thermo-Reversible Pluronic F-127 Gels in Pharmaceutical Formulations. *J. Pharm. Pharm. Sci.* **2006**, *9*, 339–358.
39. Ranch, K.M.; Maulvi, F.A.; Koli, A.R.; Desai, D.T.; Parikh, R.K.; Shah, D.O. Tailored Doxycycline Hyclate Loaded In Situ Gel for the Treatment of Periodontitis: Optimization, In Vitro Characterization, and Antimicrobial Studies. *AAPS PharmSciTech* **2021**, *22*, 1–11. [CrossRef]
40. Mortensen, K.; Pedersen, J.S. Structural Study on the Micelle Formation of Poly(Ethylene Oxide)–Poly(Propylene Oxide)–Poly(Ethylene Oxide) Triblock Copolymer in Aqueous Solution. *Macromolecules* **1993**, *26*, 805–812. [CrossRef]
41. Li, H.; Yu, G.-E.; Price, C.; Booth, C.; Hecht, E.; Hoffmann, H. Concentrated Aqueous Micellar Solutions of Diblock Copoly(Oxyethylene/Oxybutylene) E 41 B 8: A Study of Phase Behavior. *Macromolecules* **2002**. [CrossRef]
42. Kjøniksen, A.L.; Calejo, M.T.; Zhu, K.; Nyström, B.; Sande, S.A. Stabilization of Pluronic Gels in the Presence of Different Polysaccharides. *J. Appl. Polym. Sci.* **2014**. [CrossRef]
43. Abdul Rahman, M.N.; Qader, O.A.J.A.; Sukmasari, S.; Ismail, A.F.; Doolaanea, A.A. Rheological Characterization of Different Gelling Polymers for Dental Gel Formulation. *J. Pharm. Sci. Res.* **2017**, *9*, 2633–2640.
44. Goo, Y.T.; Yang, H.M.; Kim, C.H.; Kim, M.S.; Kim, H.K.; Chang, I.H.; Choi, Y.W. Optimization of a Floating Poloxamer 407-Based Hydrogel Using the Box-Behnken Design: In Vitro Characterization and in Vivo Buoyancy Evaluation for Intravesical Instillation. *Eur. J. Pharm. Sci.* **2021**, *163*, 105885. [CrossRef] [PubMed]
45. Monti, D.; Saccomani, L.; Chetoni, P.; Burgalassi, S.; Senesi, S.; Ghelardi, E.; Mailland, F. Hydrosoluble Medicated Nail Lacquers: In Vitro Drug Permeation and Corresponding Antimycotic Activity. *Br. J. Dermatol.* **2010**, *162*, 311–317. [CrossRef] [PubMed]
46. Wang, W.; Hui, P.C.L.; Wat, E.; Ng, F.S.F.; Kan, C.W.; Wang, X.; Wong, E.C.W.; Hu, H.; Chan, B.; Lau, C.B.S.; et al. In Vitro Drug Release and Percutaneous Behavior of Poloxamer-Based Hydrogel Formulation Containing Traditional Chinese Medicine. *Colloids Surf. B Biointerfaces* **2016**, *148*, 526–532. [CrossRef]
47. Akash, M.S.H.; Rehman, K.; Li, N.; Gao, J.Q.; Sun, H.; Chen, S. Sustained Delivery of IL-1Ra from Pluronic F127-Based Thermosensitive Gel Prolongs Its Therapeutic Potentials. *Pharm. Res.* **2012**, *29*, 3475–3485. [CrossRef]
48. Gupta, A.K.; Paquet, M. Improved Efficacy in Onychomycosis Therapy. *Clin. Dermatol.* **2013**, *31*, 555–563. [CrossRef]
49. Darkes, M.J.M.; Scott, L.J.; Goa, K.L. Terbinafine: A Review of Its Use in Onychomycosis in Adults. *Am. J. Clin. Dermatol.* **2003**, *4*, 39–65. [CrossRef]

polymers

Review

Gelatin-Based Hybrid Scaffolds: Promising Wound Dressings

Sindi P. Ndlovu, Kwanele Ngece, Sibusiso Alven and Blessing A. Aderibigbe *

Department of Chemistry, University of Fort Hare, Alice 5700, South Africa; 201304407@ufh.ac.za (S.P.N.); 201102901@ufh.ac.za (K.N.); 201214199@ufh.ac.za (S.A.)
* Correspondence: blessingaderibigbe@gmail.com

Abstract: Wound care is a major biomedical field that is challenging due to the delayed wound healing process. Some factors are responsible for delayed wound healing such as malnutrition, poor oxygen flow, smoking, diseases (such as diabetes and cancer), microbial infections, etc. The currently used wound dressings suffer from various limitations, including poor antimicrobial activity, etc. Wound dressings that are formulated from biopolymers (e.g., cellulose, chitin, gelatin, chitosan, etc.) demonstrate interesting properties, such as good biocompatibility, non-toxicity, biodegradability, and attractive antimicrobial activity. Although biopolymer-based wound dressings display the aforementioned excellent features, they possess poor mechanical properties. Gelatin, a biopolymer has excellent biocompatibility, hemostatic property, reduced cytotoxicity, low antigenicity, and promotes cellular attachment and growth. However, it suffers from poor mechanical properties and antimicrobial activity. It is crosslinked with other polymers to enhance its mechanical properties. Furthermore, the incorporation of antimicrobial agents into gelatin-based wound dressings enhance their antimicrobial activity in vitro and in vivo. This review is focused on the development of hybrid wound dressings from a combination of gelatin and other polymers with good biological, mechanical, and physicochemical features which are appropriate for ideal wound dressings. Gelatin-based wound dressings are promising scaffolds for the treatment of infected, exuding, and bleeding wounds. This review article reports gelatin-based wound dressings which were developed between 2016 and 2021.

Keywords: wound care; wound dressings; polymers; gelatin; hydrogels; nanofibers; sponges

Citation: Ndlovu, S.P.; Ngece, K.; Alven, S.; Aderibigbe, B.A. Gelatin-Based Hybrid Scaffolds: Promising Wound Dressings. *Polymers* **2021**, *13*, 2959. https://doi.org/10.3390/polym13172959

Academic Editors: Bramasta Nugraha and Faisal Raza

Received: 11 July 2021
Accepted: 20 August 2021
Published: 31 August 2021

1. Introduction

Wound care is a concern globally with various challenges including the increasing prevalence of type II diabetes, obesity, an aging population, and the need for cost-effective wound dressings [1,2]. The wounds are generally classified based on their healing process as acute or chronic wounds. Acute wounds are lesions that heal within the expected timeframe of approximately 2–3 months depending on the depth and size of the injury in the skin [3]. Chronic wounds fail to heal through the ordinary wound healing process over a prolonged period. Examples of chronic wounds include diabetic wounds, ulcer wounds, burn wounds, etc. [4,5]. All types of wounds require good clinical care to prevent delayed wound healing processes that may be caused by microbial infections and other negative factors. More than 300 types of wound dressing products are available in the market. However, one wound dressing is not appropriate for the treatment of all wound types [6]. In the United States of America (USA), a yearly cost of 20 billion dollars is spent on the wound care of chronic injuries [7]. The global market cost of chronic wound care was 10.12 billion dollars in 2019, and it is projected that the cost will increase to 16.36 billion dollars in 2027 [8]. These statistics demonstrate the negative socio-economic impacts of wound care globally, indicating an urgent need to develop affordable wound dressings for effective wound care.

The properties of an ideal wound dressing that make it suitable to provide a proper environment for the healing process include durability, flexibility, permeability to water vapor, adherence to the tissue, and good mechanical properties [9]. Furthermore, the dressing materials should hydrate/dehydrate the wound, maintain a moist environment, protect the wound from infections, and prevent maceration [10]. Polymer-based wound dressing materials can provide the aforementioned properties. Polymers that can be used for the fabrication of dressings are mainly classified as biopolymers and synthetic polymers [11]. Examples of biopolymers include gelatin, cellulose, chitin, alginate, hyaluronic acid, chitosan, dextran, elastin, fibrin, etc. (Figure 1) [12]. The wound dressings that are formulated from these polymers usually suffer from poor mechanical properties. The combination of biopolymers with synthetic polymers is a promising design strategy to overcome the poor mechanical properties of biopolymer-based wound dressings.

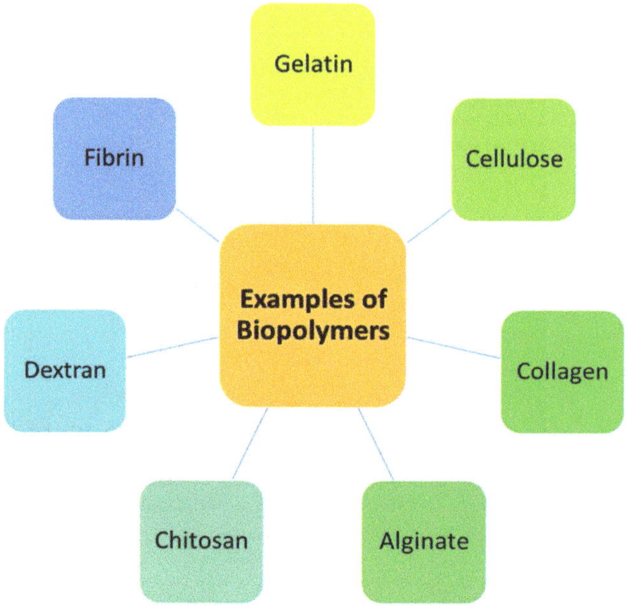

Figure 1. Examples of Biopolymers in Biomedical applications.

Gelatin is a biopolymer with interesting properties that have greatly attracted the attention of many biomedical researchers, such as low antigenicity, good biodegradability, and biocompatibility in the physiological environment [13]. The gelatin-based materials offer excellent characteristics of wound dressings. The fast degradation time and highly hydrophilic surface make gelatin inappropriate as a base material for the development of wound dressings. Thus, gelatin is combined with other polymers, especially synthetic polymers [14]. This review will discuss the outcomes of gelatin-based hybrid dressings for wound care.

2. Phases of Wound Healing Process

Wound healing is an important physiological and complex process, involving a multifaceted process, including the hemostasis phase, inflammation phase, proliferation phase, and maturation phase (Figure 2) [5]. The hemostasis phase occurs immediately after the injury and the exposed collagen, sub-endothelium, and tissue factor trigger platelet aggregation that results in degranulation and the release of growth factors (GFs) and chemokines to form the blood clot [15]. Hemostasis usually occurs concurrently with the inflammation phase. In the inflammation phase, neutrophils at the wound site cleanse the debris and remove bacteria together with reactive oxygen species (ROS), thereby offering an appropriate environment for the wound healing process [16]. The injury site tends to become red, swollen, and warm due to the presence of white blood cells [16].

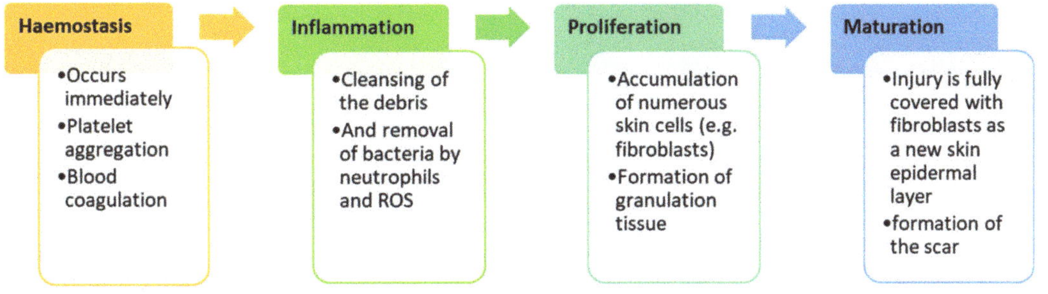

Figure 2. Sequential Phases of Wound healing.

The third phase of wound healing is the proliferation phase, and this phase is characterized by an accumulation of numerous cells and profuse connective tissue. The injury encompasses endothelial cells, keratinocytes, and fibroblasts. Extracellular matrix (ECM) components, including collagen, hyaluronic acid, proteoglycans, and elastin produce a granulation tissue to substitute the original development of blood clots [17]. Many varieties of cytokines and GFs that are involved in this phase include transforming growth factor-β family (TGF-β, including TGF-β1, TGF-β2, and TGF-β3), interleukin (IL) family, and angiogenesis factors (e.g., vascular epidermal growth factors (VEGFs)), result in the formation of new tissue [18]. The new tissue is normally pink or red when it covers the wound site. The last phase of the wound healing process is the maturation phase, which requires a precise balance between the apoptosis of the remaining cells and the formation of new cells [18]. Gradual degradation of profuse ECM and the immature type III collagen and development of mature type I collagen is critical in this phase. The surface of the injury is fully covered with fibroblasts as a new epidermal layer of the skin, and the formation of the scar occurs [19]. The maturation phase usually occurs within few months or even years. Any disruption in the wound healing phases can result in the formation of keloids or chronic wounds [18].

3. Classification of Wound Dressings

Wound dressings are materials used to protect a wound. They also act as a barrier against pathogens. An ideal wound dressing offers good features, such as good applicability, biocompatibility, stability, and flexibility, as well as ensuring a good gas barrier and biodegradability to speed up the healing process and reduce the risk of infections. Wound dressings must also be able to manage wound exudates to prevent bacterial invasion [20]. Wound dressings are categorized as primary and secondary dressings. The primary wound dressings are applied directly to the wounded area, while the secondary dressing is used to cover the primary wound dressing [21]. There are various applications of wound dressing materials. Hence, they are classified into four groups, namely traditional/passive dressings, skin substitutes, interactive/artificial dressings, and bioactive dressings (Figure 3).

Traditional/passive wound dressings are usually used in the first step of treatment to stop bleeding and prevent further interaction of the wound with the environment [22]. These dressings have disadvantages, e.g., they can cause bleeding, display poor permeation of vapor, and damage the newly formed epithelium after removal. Bacterial infections can also result from the leakage of exudates from these dressings. The traditional dressing examples are tulle, gauze, and gauze cotton composites, which are distinguished by high absorption capacity [23].

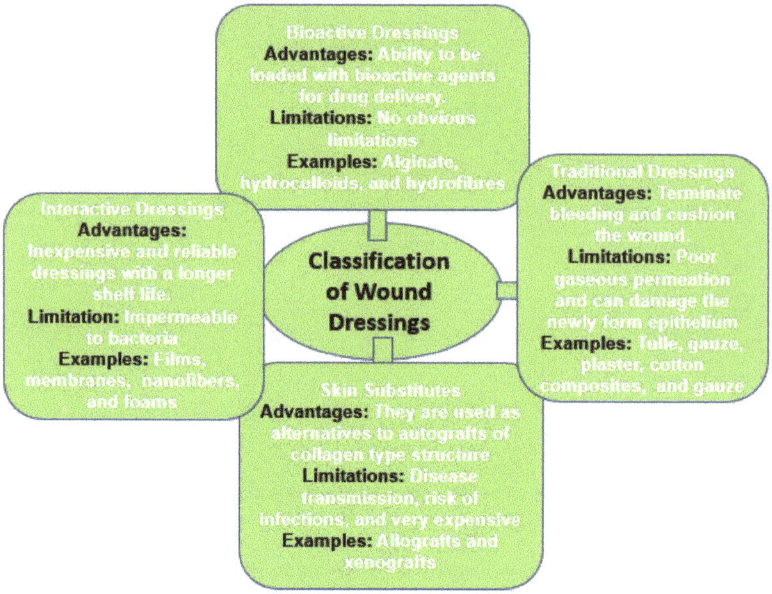

Figure 3. Classification of Wound Dressings.

Skin substitutes are biological dressings and they are additionally classified as allografts, xenografts, and tissue derivatives. Allografts are fresh or freeze-dried skin fragments collected from donors and their use is limited by immune reactions, resulting in rejection by the body. Disadvantages of allografts include disease transmission, risk of infections and they are very expensive with limited shelf life. A xenograft is a tissue graft or organ transplant from the recipient's donor of a different species (for example from animals to humans) [7].

Interactive/artificial wound dressings are frequently formulated from synthetic polymers and biopolymers. The most widely used biopolymers are gelatin, alginate, chitosan, etc. Artificial wound dressings can be classified as foams, films, composites, sprays, etc. They consist of mostly transparent polymeric films and shapes, permeable to water vapor and oxygen, but impermeable to bacteria. These dressings are suitable for less exuding wounds [23]. The advantages of interactive wound dressings are that they are inexpensive and reliable dressings with a longer shelf life [22]. Bioactive wound dressings are prepared from biopolymers and are encapsulated with bioactive agents, such as antimicrobials and growth factors, to enhance the wound healing process. Examples of biopolymers are collagens, alginate, hydrocolloids, and hydrofibres [23].

4. Properties of Gelatin in Wound Dressing Applications

Many natural polymers are frequently used in the formulation of wound dressings. These polymers include gelatin, cellulose, alginate, collagen, elastin, chitosan, chitin, dextran, etc. The common interesting properties of natural polymers are good biocompatibility and biodegradation, non-toxicity, non-immunogenicity, and affordability. In addition, some of the natural polymers exhibit strong attachment to injured tissues and stimulate blood coagulation, accelerate the wound healing process, and induce skin regeneration [12]. Gelatin is one of the biopolymers that is commonly utilized in the design of wound dressings. It is also utilized for biomedical and pharmaceutical applications [24,25]. The molecular structure of gelatin is shown in Figure 4a. It is a natural mimic of the extracellular matrix (ECM) of human tissues and organs. It is broadly utilized in the field of tissue engineering [26]. The properties of gelatin that have been attracting the attention of most biomedical researchers include excellent biocompatibility, good biodegradability, cell-interactivity, non-immunogenicity, as well as its excellent processability, ready availability, and cost-effectiveness (Figure 4b) [27]. The pretty low antigenicity of gelatin also makes it a well-established biopolymer used in numerous biological applications. However, gelatin is a hydrophilic protein, and crosslinking is normally required to enhance its mechanical performance and stability, making gelatin materials insoluble in biological environments [28]. Numerous gelatin crosslinking procedures are available, such as enzymatic using transglutaminase, or chemical using fructose, diepoxy, genipin, dextran dialdehyde, formaldehyde, diisocyanates, glutaraldehyde, or carbodiimides [13].

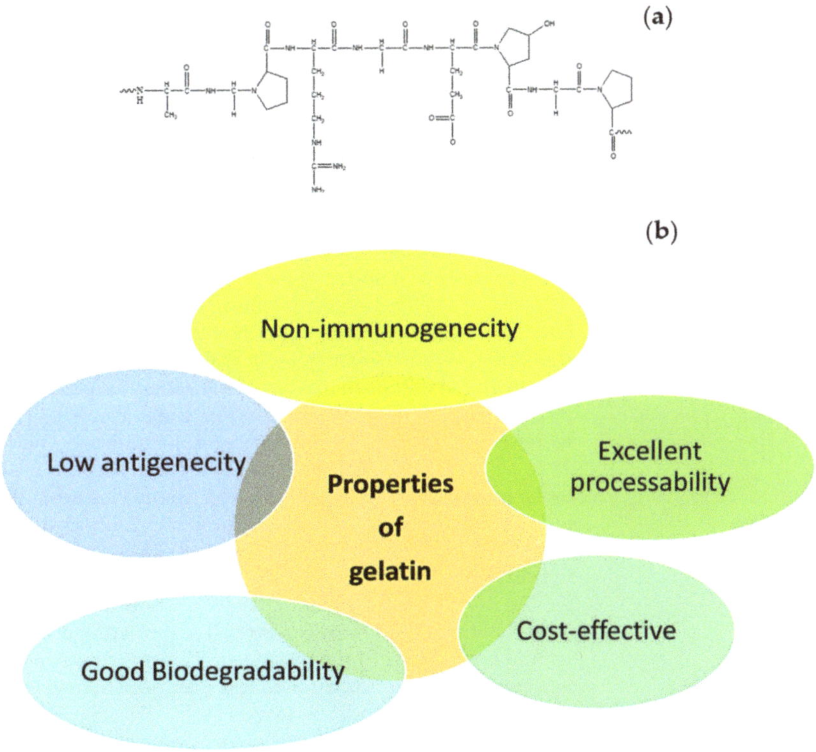

Figure 4. (**a**) Basic molecular structure of gelatin (**b**) Properties of gelatin.

In various studies, gelatin biopolymers were designed as films, gels, powders, or scaffolds for haemorrhage control in numerous surgical methods [29]. Porous gelatin matrices absorb wound exudates and maintain moisture, thus promoting the wound healing process. Gelatin-based dressings act as porous materials for cell migration and offer mechanical and structural support for the development of new tissue [30]. Although gelatin is a promising biopolymer employed as a wound dressing material, it has no antibacterial efficacy to prevent wound infections or bacterial invasion of the wound [31]. It is combined with other polymers to produce hybrid polymers with superior antibacterial effects.

Gelatin-based scaffolds can be loaded with various antimicrobial agents, such as metal-based nanoparticles, antibiotics, phytochemicals (e.g., curcumin), plant extracts (e.g., Aloe vera), etc., to overcome their poor bactericidal effects [31]. To the best of our knowledge, only two gelatin-based wound dressing materials are commercially available: Gelfoam and Surgifoam. Gelfoam and Surgifoam are composed of porcine gelatin and collagen. Gelfoam and Surgifoam are in the form of compressed sponge and sponge, respectively [32,33].

These commercially available gelatin dressings demonstrate outstanding hemostatic effects. Hence, they are very suitable for bleeding wounds. However, they suffer from some shortcomings, including non-elasticity, etc. [33].

5. Gelatin-Based Hybrid Wound Dressings

5.1. Hydrogels

Hydrogels are polymeric materials with a good hydrophilic composition that enables their high retention of a significant quantity of water and other biological fluids within their three-dimensional network (Figure 5) [34]. They can be modified for enhanced stability or degradation in the event of contact with biological fluids over an extended period. These polymeric materials have been used in wound healing applications due to their biodegradation, biocompatibility, porosity, ability to encapsulate and release bioactive agents, flexibility, and high-water content [35]. The other advantages of polymer-based hydrogels that have attracted a lot of attention among biomedical researchers in the field of wound management include patient compliance, accelerated wound healing mechanism, the high adsorption capacity of biological fluids which provide moisture to the wound bed, their capability to protect the wound from microorganisms, and specific environmental stimuli-responsiveness (e.g., pH, temperature, and ionic strength). The environmental stimuli-responsive nature of the wound dressings promotes drug release into the infected wound area in a sustained profile, thereby reducing the dosing frequency [36,37]. Several researchers have reported gelatin-based hybrid hydrogels (Table 1).

Hsu et al., formulated gelatin-hyaluronic acid (HA) hybrid hydrogels encapsulated with recombinant thrombomodulin by chemical cross-linking followed by freeze-drying for diabetic wound management [38]. The scanning electron microscopy (SEM) images demonstrated porous morphology, indicating the porosity of the hydrogels was decreased by an increase in the HA content. The water absorption of the hybrid hydrogels rapidly increased within the first 30 min, and the hydrogels swelled more than 11-fold within 24 h, which is beneficial for drug absorption, absorbing wound exudates, and offering a moist environment for injury bed. The wound closure studies in vivo using streptozotocin-induced mice showed that the thrombomodulin-loaded hybrid hydrogels significantly accelerated wound contraction after two days of wounding when compared to pristine hybrid hydrogels [38]. Mao et al., fabricated gelatin-oxidized starch hybrid hydrogels for wound healing applications. The in vitro cytotoxicity studies demonstrated the high cell viability of skin fibroblasts (L929 cells) of the hydrogels, indicating the good biocompatibility and non-toxicity of the hydrogels. The in vivo wound healing studies demonstrated a fast wound healing process with less scar formation when the wounds in the rabbit model were treated with hybrid hydrogels [39].

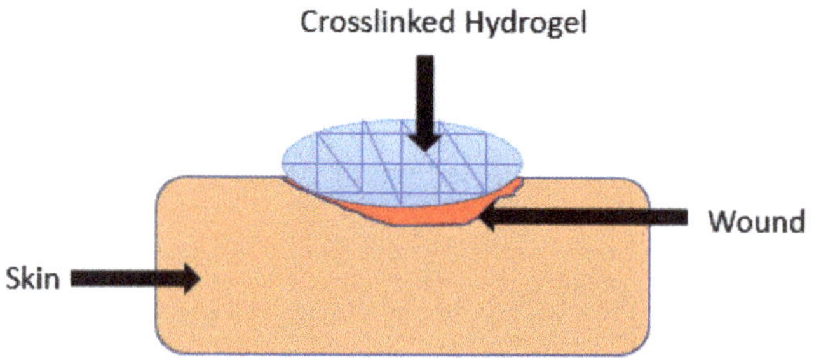

Figure 5. Crosslinked Hydrogel on Skin Wound.

Table 1. Summary of Gelatin-based Hydrogel Wound Dressings.

Types of Wound Dressings	Polymers Combined with Gelatin	Loaded Bioactive Agents	Outcomes	References
Hydrogels	HA	Recombinant thrombomodulin	High swelling capacity and accelerated diabetic wound closure.	[38]
Hydrogels	Oxidized Starch	_	Good cytocompatibility and fast wound healing mechanism with less scar development.	[39]
Hydrogels	Pluronic	Nanocurcumin	Accelerated burn wound reduction.	[40]
Hydrogels	Gellan	Tannic acid	Superior antimicrobial activity and fast full-thickness wound healing.	[41]
Hydrogels	PEG	ASCs	Non-toxicity on skin cells and fast wound contraction.	[42]
Hydrogels	Bacterial cellulose	Curcumin	Good mechanical properties and controlled drug release.	[43]
Hydrogels	Bacterial cellulose	Methylene blue	Good mechanical performance and high swelling capacity.	[44]
Hydrogels	PEG and CMC	_	Excellent swelling behavior	[45]
Hydrogels	PVA and chitosan	_	Excellent mechanical properties and good hemostatic effects.	[46]

Dang et al., developed injectable hybrid hydrogels that are based on gelatin and pluronic. They were loaded with nanocurcumin for burn wound care. The in vitro cytocompatibility analysis demonstrated that all the hydrogel formulations presented no toxic effect on the fibroblasts after 48 h of incubation, suggesting good cytocompatibility of the hybrid hydrogels. The burn wounds on mice models were almost closed on day 10 when treated with nanocurcumin-loaded gelatin-pluronic hydrogels compared to the pristine hydrogels and other commercial dressings [40]. Zheng et al., prepared injectable hydrogels using gelatin and gellan loaded with tannic acid for antibacterial wound dressing. The in vitro antimicrobial analysis of tannic acid-loaded hybrid hydrogels using agar disc diffusion showed superior antibacterial efficacy against *S. aureus*, *E. coli*, and drug-resistant bacteria (methicillin-resistant *S. aureus* [MRSA]). The in vivo studies on full-thickness wounds on mice model showed that the wounds treated with tannic acid-loaded hydrogels were significantly healed faster and they were fully closed on the 12th-day post-surgery without scar development [41]. Dong et al., designed injectable PEG-gelatin hydrogels encapsulated with adipose-derived stem cells (ASCs) for cutaneous wound management. The cytotoxicity analysis revealed more than 85% cell viability of ASCs when encapsulated in hybrid hydrogels, suggesting that the hydrogels can be useful for the delivery of numerous cells for in vivo and clinical application. The in vivo studies using murine excisional wound healing model demonstrated that the wounds treated with ASC-loaded hydrogels were completely closed on day 10 while the wounds treated with plain ASCs and plain hydrogels were closed on days 12 and 16, suggesting that the encapsulation of ASCs in the hydrogels significantly accelerated the wound healing process [42].

Khamrai et al., prepared a gelatin-based polyelectrolyte hydrogel patch loaded with curcumin for wound healing using a sequential solution mixing and casting method. The prepared hydrogel displayed self-healing capability at a physiological pH of 7.4 and acted as a transdermal drug delivery system of curcumin [43]. The gelatin-based hydrogel patch was loaded with ionically self-assembled bacterial cellulose obtained from *Glucanoacetobacter xylinus* bacterial strain. The mechanical properties exhibited by the gelatin-based hybrid hydrogel showed an increased elongation of 4.8% and a decreased modulus of 4.6 MPa, stating that the loaded bioactive agent had a positive effect on the elongation and a negative effect on the modulus. Atomic force microscopy (AFM) depth profilometry analysis showed complete healing after application in a buffer of pH 7.4 after damage [43]. The in vitro drug release profile displayed a controlled release of curcumin from the prepared gelatin-based hydrogel, which contributed to the antimicrobial activity of the hydrogel, enhancing wound healing. The in vitro antimicrobial studies demonstrated that curcumin-loaded hydrogels possessed enhanced antibacterial activity against *E. coli* and *S. aureus* when compared to plain hydrogels, indicating their potential use for the treatment of bacterial-infected wounds [43].

Treesuppharat et al., formulated gelatin-bacterial cellulose hydrogels encapsulated with methylene blue via a copolymerization process and were cross-linked using glutaraldehyde [44]. The hydrogel composites were malleable and flexible. The SEM images of hybrid hydrogels revealed a porous morphology, suggesting good porosity for effective drug delivery. The results from AFM agreed with the SEM morphology. The prepared hybrid hydrogel showed good thermal stability, mechanical properties, and chemical resistance before the loading of bacterial cellulose. After loading the hydrogels with bacterial cellulose, their porosity changed from macro-porous to mesoporous pores. The swelling studies demonstrated the hydrogel network swelling capacity in the range of 400–600% [44].

Li et al., prepared gelatin-based composite hydrogel by gels spinning with PEG6000 as a modifier and cross-linked with dialdehyde carboxymethyl cellulose (DCMC) [45]. The prepared samples of the gelatin-based hydrogels were named as follows GeP, GeP-D1000, GeP-D500, GeP-D100, and GeP-D50 when the ratio of DCMC to gelatin was 0, 1/1000, 1/500, 1/100, and 1/50, respectively. The mechanical properties for the gelatin-based hydrogel fibres showed the highest tensile strength of 2.15 + 0.21 MPa and a reduced elongation at a break of 10.2 + 0.8% for GeP-D50. The increase in the tensile strength was attributed to an increase in DCMC in the hydrogel, resulting in a decrease in the elongation at break. The gelatin-PEG hydrogel fiber showed excellent swelling behavior in the range of 89–93%, stating that it can absorb wound exudates, and provide a moist environment to accelerate the wound healing process. The DCMC cross-linker reduced the swelling degree of hydrogels, which is advantageous to the hydrogel fibres to prevent the undesired reduction of the mechanical properties. The SEM of the prepared hydrogel fibres displayed a porous network and 3-D morphology which indicates that the hydrogel will aid in cell adhesion and proliferation. The hydrogel with a more porous network was observed to be GeP-D1000, meaning it can hold free water compared to GeP-D50 because it is more compact. The hydrogel fibers GeP-D500, and GeP-D1000 were biocompatible when evaluated in normal fibroblasts with no visible dead cells. However, GeP-D50 and GeP-D100 were not biocompatible [45].

Fan et al., fabricated gelatin-PVA-chitosan hybrid hydrogels using the gamma irradiation method for wound dressing application [46]. The swelling analysis revealed that gelatin-PVA-chitosan hydrogels showed excellent swelling behavior, which was attributed to an increase in the ratio of gelatin and chitosan. Their good swelling property was attributed to the hydrophilic nature of gelatin and PVA polymers. The hybrid hydrogels demonstrated good capability to maintain a moist environment by retaining 10-20% of water, meaning it has a good water evaporation rate. The mechanical properties for the gelatin-PVA-chitosan hydrogels revealed that the highest tensile strength was 2.2 MPa for the hydrogel with a ratio weight of chitosan: gelatin (1:3). The elongation of the prepared hydrogel decreased with an increase in gelatin, while the tensile strength increased with an increase in gelatin, which enhanced the mechanical properties of the hybrid hydrogels. The SEM images showed a porous morphology for the gelatin-PVA-chitosan hydrogels, revealing that the hydrogels are permeable to wound exudates and water vapor. The gelatin-PVA-chitosan hydrogel displayed a good blood clotting with the lowest BCI index of 0.032 for the hydrogel with a ratio weight of chitosan: gelatin (1:1) [46].

The gelatin-based hybrid hydrogels display interesting features, as reported in a series of in vitro and in vivo studies by some researchers. Their interesting features make them promising scaffolds for wound dressings. The blending of gelatin with other polymers, especially synthetic polymers, for the fabrication of hydrogels resulted in an excellent mechanical performance which is beneficial for easy handling and application during wound care. The mechanical properties of gelatin-based hybrid hydrogels imitate those of human skin, suggesting their compatibility with the skin. SEM micrographs of hybrid hydrogel scaffolds showed a porous morphology that can improve hydrogel swelling capacity, absorption of wound exudates, and proliferation and adhesion of skin cells that are essential during the wound healing process. The loading of bioactive agents (e.g., antibiotics and antioxidant agents) into the gelatin hybrid hydrogels significantly improved their biological activities, resulting in accelerated wound healing in vivo. These hydrogels displayed controlled drug release that can further enhance their biological activities and reduce drug toxicity.

5.2. Films and Membranes

Films are semi-permeable dressings with a translucent and adhesive nature (Figure 6). Films provide a moist environment, ease cell migration, promote autolysis, are partially permeable to water vapor and oxygen, and inhibit bacteria proliferation [47]. They are suitable for treating chronic wounds (on the heels, elbow, and a flat surface of the body), moderate exuding wounds, and superficial wounds. Films are cost-effective, clear necrotic debris, are waterproof, and permit cyclic inspections of a wound [48]. The disadvantage of film dressings is that they cause skin maceration upon removal and most of them are non-absorptive or less absorptive. The film dressings are not frequently changed, depending on the amount of exudates, they can be changed once a week [46]. Gelatin-based hybrid film wound dressings have been reported by several researchers (Table 2). Taheri et al., formulated gelatin-chitosan hybrid films encapsulated with tannic acid and/or bacterial nanocellulose for wound healing applications [49]. The FTIR and XRD analysis confirmed the successful preparation of hybrid films by displaying the expected peaks. The SEM images exhibited scattered white spots, indicating the desired dispersion of nanocellulose particles on the surface of the films. The water vapor transmission experiments demonstrated that the addition of tannic acid and nanoparticles in the films significantly decreased the WVTR, providing sufficient moisture for wound healing. The results from the mechanical analysis showed that all the films possessed a tensile strength of more than 80 MPa. The in vivo studies using Wistar rats demonstrated that the full-thickness skin wounds treated with the dual drug-loaded films and nanoparticle-loaded films were healed with a closure faster than the tannic acid-loaded films and plain hybrid films [49]. Sakthiguru and Sithique designed gelatin-chitosan biocomposite films incorporated with allantoin for wound healing application [50]. The water absorption tests showed enhanced water absorption capacity of allantoin-incorporated hybrid films. The in vitro cytotoxicity experiments of all the films assessed using the MTT assay demonstrated more than 80% cell viability when incubated with L929 fibroblasts, revealing excellent biocompatibility and non-toxicity. The antimicrobial studies demonstrated that allantoin-loaded films had superior antibacterial activity against *S. aureus* and *E. coli* when compared to the free allantoin and plain films, indicating that the allantoin-incorporated dressings are potential antibacterial wound dressing materials [50].

Akhavan-Kharazian and Izadi-Vasafi developed hybrid films that are prepared from gelatin and chitosan. The films were incorporated with nanocrystalline cellulose and calcium peroxide for wound healing [51]. The swelling analysis demonstrated high swelling behavior at pH 5, 7, and 9, simulating wound exudate, physiological condition, and an infected wound, respectively. The water vapor permeation studies of the hybrid films prepared exhibited WVTR values in the range of 35 to 45 $g/m^2/h$ which is appropriate for maintaining suitable fluid balance on the wound bed. The in vitro cytotoxicity analysis using the MTT assay showed almost 100% cell viability of the human fibroblast cells when immersed with dual-loaded film/ plain films for seven days, showing that the prepared gelatin-based hybrid films are non-toxic [51]. Patel et al., prepared gelatin-chitosan films for drug delivery of lupeol for wound dressing application. The SEM micrograph images of the hybrid films showed relatively smooth, fibrous, and porous morphology appropriate for increasing the oxygen supply to the injury for accelerated wound healing. The in vitro drug release studies showed that the release of lupeol from the films followed a biphasic release pattern with an initial burst release followed by a sustained release of 90.99 ± 1.27% lupeol after 24 h. The in vitro antioxidant experiments demonstrated that the incorporation of lupeol in the films significantly enhanced the free radical-scavenging effects of the gelatin-based hybrid films, revealing the wound healing properties of lupeol-loaded films at the inflammation phase of the wound healing [52].

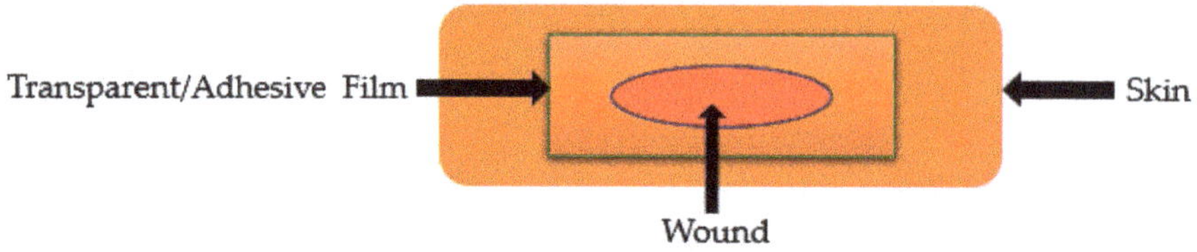

Figure 6. Transparent Film Dressing on Skin Wound.

Türe reported gelatin-alginate composite films loaded with hydroxyapatite for wound management. The in vitro antimicrobial studies of the drug-loaded films using agar disc diffusion assay demonstrated that the drug-loaded films were effective in inhibiting the growth of *S. aureus* and *E. coli* while the films not loaded with the drug did not exhibit any inhibitory effect, suggesting that the drug-loaded hybrids are potential dressings for the treatment of bacteria-infected wounds [53]. Cahú et al., developed gelatin-chitosan-chondroitin 4-Sulfate hybrid films incorporated with zinc oxide (ZnO) nanoparticles. The nanoparticles-loaded films did not show any toxicity towards the skin fibroblasts (3T3) or keratinocytes (HaCaT) cell lines, indicating excellent biocompatibility with good antibacterial effect against *S. aureus* and *E. coli* in vitro. The in vivo wound healing experiments using the rat model demonstrated that gelatin-based hybrid films significantly increased the percentage of wound reduction from 65% to 86% in full-thickness excision compared with only 51% for the control, after six days [54]. Evranos et al., prepared bone ash-incorporated gelatin-chitosan film wound dressings loaded with ciprofloxacin. The in vitro drug release studies at physiological conditions showed a controlled release of ciprofloxacin from the films due to the incorporation of bone ash into the hybrid films. These films demonstrated superior antimicrobial effects against *E. coli* and *Bacillus subtilis* (*B. subtilis*) [55].

Baek et al., developed gelatin-PCL-(+)-catechin films for wound care. The FTIR data confirmed the successful formulation of films, while the in vitro cytotoxicity analysis demonstrated good cell viability and proliferation of NIH/3T3 cells, indicating good biocompatibility that is appropriate for an ideal wound dressing [56]. Garcia-Orue reported gelatin-chitosan bilayer hydrofilms for wound healing application. The water uptake studies of the hybrid hydrofilms displayed a significantly higher swelling ability of approximately 700% in equilibrium. The water vapor transmission of the films demonstrated a WVTR value of 787.0 ± 50.9 $g/m^2 \cdot day$. The cytotoxicity studies demonstrated more than 70% cell viability of fibroblast cells when immersed with the hydrofilms, revealing good biocompatibility. The ex vivo experiments using human skin demonstrated accelerated wound contraction of the wounds treated with the hydrofilms [57].

Bhowmik et al., prepared gelatin-based biocomposite films incorporated with crystalline cellulose (CCs) for wound healing application [58]. The SEM images of the gelatin-CCs films displayed a rough morphology with a lot of crystals on the surface of the films. The mechanical characterization of the gelatin-CCs films in the ratio of 10:10 showed the highest tensile strength of 64.16 MPa with a tensile modulus of 2.64 MPa. The tensile strength and tensile modulus increased with an increase in the concentration of CCs. The gelatin-CCs films demonstrated an excellent fluid absorbing capability, making the films suitable for maintaining a moist environment on the wound area, which is essential for wound healing. The gelatin-CCs films were biocompatible and non-toxic. The in vivo wound healing studies and histological analysis studies using the mice model demonstrated that, on the 10th day, the wound dressed with gelatin-CCs films contracted with re-epithelization on the wound bed without inducing trauma on the wound bed [58].

On the other hand, membranes display similar properties as film wound dressings. The advantages of polymer-based membranes in wound dressing include their ability to absorb excess exudates, maintain appropriate moisture for the wound healing process, retain biological fluids under pressure, do not require frequent dressing changes, reduces the disruption of the wound bed, and present potential cleaning activity [59]. Furthermore, membranes demonstrate good mechanical properties, such as softness, comfortability, flexibility, and stretchability [59].

Table 2. Summary of Gelatin-based Hybrid Film and Membrane Wound Dressings.

Types of Wound Dressings	Polymers Combined with Gelatin	Loaded Bioactive Agents	Outcomes	References
Films	Chitosan	Tannic acid and bacterial nanocellulose	Good mechanical performance and faster full-thickness wound closure.	[49]
Films	Chitosan	Allantoin	Excellent biocompatibility and non-toxicity with superior antibacterial efficacy.	[50]
Films	Chitosan	Nanocrystalline cellulose and calcium peroxide	Moderate WVTR and excellent cytocompatibility	[51]
Films	Chitosan	Lupeol	Initial rapid drug release followed by sustained release, and good antioxidant efficacy.	[52]
Films	Alginate	Hydroxyapatite	High antibacterial activity.	[53]
Films	Chitosan	ZnO nanoparticles	Good antibacterial effects and increased full-thickness wound contraction rate.	[54]
Films	Chitosan	Bone ash and ciprofloxacin	Superior antimicrobial effects	[55]
Films	PCL	Catechin	High cell and proliferation of skin cells.	[56]
Films	Chitosan	–	High swelling capacity and accelerated wound healing.	[57]
Films	Cellulose	–	Excellent fluid absorbing effect and fast wound closure.	[58]
Membranes	CM chitosan and HA	–	High cell viability and proliferation	[60]
Membranes	Chitosan	–	High growth inhibition against several bacterial strains	[61]
Membranes	Polymyxin B sulfate	Ciprofloxacin and HNTs	High swelling capacity, non-toxic, and good antibacterial activity.	[62]

Xu et al., designed gelatin-CM and chitosan-HA membranes for corneal wound healing applications. The cytocompatibility analysis of the membranes revealed high cell viability and proliferation of the primary rabbit corneal epithelial cells, revealing good cytocompatibility. The in vivo studies using alkali-induced corneal damage in rabbits demonstrated that these hybrid membranes could significantly enhance corneal epithelial reconstruction and restore cornea transparency and thickness [60]. Kenawy et al., prepared biodegradable cinnamaldehyde-crosslinked gelatin-chitosan membranes for wound healing applications. The wettability studies demonstrated a water contact angle of about 29°, indicating the hydrophilic nature of the membranes. The in vitro antimicrobial experiments demonstrated a higher growth inhibition against *Pseudomonas aeruginosa (P. aeruginosa)*, *Salmonella*, *E. coli*, and *S. aureus* for cinnamaldehyde-crosslinked gelatin-chitosan membranes than the uncrosslinked hybrid membranes [61].

Shi et al., prepared a gelatin elastomer nanocomposite membrane incorporated with polymyxin B sulfate and ciprofloxacin, loaded with halloysite clay nanotubes (HNTs) using a simple gelling method and a hot melt blending technique [62]. The mechanical analysis showed a tensile strength of 1 MPa, while the increase in the amounts of HNTs led to an increased tensile strength of 2 MPa. The prepared elastomer nanocomposite membranes were capable of protecting and promoting wound healing. The elastomer nanocomposite membranes displayed a good water uptake of over eight times its swelling weight. The HNTs enhanced the properties of the prepared membrane and affected the water absorption of the samples. The in vitro cytotoxicity studies of the nanocomposite membranes displayed biocompatibility and non-toxicity on L929 cells. The elastomer nanocomposite membrane displayed a sustained release of HNTs. The bacterial zone of inhibition of all the elastomer membranes was significant against *P. aeruginosa* and *S. aureus* [62].

Gelatin-based hybrid films and membranes exhibit good mechanical properties that make them easy for application on wounds. Most of the films demonstrated moderate WVTR appropriate to prevent wound dehydration and provided a suitable moist environment for the wound healing process. The high cell viability and proliferation of various skin cells, when incubated with gelatin films or membranes, confirmed the excellent biocompatibility and non-toxicity of the gelatin-based hybrid materials. The combination of gelatin with other polymers such as chitosan for the fabrication of films and membranes resulted in high growth inhibition of various bacterial strains that are responsible for bacteria-infected wounds. Generally, films display low absorption capacity, making them inappropriate for exuding wounds. However, gelatin-based hybrid films exhibited higher absorption capability due to the hydrophilic nature of gelatin. The drug-loaded gelatin films and membranes significantly resulted in good biological effects, such as antibacterial and antioxidant activities, that are required in wound treatment, especially for chronic wounds.

5.3. Sponges

Sponges are soft and flexible materials with a well interconnected micro-pore structure (Figure 7). Due to their unique structural features, they have good fluid absorption capability, cell interaction, and hydrophilicity [63]. Their high swelling capacity and quick hemostatic capability make them suitable to prevent the accumulation of exudates. The sponges that absorb a sufficient amount of wound exudates provide a moist environment and also protect the wound bed from bacterial invasion [64]. The porous sponges based on natural as well as synthetic biopolymer have been widely used for biomedical dressings. Sponges with pore sizes between 10 and 100 microns in diameter and interconnected channels increased tissue growth [65]. Gelatin is one of the biopolymers widely reported for the preparation of sponges (Table 3).

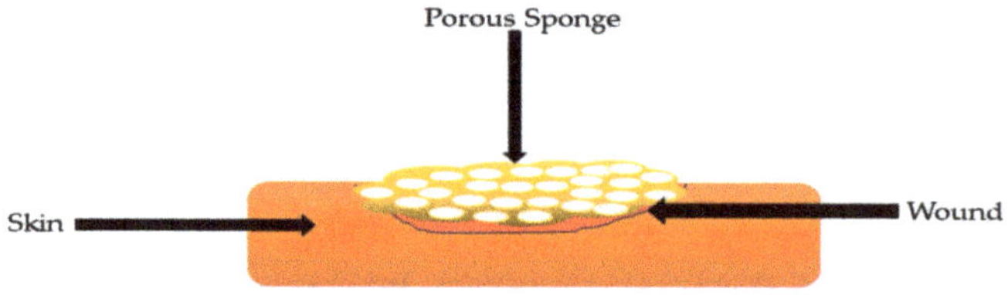

Figure 7. Microporous Sponge on Skin Wound.

Table 3. Summary of Gelatin-based hybrid Sponge Wound Dressings.

Types of Wound Dressings	Polymers Combined with Gelatin	Loaded Bioactive Agents	Outcomes	References
Sponges	Konjac glucomannan	Au nanoparticles and gentamicin	Non-toxic and superior antibacterial activity with accelerated full-thickness wound healing.	[66]
Sponges	Collagen	bFGF	The faster full-thickness wound healing process.	[67]
Sponges	Gelatin	Ag nanoparticles	High porosity and high antibacterial efficacy.	[68]
Sponges	Chitosan	Curcumin	Initial burst drug release followed by sustained slowly release with fast wound healing and no scar formation	[69]
Sponges	Chitosan	Tannis and PRP	Accelerated wound healing	[70]
Sponges	Keratin and fibrin	Mupirocin	Initial burst drug release followed by sustained slow release with good antibacterial efficacy.	[71]
Sponges	Bacterial cellulose	Ampicillin	Sustained drug release and excellent antibacterial activity.	[72]
Sponges	Sodium alginate	Tetracycline hydrochloride	Good swelling behavior and controlled drug release with high antibacterial effects.	[73]

Zou et al., reported gelatin-konjac glucomannan hybrid sponges loaded with gold (Au) nanoparticles and gentamicin sulfate for the treatment of bacteria-infected wounds [66]. The transmission electron microscope (TEM) images displayed the shape of Au nanoparticles which was spherical or elliptical in a single dispersed modality with an average particle size of 3.55 $\pm$ 0.26 nm. The in vitro cytotoxicity analysis of the hybrid sponges demonstrated a cell viability value of more than 88% on L929 cells, indicating that these dual drug-loaded sponges were non-toxic. The in vitro antimicrobial experiments demonstrated that the dual drug-loaded sponges possessed higher antibacterial efficacy against *E. coli*, *S. aureus*, and MRSA while the plain hybrid sponges did not possess any antibacterial effect against these bacterial strains. The in vivo studies using the rabbit model showed that the full thickness wounds dressed with dual drug-loaded hybrid sponges were almost completely healed on day 14 when compared to other groups [66].

Jinno et al., performed comparison studies of bFGF-loaded gelatin-collagen sponges and collagen sponges in wound healing application. The in vivo wound healing studies using full-thickness skin lesions in rats demonstrated that there were enhancement observed in the dermis-like tissue area, the neoepithelial length, and the angiogenesis rates in the group of animal models treated with bFGF-incorporated sponges compared to collagen sponges and plain gelatin-based hybrid sponges [67].

Ye et al., fabricated tannic acid-crosslinked gelatin-gelatin sponges loaded with Ag nanoparticles for wound healing application. The porosity analysis displayed that the addition of Ag nanoparticles significantly increased the porosity of the sponges from 43.25 $\pm$ 3% to 85.13 $\pm$ 2%, and this can stimulate the absorption of exudates and allow the exchange of substances between the skin cells. The antimicrobial studies showed that the addition of Ag nanoparticles enhanced the antibacterial effects of the sponges against *S. aureus* and *E. coli*. The in vivo studies using the rabbit model demonstrated that the *S. aureus*-infected full-thickness wounds possessed wound closure rates of 100%, 97%, 90%, and 80% on the 15th day for Ag nanoparticle-loaded sponges, Aquacel® Ag, pristine gelatin-chitosan sponges, and control, respectively [68]. Naghshineh et al., formulated hybrid sponges that are based on gelatin and chitosan. The wound dressings were loaded with curcumin for the treatment of wounds. The in vitro drug release profile showed an initial burst release of curcumin from the sponges followed by a sustained and slow release for 48 h. The in vivo wound closure studies using the rat model showed that the lesions covered with curcumin-loaded sponges were completely healed on day 10 without the formation of scars [69].

Lu et al., examined the effects of chitosan-gelatin sponges loaded with tannins and platelet-rich plasma (PRP) on the rate of wound healing [70]. The FTIR spectra showed that the chitosan and gelatin were crosslinked via chemical bonds, providing the hybrid sponges with good thermostability and appropriate mechanical properties. The porous structure of the sponges conferred the material with good water-absorbing quality. The hybrid sponges inhibited the growth of *E. coli* and *S. aureus* with low toxicity. The wounds covered with the tannins-PRP-loaded sponges healed quicker than the wound covered with pristine gelatin or chitosan sponge in vivo. The addition of PRP to the hybrid sponges accelerated wound healing significantly [70]. Singaravelu et al., formulated gelatin-keratin–fibrin 3D sponges loaded with mupirocin for wound healing. The SEM images of the sponges showed highly porous morphology with randomly interconnected pores that can promote gaseous exchange and cell growth. The in vitro drug release studies demonstrated initial rapid drug release of mupirocin from the sponges followed by a slow and sustained release. The in vitro antimicrobial studies of the drug-loaded sponges against *E. coli* and *S. aureus* displayed a clear zone of inhibition with 8 and 6 mm, respectively, while sponges without mupirocin did not show any inhibition zone [71].

Ye et al., fabricated novel honeycomb-like gelatin-bacterial cellulose composite sponges. The SEM cross-sectional morphology of the fabricated hybrid sponges was a combination of a continuous micrometer-size honeycomb structure with fairly regular, aligned, and straight channels. These hybrid composite sponges had a large surface area and uniform pore distribution, and high porosity with excellent swelling capability. The in vitro drug release studies displayed a sustained release of ampicillin for 48 h that follows a non-Fickian diffusion. The obtained gelatin-based hybrid sponges exhibited excellent antibacterial activity, and good biocompatibility, making them useful in various antibacterial applications [72]. Wen et al., incorporated gelatin into sodium alginate to enhance the shape-forming properties and tetracycline hydrochloride (TCH) was loaded to the fabricated antibacterial gelatin-sodium alginate composite sponges. The swelling analysis of the hybrid sponges displayed good swelling behavior due to their high porosity. The in vitro studies showed that the TCH-loaded sponges exhibited a controlled release profile with good antibacterial efficacy against *E. coli* ATCC25, ATCC922, as well as *B. subtilis* ATCC 9372 and *S. aureus* ATCC 6538. The fabricated gelatin-sodium alginate sponges are potential wound dressings for treating bacteria-infected wounds [73].

Gelatin-based hybrid sponges demonstrate excellent swelling behavior due to their high porosity. The sponges with good swelling behavior are suitable for high exuding wounds. Most of the in vitro drug release profiles of the drug-loaded gelatin-based sponges showed initial burst release followed by a sustained and a slow-release. This mechanism is useful in killing the bacterial strains in the wound bed with continuous protection of the injury from further microbial invasion. Furthermore, the gelatin sponges loaded with bioactive agents exhibited a superior wound healing process without the formation of scars in vivo when compared with some of the commercially available products and pristine gelatin sponges, revealing the efficacy of gelatin-based sponges as potential wound dressings.

5.4. Nanofibers and Nanofibrous Materials

Nanofibers are wound dressing materials that possess diameter sizes that range from nanometers to a few microns [74]. The popularly used technique for the preparation of these materials is electrospinning (Figure 8) [75]. The electrospun nanofibers are considered appropriate wound dressings for chronic wounds because of their drug delivery capability. Nanofibers imitate the ECM, thereby promoting the proliferation of epithelial cells and the development of new tissues in the wound environment [76]. The advantages of the nanofibers and nanofibrous dressings include their ability to stimulate hemostasis of damaged tissues, promote dermal drug delivery, improve fluid absorption, high-gas permeation, cell respiration, high surface area to volume, high porosity, maintaining of the moist environment, thereby inhibiting microbial infections [77,78]. Many gelatin-based hybrid nanofibers have been reported by researchers for the treatment of different wounds (Table 4). Ajmal et al., formulated gelatin-PCL hybrid nanofibers co-loaded with quercetin and ciprofloxacin hydrochloride for wound healing application. The SEM micrographs of dual drug-loaded nanofibers displayed uniform size distribution, randomly oriented and beadless morphology mimicking the ECM, with an average diameter of approximately 234.172 ± 98.234 nm. The porosity of the nanofibers was in the range of 60–90%, suggesting that these nanofibers are suitable for sufficient exchange of gases and nutrients during the skin wound healing process. The FTIR and XRD data confirmed the successful formulation of gelatin-based nanofibers loaded with quercetin and ciprofloxacin [79].

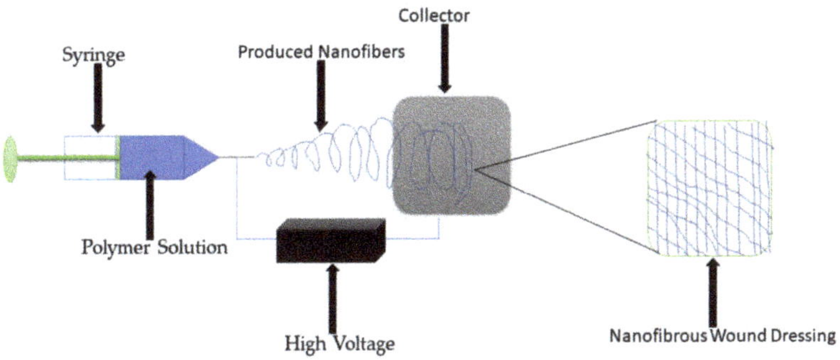

Figure 8. Preparation of Nanofibrous Using Electrospinning Technique.

The in vitro drug release studies at physiological conditions (pH 7.4 and 37 °C) showed that the release of the loaded drugs from gelatin-based hybrid nanofibers was biphasic in nature, with an initial rapid drug release followed by a slow and sustained release. The antioxidant experiments of the dual drug-loaded nanofibers using DPPH reduction methods showed significantly high antioxidant effects with more than 100% cell viability of 3T6-Swiss albino fibroblasts, indicating good biocompatibility. The in vitro antibacterial analysis showed a wide zone of inhibition against *S. aureus* resulting from the initial rapid release of ciprofloxacin. The plain nanofiber did not exhibit any significant antibacterial activity. The in vivo wound healing studies using Wistar rats showed that the full-thickness wounds treated with dual drug-loaded nanofibers provided 100% wound closure on day 16, whereas the wound closure for the plain PCL-GE and gauze was 78.85 and 71.32%, respectively [79].

Bakhsheshi-Rad et al., developed electrospun hybrid nanofibers that are based on gelatin cephalexin and PCL. The nanofibers were loaded with cephalexin for antimicrobial wound management [80]. The SEM micrographs of the nanofibers displayed a continuous, uniform, and smooth morphology with mean fiber diameters that ranged between 280 and 330 nm. The mechanical characterization of the nanofibers demonstrated a tensile strength of 3.05 MPa and a tensile strain of 89% simulating human skin. The water contact angle studies showed the hydrophilic nature of hybrid nanofibers with a contact angle of about 57 ± 1°. The in vitro antibacterial studies of cephalexin-loaded hybrid nanofibers showed a high size of inhibition of 6.1 mm for *E. coli* and 6.9 mm for *S. aureus*. The in vivo wound closure experiments employing BALB/c mice showed enhanced wound healing with the cephalexin-loaded hybrid nanofibers [80]. Adeli-Sardou et al., synthesized gelatin-PCL nanofibers loaded with Lawsone for skin regeneration. The mechanical studies of the nanofibers showed the highest tensile strength, Young's modulus, and strain 2.14 ± 0.3 MPa, 2.12 ± 0.9 MPa, and 37 ± 6.6%, respectively. The in vitro drug release studies at physiological conditions showed prolonged release of lawsone from the hybrid nanofiber for 20 days. The in vivo wound healing studies showed that the wounds treated with lawsone-loaded nanofibers were 100% closed at the end of 14 days, while those dressed with the plain nanofibers induced 71% wound closure [81].

İnal and Mülazımoğlu reported electrospun nanofibers prepared from gelatin and poly([2-(methacryloyloxy)ethyl] trimethylammonium chloride) (PMETAC) for wound care. The degradation experiments using an environment simulating the skin demonstrated fast biodegradation of over 80% of the gelatin-PMETAC nanofibers in the first week. The in vitro cytotoxicity studies using MTT assay showed low toxicity of nanofibers when incubated with L929 fibroblast cells. The in vitro antibacterial studies of nanofibers showed high inhibition of more than 90% against *E. coli*, *S. aureus*, and *Acinetobacter baumannii*, while the inhibition for *methicillin-resistant Staphylococcus aureus* (MRSA) was 75%. These excellent antibacterial effects were induced by the presence of PMETAC [82]. Cam et al., formulated gelatin-bacterial cellulose nanofibers loaded with glibenclamide and metformin for diabetic wound care. The cytotoxicity studies showed a high cell viability of L929 mouse fibroblast cells when immersed with the nanofibers, suggesting non-toxicity and good biocompatibility. The wound contraction experiments in vivo using wounds in type-1 diabetic rats showed that the drug-loaded nanofibers exhibited superior wound healing than the pristine nanofibers on day 14, suggesting that the loading of glibenclamide and metformin into the wound dressing significantly accelerated diabetic wound healing [83].

Rather et al., prepared electrospun gelatin-PCL nanofibers functionalized with cerium oxide (CeO_2) nanoparticles for wound healing applications. The FTIR and XRD data confirmed the successful formulation of nanofibers. The cell proliferation assay of the hybrid nanofibers exhibited high proliferation and viability of 3T3-L1 cells, indicating their good biocompatibility. The gelatin-PCL nanofibers functionalized with cerium oxide nanoparticles showed better scavenging potential when compared to the pristine nanofibers, confirming excellent antioxidant efficacy useful in the inflammatory phase of wound healing [84]. Alishahi et al., designed glucantime-loaded electrospun hybrid nanofibers that are based on gelatin and PVA/PEO/chitosan for wound care of cutaneous *Leishmania* wounds. The results from this study showed that 4 and 6 cm^2 of drug-loaded hybrid nanofibers destroyed leishmania promastigotes up to 78% with high cell viability of fibroblast cells, indicating that the scaffolds are promising scaffolds for the management of Leishmania wounds [85].

Zhang et al., prepared gelatin-silk fibroin electrospun nanofibers encapsulated with astragaloside IV for wound management [86]. The porosity of the plain hybrid nanofibers and drug-loaded hybrid nanofibers was 88% and 89%, respectively, which are appropriate for an ideal wound dressing. The drug release profile of astragaloside IV-loaded nanofibers was rapid in the first 12 h followed by a slow-release, which is suitable for wound healing. The wound healing studies showed that the drug-encapsulated nanofiber dressings promoted a significantly higher rate of healing at the early stage of trauma than the blank nanofiber dressing and pure astragaloside IV solution group. The above-mentioned findings result from the good biocompatibility and efficient barrier against microorganisms by the astragaloside-loaded hybrid nanofibers [86]. Xia et al., designed gelatin-PCL nanofibers loaded with ciprofloxacin using centrifugal spinning for antimicrobial wound management. The water contact angle study showed the average contact angles of hybrid nanofibers were 75°, 72°, 68°, and 47° when ciprofloxacin concentration was 6%, 8%, 10%, and 12%, respectively, showing that the nanofibers become significantly more hydrophilic as the concentration of the antibiotic increased. The in vitro drug release experiments under physiological conditions showed a sustained release of ciprofloxacin from the hybrid nanofibers with a high zone of inhibition in vitro against *S. aureus* and *E. coli*. The pristine nanofiber did not display any significant antimicrobial activity [87].

Fallah et al., formulated electrospun gelatin-PCL hybrid nanofibers loaded with curcumin for antibacterial wound healing. The antimicrobial studies showed that the nanofibers displayed almost 100% antibacterial activity against MRSA and 82.56% against extended-spectrum β lactamases (ESBL), dangerous nosocomial bacterial strains. These results suggest that curcumin-loaded hybrid nanofibers are potential materials for the management of bacteria-infected wounds [88]. Gharaie et al., formulated gelatin-chitosan-PU nanofibers via the electrospinning method. The FTIR data showed the expected functional groups of the hybrid nanofibers confirming the successful formulation of the nanofiber. The SEM micrographs of the hybrid nanofibers displayed uniform and beadless morphology that mimic the ECM [89]. Pavliňáková et al., prepared hybrid nanofibers from gelatin and PCL and reinforced them with halloysite nanotubes HNTs for wound healing application. The mechanical characterizations showed that the incorporation of HNTs significantly improved the mechanical properties of hybrid nanofibers. The in vitro cytocompatibility studies showed high cell viability and proliferation of NIH-3T3 fibroblasts when incubated with HNT-reinforced nanofibers, suggesting that these scaffolds are biocompatible [90].

Jiang et al., prepared electrospun gelatin-PCL nanofibers loaded with palmatine for wound management. The in vitro experiments of the palmatine-loaded nanofibers exhibited good antioxidant and antibacterial activity. The in vivo examinations and histological studies showed that palmatine-loaded nanofibers accelerated the healing process of the full-thickness wounds and hindered hypertrophic scar development in the rabbit ear model [91].

Yang et al., reported gelatin-PCL nanofibers incorporated with Au nanoparticles for bacteria-infected wound care. The in vitro antimicrobial analysis of the nanoparticle-loaded hybrid nanofibers demonstrated excellent antibacterial efficacy against multi-drug resistant (MDR) *S. aureus* and *E. coli*. The in vivo wound healing experiments using full-thickness wounds treated with MDR *E. coli* and MDR *P. aeruginosa* on Wistar rats showed that the levels of bacteria in the bacteria-infected injuries treated with Au nanoparticle-loaded nanofibers significantly decreased with superior wound healing mechanism when compared to the pristine nanofibers and gauze [92]. Ong et al., reported Tegaderm-gelatin-PCL nanofibers for the management of wounds. The in vivo wound healing experiments using full-thickness wound on pig model demonstrated that the wounds treated with Tegaderm-gelatin-PCL nanofibers significantly accelerated reepithelization with complete lesion closure on day 28 [93]. Hivechi et al., formulated biaxially electrospun gelatin-PCL nanofibers reinforced with cellulose nanocrystals for wound healing applications [94]. The FTIR and XRD spectrums confirmed the successful formulation of nanocrystal-loaded hybrid nanofibers by displaying expected functional groups and amorphous nature, respectively. The mechanical studies showed that the incorporation of cellulose nanocrystals significantly increased the tensile strength from 14.5 ± 1.9 MPa to 23.6 ± 5.6 MPa and modulus from 112.4 ± 32.0 MPa to 206.0 ± 27.7 MPa. The wound healing analysis in vivo displayed $98 \pm 3\%$ wound closure on the 14th day for cellulose nanocrystal-loaded nanofibers while the control induced only $82 \pm 6\%$ wound closure [94].

Jafari et al., formulated bilayer gelatin-PCL nanofibers co-loaded with amoxicillin and ZnO nanoparticles for full-thickness wound management. The in vitro drug release profile showed a sustained release of amoxicillin for six days. The cytocompatibility studies in vitro using the MTT assay displayed a high cell proliferation and viability of Wharton's jelly derived mesenchymal stromal cells (WJ-MSCs) when seeded with the nanofibers confirming good biocompatibility of the bilayered scaffolds. The in vivo wound healing studies showed a high wound closure percentage for the wounds treated with dual drug-loaded nanofibers when compared to the control [95]. Bazmandeh et al., developed formulated electrospun gelatin-chitosan-HA hybrid nanofibers for wound care.

The in vitro cytotoxicity studies of the nanofibers using MTT assay demonstrated 96% cell viability of the normal human dermal fibroblasts (NHDFs) with high cell proliferation and adhesion, revealing excellent biocompatibility and non-toxicity of the nanofibers. The in vivo wound healing studies employing Wistar rats with surgical operated full-thickness incision wounds demonstrated that the wound closure in gelatin-chitosan-HA nanofibers was significantly high when compared to the gelatin-chitosan scaffolds. On day 14 post-treatment, the wounds were almost completely closed in the animal group treated with gelatin-chitosan-HA nanofibers [96].

Yao et al., developed gelatin-collagen bilayer nanofibers enriched with *Lithospermi radix* plant extract for the treatment of wounds. The in vitro drug release profile showed that the *Lithospermi radix* extract was effectively released slowly from the hybrid nanofibers. The examination of the wound-healing efficacy of the bilayer nanofibers showed the highest wound recovery rate in vivo in SD rats [97]. Hadisi et al., formulated gelatin-oxidized starch loaded with *Lawsonia Inermis* (henna) for the treatment of burn wounds [98]. The SEM images of the hybrid nanofibers displayed continuous, uniform, bead-free fibers with an average fiber diameter of about 87.01 $\pm$ 2.044 nm. The in vitro antimicrobial studies exhibited a high inhibition zone around the henna-loaded hybrid nanofibers against *S. aureus* and *E. coli*. In contrast, the plain hybrid nanofibers did not exhibit significant antibacterial effects. The in vivo wound healing studies revealed accelerated wound closure for henna-loaded nanofibers with the absence of detrimental suppurative reaction at the burn wound site. The gauze and plain nanofiber did not accelerate the wound reduction [98]. Ahlawat et al., formulated gelatin-PVA nanofibers loaded with *Carica papaya* plant extracts for microbial wound healing applications [99]. The in vitro cytotoxicity experiments showed an 80% cell viability of NIH 3T3 fibroblast cells when immersed with *Carica papaya*-loaded nanofibers revealing that hybrid nanofiber did not induce toxicity. The antimicrobial studies using the agar disc diffusion method demonstrated that the *Carica papaya*-enriched nanofibers possessed a higher zone of inhibition on agar plate against *E. coli* and *S. aureus*, suggesting good antibacterial effects of the plant extract [99].

Sobhanian et al., formulated collagen-grafted PVA-gelatin-alginate nanofibers via the electrospinning method for wound treatment. The swelling percentage of collagen-grafted hybrid nanofiber was 624.08 $\pm$ 110% and 801.25 $\pm$ 41% for 1 and 24 h, respectively, which is appropriate for cell attachment. The mechanical analysis of nanofibers displayed an ultimate tensile strength of 4.3 MPa and Young's modulus of 150 MPa, which are in the range of the human skin. The in vitro cell proliferation evaluation of the collagen-grafted PVA-gelatin-alginate nanofibers showed high proliferation and adhesion of the fibroblasts [100]. Vázquez et al., reported gelatin-PLGA nanofiber wound dressings. The in vitro studies showed non-toxicity and high proliferation of mesenchymal stem cells (MSCs) [101]. The Ag sulfadiazine-loaded gelatin-PU nanofibers formulated by Heo et al., exhibited accelerated wound healing of burn injury in Sprague Dawley (SD) rats with good antibacterial efficacy than the gauze [101].

Other various nanofibrous scaffolds display the same properties as nanofibers. Those scaffolds include nanofibrous mats, nanofibrous membranes, nanofiber patches, nanofibrous films, nanofibrous bandages, etc. They also mimic ECM, making them suitable for wound healing and tissue regeneration applications [102]. Farzamfar et al., developed electrospinning gelatin-PCL nanofibrous mats encapsulated with taurine for wound dressing [103]. The SEM micrograph images of taurine-loaded nanofiber mats showed non-woven porous morphology with bead-free fibers. The mechanical analysis of the nanofiber mats showed ultimate tensile strengths that ranged between 2.36 $\pm$ 0.10 MPa and 2.58 $\pm$ 0.40 MPa, revealing that these scaffolds can withstand the forces exerted to the dressings during their wound healing applications. The in vitro cell proliferation studies using the MTT assay showed the high proliferation of L929 fibroblast cells when incubated with nanofiber mats, indicating good biocompatibility. The in vivo wound healing experiments using Wistar rats showed that full-thickness excisional wounds dressed with the taurine-loaded nanofibrous mats achieved a significant injury closure of 92% after 14 days when compared to the gauze that achieved 68% of wound closure [103].

Table 4. Gelatin-based hybrid nanofiber Wound Dressings.

Types of Wound Dressings	Polymers Combined with Gelatin	Loaded Bioactive Agents	Outcomes	References
Nanofibers	PCL	Ciprofloxacin	Good porosity, sustained drug release, and accelerated full-thickness wound closure.	[79]
Nanofibers	PCL	Cephalexin	Good mechanical properties and high antibacterial activity.	[80]
Nanofibers	PCL	Lawsone	Prolonged drug release and accelerated wound reduction	[81]
Nanofibers	PMETAC	–	Non-toxicity and excellent antibacterial activity	[82]
Nanofibers	Bacterial cellulose	Glybenclamide and metformin	Good biocompatibility and quickly diabetic wound healing.	[83]
Nanofibers	PCL	CeO_2 nanoparticles	High cell viability and proliferation with good antioxidant efficacy.	[84]
Nanofibers	PVA/PEO/chitosan	Glucantime	Destroyed leishmania promatigotes with high cell viability of skin cells	[85]
Nanofibers	Silk fibroin	Astragaside IV	High porosity and high wound closure rate	[86]
Nanofibers	PCL	Ciprofloxacin	Good antibacterial efficacy	[87]
Nanofiber	PCL	Curcumin	Excellent antibacterial activity	[88]
Nanofiber	Chitosan and PU	–	Bead-free morphology biomimicking ECM.	[89]
Nanofibers	PCL	HNTs	Enhanced mechanical properties and good cytocompatibility.	[90]
Nanofibers	PCL	Palmatine	Good antioxidant and antibacterial effects with accelerated wound healing.	[91]
Nanofibers	PCL	Au nanoparticles	Excellent antibacterial activity	[92]
Nanofibers	PCL	–	Accelerated wound healing process	[93]
Nanofibers	PCL	Cellulose nanocrystals	Excellent mechanical properties and fast wound closure rate.	[94]
Nanofibers	PCL	Amoxicillin and ZnO nanoparticles	Sustained drug release and high cell proliferation.	[95]
Nanofibers	Chitosan and HA	–	Accelerated full-thickness wound contraction.	[96]
Nanofibers	Collagen	Lithospermi radix plant extract	Higher wound recovery rate	[97]
Nanofibers	Oxidized starch	Lawsonia Inermis	Good antibacterial activity and accelerated burn wound healing.	[98]
Nanofibers	PVA	Carica papaya	Non-toxicity and good antibacterial efficacy.	[99]
Nanofibers	Collagen, alginate, and PVA	–	Good mechanical performance and high cell proliferation and adhesion	[100]
Nanofibers	PLGA	–	Non-toxicity and high cell proliferation.	[101]
Nanofibrous mats	PCL	Taurine	Good mechanical properties and accelerated wound closure.	[103]
Nanofibrous mats	PCL	Clove essential oil	High cell proliferation and good antibacterial efficacy.	[104]

Table 4. Gelatin-based hybrid nanofiber Wound Dressings.

Types of Wound Dressings	Polymers Combined with Gelatin	Loaded Bioactive Agents	Outcomes	References
Nanofibrous mats	PCL	Gymnema sylvestre plant extract	Promoted skin cellular adhesion, migration, and proliferation with good antimicrobial effects	[105]
Nanofibrous mats	PCL	Cinnamon	Accelerated full-thickness wound closure rate.	[106]
Nanofibrous mats	Cellulose	Hydroxyapatite	High wound closure percentage	[107]
Nanofibrous mats	PCL	Curcumin and chitosan nanoparticles	Sustained drug release and a high rate of wound healing.	[108]
Nanofibrous mats	Keratin	–	High cell attachment and proliferation with accelerated wound contraction.	[109]
Nanofibrous mats	PCL	Ketoprofen	Sustained drug release profile and enhance cell adhesion and proliferation.	[110]
Nanofibrous mats	PVA	Ag nanoparticles	Accelerated full-thickness wound closure	[111]
Nanofibrous membranes	PCL	Fe_3O_4	Good mechanical properties and potential antibacterial efficacy.	[112]
Nanofibrous membranes	PCL	QAS	Excellent biocompatibility and superior antibacterial efficacy	[113]
Nanofibrous membranes	PVP	Ag sulfadiazine	Excellent mechanical performance and superior antibacterial efficacy	[114]
Nanofibrous membranes	PCL and PU	Propolis	Accelerated wound healing	[115]
Nanofibrous films	Chitin	–	Good transparency and non-toxicity	[116]
Nanofibrous films	PCL	CeO_2 nanoparticles	Accelerated wound closure	[117]
Nanofibrous patches	PCL	bFGF and VEGF	Fast skin regeneration skin with scar formation	[118]
Nanofibrous composite materials	PCL	Silicate-based bioceramic particles	Fast diabetic wound healing	[119]

Unalan et al., reported electrospun gelatin-PCL nanofibrous mats loaded with clove essential oil for antibacterial wound care management. The successful incorporation of essential oil was confirmed by FTIR analysis and gas chromatography-mass spectrometry (GC-MS). The in vitro cytotoxicity studies showed high cell viability and growth of NHDFs when incubated with the nanofiber mats for two days, suggesting non-toxicity and excellent biocompatibility of the mats. The antimicrobial studies of nanofibrous mats loaded with clove essential oil showed high inhibition effects against *E. coli* and *S.aureus* than the pristine hybrid nanofiber mats, revealing nanofibrous as potential antibacterial wound dressing material. Furthermore, the in vitro wound healing studies of the essential oil-loaded nanofiber mats using scratch assay showed an accelerated wound closure mechanism [104]. Ramalingam et al., fabricated electrospun nanofibrous gelatin-PCL mats enriched with *Gymnema sylvestre* plant extract [105]. The in vitro drug release profile showed an initial burst release of plant extract that can result in preventing the colonization of bacteria. The in vitro experiments showed that the electrospun hybrid mats stimulated cellular adhesion, migration, and proliferation of human dermal fibroblasts and keratinocytes, which are vital cell types involved in the skin healing process. The in vitro antimicrobial studies using the Kirby-Bauer disc diffusion assay showed no zone of inhibition around the plain nanofibrous mats, whereas the mats loaded with *Gymnema sylvestre* extracts showed a clear zone of inhibition against *E. coli*, *S. aureus*, MRSA, and *P. aeruginosa* [105].

Salehi et al., reported nanofibrous mats prepared from gelatin, PCL and enriched with cinnamon for wound treatment. The in vivo wound healing study using a full-thickness model on Wistar rats showed an accelerated wound healing process when injuries were dressed with cinnamon-loaded mats compared to the plain mats [106]. The electrospun cellulose acetate-gelatin-hydroxyapatite nanofiber mats reported by Samadian et al., demonstrated that all the fabricated mats possessed a higher wound closure percentage on the full-thickness excision wound model in male Wistar rats than the sterile gauze [107].

Zahiri et al., prepared nanofiber gelatin-PCL mats incorporated with curcumin-loaded chitosan nanoparticles for application in wound treatment. The in vitro drug release studies at physiological conditions showed sustained and controlled release of nanocurcumin from the hybrid nanofibers. The in vivo wound healing studies of curcumin-loaded hybrid nanofibers showed high degrees of wound healing with more than 62% and 82% wound closure on days 7 and 14, respectively [108]. Yao et al., formulated gelatin-keratin nanofibrous mats for wound dressing. The SEM images of the hybrid mats exhibited a uniform morphology and bead-free structure with a mean fiber diameter of 160.4 nm. The in vitro cell proliferation studies showed high proliferation and adhesion of L929 fibroblasts when incubated with the nanofiber mats, indicating non-toxicity. The in vivo experiments using full-thickness wounds in rats showed a 97.9 $\pm$ 1.6% closure in wound area on day 14 post-surgery, whereas the gauze displayed only 85.8 $\pm$ 6.0% wound closure [109]. Basar et al., formulated gelatin-PCL nanofiber mats for the controlled release of ketoprofen. The in vitro drug release data demonstrated a burst release of ketoprofen that reached a plateau from the nanofibrous mats followed by a slow and sustained release [110].

Amer et al., fabricated gelatin-PVA nanofibrous mats incorporated with Ag nanoparticles for wound healing application. The FTIR data confirmed the successful preparation of Ag nanoparticle-loaded mats by showing the expected functional groups. The SEM images of the hybrid nanofiber mats showed a combination of smooth, beads-free, and uniform fibrous morphologies. The in vivo studies showed an accelerated wound healing process when the full-thickness skin wounds in rabbits were treated with both hybrid nanofiber mats incorporated with nanoparticles and pristine hybrid nanofiber mats [111]. Cai et al., prepared nanofibrous membranes that are based on gelatin and PCL. The membranes were loaded with Fe_3O_4 nanoparticles for microbial-infected wound care [112]. The SEM morphology of hybrid fiber membranes was smooth without noticeable beads with a diameter of 435 nm, suggesting that all the Fe_3O_4 nanoparticles were successfully loaded in the nanofibrous membranes. The mechanical analysis of 1 wt% nanoparticle-loaded nanofibrous scaffolds showed a tensile strength of 6.4 $\pm$ 0.2 MPa, Young's modulus of 124.9 $\pm$ 4.8 MPa, Elongation at break of 8.2 $\pm$ 0.3%, and toughness of 0.26 $\pm$ 0.03 MJ/m^3. The in vitro antimicrobial experiments of nanoparticle-incorporated nanofibers demonstrated a high zone of inhibition against *S aureus* and *E. coli*, indicating that these scaffolds could be effective antibacterial wound dressings [112].

Shi et al., developed gelatin-PCL nanofiber membranes encapsulated with Trimethoxysilylpropyl octadecyldimethyl ammonium chloride (QAS) for antibacterial wound management [113]. The physicochemical properties of QAS-loaded hybrid nanofibrous membranes were confirmed by FTIR and X-ray photoelectron spectroscopy (XPS). The water uptake studies showed that all the formulated membranes have a mean water absorption of above 400% that meets the condition of an ideal wound dressing. The mechanical analysis showed that the nanofiber membrane tensile strength ranged between 9 and 12 MPa [113]. The in vitro antibacterial studies of QAS-loaded hybrid nanofibrous membranes showed a 99.9% reduction of both *S. aureus* and *E. coli* after 6 h with a high cell viability of more than 90% when incubated with L929 fibroblast cells. These results revealed that QAS-loaded nanofibrous membranes are potential materials for the treatment of bacteria-infected wounds with excellent biocompatibility and non-toxicity [113].

Semnani et al., formulated gelatin-PVP nanofibrous membranes loaded with Ag sulfadiazine for bacteria-infected wound treatment. The mechanical analysis of Ag sulfadiazine-loaded nanofiber membranes showed Young's modulus of 22.58 MPa that was in the same range as human skin. The in vitro antimicrobial experiments showed high inhibition zone against *E. coli* and *S. aureus* when incubated with Ag sulfadiazine-loaded nanofiber membranes while pristine membranes did not demonstrate any antibacterial effects as expected. Moreover, the in vitro drug release profile under physiological conditions showed that Ag sulfadiazine release behavior from the fabricated membranes was short-term [114]. Eskandarinia et al., fabricated nanofibrous gelatin-PCL-PU membrane scaffolds loaded with propolis for wound management. The in vitro antibacterial studies of propolis-loaded nanofibrous membranes showed superior antibacterial effects against *E. coli* (1.9 ± 0.4mm), *S. epidermidis* (1.0 ± 0.2 mm), and *S. aureus* (5.4 ± 0.3 mm). The wound healing analysis demonstrated that the nanofibrous membranes significantly accelerated the wound reduction and collagen deposition in the Wistar rats' skin wound model [115].

Ogawa et al., formulated nanofibrous films that are based on gelatin and chitin for wound management. The nanofiber films displayed transmittances that are greater than 75% at 600 nm, indicating good transparency that is appropriate for wound monitoring without removing the nanofibrous film. The biocompatibility studies in vivo showed many neutrophils in the subcutaneous layer of mice when treated with the films, suggesting non-toxicity [116]. Naseri-Nosar et al., formulated gelatin-PCL hybrid nanofibrous films incorporated with CeO_2 nanoparticles for wound treatment. The in vivo studies using the rat model showed that the full-thickness wounds dressed with the CeO_2 nanoparticle-loaded film dressings achieved a more significant wound closure of almost 100% after two weeks than the sterile gauze with only 63% wound closure [117].

Josh et al., developed heparin-functionalized nanofibrous patches from gelatin and PCL co-loaded with bFGF and VEGF for skin regeneration [118]. The SEM micrograph images of nanofiber patches showed a beadless uniform nanofiber structure with an average fiber diameter of approximately 370 nm. The water vapor transmission studies of gelatin-PCL nanofiber patches exhibited a WVTR value of about 2467 ± 243 $g/m^2/day$, indicating that the formulated materials are ideal wound dressings. The in vivo wound healing experiments using the rat model demonstrated that the heparin-functionalized dual GF-loaded nanofiber patches significantly accelerated the wound healing process with complete regeneration of the skin and the absence of scarring at the end of 14 days. The pristine patches wounds were not completely healed [118]. Lv et al., prepared gelatin-PCL nanofibrous composite materials loaded with silicate-based bioceramic particles for diabetic wound management [119]. The in vivo wound healing experiments using the diabetic mice model demonstrated that the diabetic wounds treated with bioceramic particle-loaded nanofibrous composite healed significantly faster after seven days than the plain nanofibrous composites and control.

The electrospinning technique was used to fabricate gelatin-based hybrid nanofibrous scaffolds due to its simplicity and cost-effectiveness when compared to other known methods. The SEM micrographs of gelatin nanofibers exhibited a randomly oriented and beadless morphology mimicking the ECM, indicating that these nanofibers can provide an appropriate environment for the wound healing process. Loading gelatin nanofibers with bioactive agents also promote their antibacterial efficacy, making them ideal wound dressings. The drug-loaded gelatin-based hybrid nanofibers demonstrated sustained drug release profiles with excellent biological effects (e.g., antibacterial activity) and accelerated the wound healing process of chronic injuries. The biological outcomes of gelatin-based nanofibers demonstrate that they are suitable for the management of chronic wounds, such as diabetic wounds, full-thickness wounds, etc.

5.5. Gelatin-Based Microspheres

Microspheres are spherical shells that are commonly formulated from biodegradable or resorbable polymers. They possess a very small diameter, generally in the micrometre range [120]. This type of system displays unique features, such as high drug load capacity, site-specific action, controlled drug release, and good stability (thermally, physically, and chemically). They are also non-toxic, cost-effective, and easy to prepare [121,122]. Gelatin-based microspheres have been reported to display distinct properties appropriate for wound dressings (Table 5). The advantages of gelatin-based wound dressings are summarized in Table 5. These microspheres can be further loaded in various types of wound dressing scaffolds (Figure 9). Che et al., incorporated gelatin microspheres into a composite hydrogel for improved mechanical properties. The gelatin microspheres were developed by an emulsion cross-linking method before incorporation into the hydrogel. Increasing the ratios of microspheres to 40 mg/mL resulted in a short gelation time and low swelling capability of the hydrogel with high mechanical strength. However, the hydrogel incorporated with 30 mg/mL of the gelatin microspheres displayed good stability and mechanical properties appropriate for wound healing with potent bacteria growth inhibition effects against *Escherichia coli* and *S. aureus* [123].

Table 5. Summarizing the Advantages and Disadvantages of Gelatin-based Hybrid Wound Dressings.

Types of Gelatin-Based Hybrid Wound Dressings	Advantages	Disadvantages
Hydrogels	• Ability to be loaded with bioactive agents. • Accelerate wound healing process and formation of less scar. • Good biocompatibility and non-toxicity. • Excellent mechanical properties. • Sustained and controlled drug release	• The high content of gelatin can decrease hydrogel porosity. • Less antibacterial activity if not loaded with bioactive agents.
Films and Membranes	• Transparent • Appropriate WVTR for the wound healing process. • Excellent mechanical performance. • Non-toxicity • Sustained drug release kinetics.	• Low content of gelatin can result in low absorption capacity.
Sponges	• Good cytocompatibility • High porosity • Ability to be loaded with drugs. • Capacity to accelerate wound healing process without the formation of scars. • Good biological activities	• Delayed wound healing process if they are not loaded with antibacterial drugs. • They are not suitable for low exuding injuries due to the high swelling capacity.
Nanofibers	• They possess a structure that mimics ECM. • High porosity • Ability to be used as drug delivery systems. • Easily formulated by the most popular technique called electrospinning. • Excellent biocompatibility	• Poor antibacterial activity if not loaded with antibacterial drugs.
Microspheres	• They can be loaded with bioactive agents. • Display good antibacterial activity. • They can be loaded onto other wound dressings to improve biological activities. • They are suitable for bleeding, infected, and burn wounds.	There are no reported shortcomings

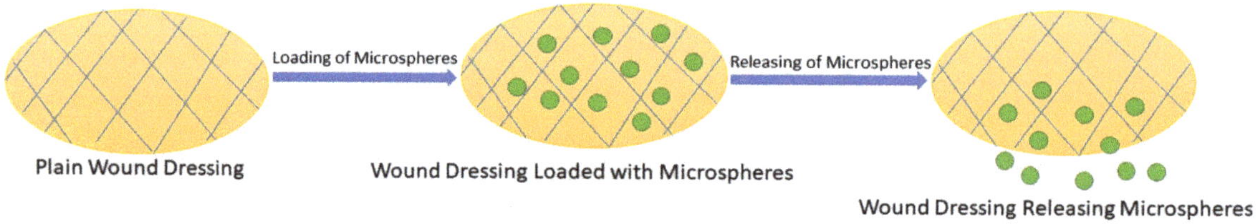

Figure 9. Schematic Diagram of Wound Dressing loaded with Microspheres.

Koslowska et al., prepared microspheres from gelatin and a combination of collagen and gelatin. The microspheres were loaded into collagen/gelatin/hydroxyethyl cellulose composites. The composites were loaded with *calendula officinalis* flower extract. The incorporation of the microspheres into the composites enhanced the porosity, drug loading capability, and drug release of the composites [124]. Fang et al., incorporated gelatin microspheres loaded with ciprofloxacin hydrochloride into chitosan/gelatin composites. The wound dressings displayed appropriate porosity, excellent mechanical properties, high water absorption ability, and biocompatibility. The drug release profile was sustained with a good antibacterial effect against *E. coli*, *P. aeruginosa*, and *S. aureus*, in vitro and in vivo. The deposition of collagen was accelerated revealing microspheres as potential wound dressing for the treatment of bacterial-infected wounds and wounds with seawater immersion [125]. Thyagarajan et al., prepared wound dressings that will inhibit overexpression of matrix metalloproteinase, a family of endopeptidases involved in the remodelling of ECM, which is also capable of degrading ECM when over-expressed. Microspheres were prepared from gelatin and siderophore. Siderophores are iron chelators that inhibit matrix metalloproteinase at the wound site and also reduce bacterial load. The microspheres were rigid with high porosity, and a mean diameter in the range of 7.0 ± 0.52–25.3 ± 0.31 μm. The microspheres were non-toxic, biocompatible on NIH 3T3 fibroblast cell lines with a rapid drug release profile, and supported cell attachment and proliferation [126]. Yang et al., loaded platelet-rich plasma into gelatin microspheres prepared by an emulsion cross-linking method. The average particle size of the microspheres was 15.95 ± 3.79 μm. The drug release profile of the microsphere was sustained for seven days. The microspheres promoted cell proliferation and migration of L929 mouse fibroblast cells in vitro [127].

Li et al., reported gelatin-based injectable microspheres for bleeding wounds. The microspheres were prepared by a water-in-oil emulsion method, followed by crosslinking with glutaraldehyde. The microspheres were negatively charged and the blood clotting time of the microspheres occurred within 60 s. In vivo hemostatic studies on a deep liver wound bleeding model showed a good hemostatic effect of the microspheres. The formulations are suitable for deep wound bleeding in surgery [128]. Zhu et al., prepared collagen/cellulose nanocrystals incorporated with gentamycin sulfate loaded in gelatin microsphere. The in vitro release profile of the drug was sustained for 144 h. The scaffold displayed good compatibility with NIH-3T3 cells in vitro and was effective against *E. coli* and *S. aureus* [129]. The wound dressings are potential wound dressings for the treatment of microbial-infected burn wounds. Kirubanandan et al., developed porous collagen scaffolds incorporated with ciprofloxacin-loaded gelatin microspheres. The delivery of ciprofloxacin from the scaffolds was controlled for two days with 27% drug burst release within the first 5 h. The scaffolds inhibition effect against pseudomonas pathogens was significant in vitro. In vivo study of the scaffolds in full-thickness wounds revealed accelerated healing in 20 days. The wound closure was confirmed by epidermis and dermis regeneration at the wound site. The ciprofloxacin-loaded gelatin microspheres in the scaffold promoted a sustained release profile of the drug via degradation of gelatin in the infected wound environment [130].

Gelatin-based microspheres were prepared and loaded with bioactive agents, such as antibiotics and growth factors before incorporation into the scaffolds. The biodegradable nature of gelatin promoted a sustained release profile, as well as increased the water absorption capacity and the hemostatic effect of the wound dressing. Based on the different research reports, gelatin-based microspheres are suitable for the treatment of burn and infected wounds, and also appropriate for skin regeneration.

6. Gelatin-Based Hybrid Wound Dressings vs. Traditional Wound Dressing Technology

The currently used traditional dressings include plasters, gauze, cotton wool, tulle, bandages, and lint, which are utilized as primary or secondary dressings to protect injuries from contaminations [131]. The other advantages of traditional wound dressings include their ability to absorb wound exudate, offer a dry environment for the wound, and cushion the wound [131,132]. Gauze products that are formulated from non-woven and woven fibers of rayon, polyesters, and cotton can provide a limited barrier against bacterial invasion. Cotton bandages are usually employed for the retention of light wound dressings, short-stretch compression, and high compression bandages offer continuous compression in venous ulcers. Tulle wound dressings (e.g., Paratulle, and Jelonet) are commercially available and are appropriate for superficial clean injury [3]. Although traditional wound dressing products exhibit these interesting advantages, they suffer from several limitations. The disadvantages of traditional dressings include their inability to provide moisture to the wound bed for accelerated wound healing and the capability to cause further skin damage or pain during removal resulting from their high adherent when used in high exuding wounds [133]. They display poor vapor transmission, cause bleeding, and harm the newly formed epithelium during removal. The leakage of wound exudates from traditional wound dressings promotes bacterial invasion [134].

The gelatin-based hybrid wound dressings can be used as ideal dressings to replace the traditional wound dressing products because of their interesting features when compared to the traditional dressings. Gelatin hybrid dressings provide a moist environment for injuries to recover quickly. The suitably moist environment that is offered by gelatin hybrid dressings is due to their moderate WVTR. Interestingly, gelatin-based wound dressings can be loaded with various types of bioactive agents (e.g., antibiotics, nanoparticles, microspheres, antioxidants, etc.) to improve their biological activities and speed up the wound healing process that is essential in the treatment of chronic wounds. Gelatin-based hybrid wound dressings also display good mechanical properties, excellent biocompatibility, non-toxicity, good biodegradation, high porosity, and good absorption and swelling capacity. Nevertheless, gelatin dressings suffer from poor antibacterial activity that is overcome by encapsulating selected antimicrobial agents (such as ciprofloxacin, essential oils, and metal-based nanoparticles) into them. Gelatin-based hybrid wound dressings demonstrate many distinct advantages when compared to the traditional dressings, making them promising scaffolds for the treatment of chronic and high exuding wounds.

7. Conclusions and Future Perspectives

Gelatin-based hybrid wound dressings promote accelerated wound healing and also exhibit ideal properties, such as moderate WVTR, high porosity, good mechanical performance, high water uptake and swelling behavior, good biocompatibility, antigenicity, and non-toxicity. However, the application of gelatin alone for the development of wound dressings is hampered by its poor antibacterial activity and weak mechanical performance. It is used in combination with other polymers, resulting in excellent mechanical properties that are required for ideal wound dressings. To further improve the therapeutic outcomes of gelatin-based hybrid scaffolds, they are loaded with bioactive agents. The in vitro and in vivo studies have demonstrated that the poor antimicrobial properties of gelatin are overcome by combining this biopolymer with other polymers and loading them with antibacterial agents. The loading of two bioactive agents into gelatin-based hybrid scaffolds resulted in superior biological efficacy due to synergistic effects. Interestingly, the hydrophilic nature of gelatin-based hybrid dressings does not only promote cell adhesion but also stimulates cell differentiation and proliferation, which offers a good environment for wound healing and skin regeneration. There are very few gelatin-based hybrid dressings that are under clinical trials, but many reports of in vitro and in vivo studies have shown that these hybrid dressings are promising wound dressings. Most of the reported gelatin-based wound dressings are still in the preclinical phase.

Different strategies, such as incorporating bioactive agents (such as nanoparticles, plant extracts, antibiotics, growth factors, etc.) into the prepared wound dressings, enhanced their bactericidal activity and wound healing effects. Despite the level of development of gelatin-based wound dressings attained so far, there is a pressing need for further improvements of these dressings, such as the incorporation of antibacterial agents, nanoparticles with antibacterial agents, growth factors with antibacterial agents, etc., to afford improved therapeutic outcomes. The use of gelatin biopolymers in combination with selected synthetic polymers for 3D printing to produce new wound dressing products is an alternative approach that should be explored for the preparation of effective wound dressings. The incorporation of sensors into these wound dressings for monitoring infected wounds and the healing phases is also a potential approach to developing effective wound dressings. The knowledge acquired by researchers so far on wound healing and the trend of research, together with the use of nanotechnology, represent tools that will result in effective wound dressings for treating chronic wounds.

Author Contributions: Conceptualization: S.P.N., K.N., S.A. and B.A.A.; methodology: S.P.N., K.N., S.A. and B.A.A.; investigation: S.P.N., K.N., S.A. and B.A.A.; writing—original draft preparation: S.P.N., K.N. and S.A.; writing—review and editing: S.P.N., K.N., S.A. and B.A.A.; supervision: B.A.A.; funding acquisition: B.A.A. All authors have read and agreed to the published version of the manuscript.

Funding: The financial assistance of the Govan Mbeki Research and Development Council, University of Fort Hare, Medical Research Council, and National Research Foundation, South Africa, towards this research are hereby acknowledged. The views and opinions expressed in this manuscript are those of the authors and not of MRC or NRF.

Institutional Review Board Statement: Not applicable.

Informed Consent Statement: Not applicable.

Data Availability Statement: The data presented in this study are available on request from the corresponding author.

Conflicts of Interest: The authors declare no conflict of interest.

References

1. Majd, S.A.; Khorasga, M.R.; Moshtaghian, S.J.; Talebi, A.; Khezri, M. Application of Chitosan/PVA Nanofiber as a potential wound dressing for streptozotocin-induced diabetic rats. *Int. J. Biol. Macromol.* **2016**, *92*, 1162–1168. [CrossRef]
2. Grip, J.; Engstand, R.E.; Skjaeveland, I.; Skalko-Basnet, N.; Isaksoon, J.; Basnet, P.; Holsaeter, A.M. Beta-glucan-loaded nanofiber dressing improves wound healing in diabetic mice. *Eur. J. Pharm. Sci.* **2018**, *121*, 269–280. [CrossRef] [PubMed]
3. Dhivya, S.; Padma, V.V.; Santhin, E. Wound dressings—A review. *BioMedicine* **2015**, *5*, 24–28. [CrossRef] [PubMed]
4. Boateng, J.; Matthews, K.; Steven, H.; Eccleston, G. Wound healing dressings and drug delivery systems: A review. *J. Pharm. Sci.* **2008**, *97*, 2892–2923. [CrossRef] [PubMed]
5. Patel, S.; Srivastava, S.; Singh, M.R.; Singh, D. Mechanistic insight into diabetic wounds: Pathogenesis, molecular targets and treatment strategies to pace wound healing. *Biomed. Pharmacother.* **2019**, *112*, 108615. [CrossRef] [PubMed]
6. Gaspar-pintiliescu, A.; Stanciuc, A.; Craciunescu, O. Natural composite dressings based on collagen, gelatin and plant bioactive compounds for wound healing: A review. *Int. J. Biol. Macromol.* **2019**, *138*, 854–865. [CrossRef]
7. Aderibigbe, B.A.; Buyana, B. Alginate in Wound Dressings. *Pharmaceutics* **2018**, *10*, 42. [CrossRef]
8. Chronic Wound Care Market. Available online: https://www.fortunebusinessinsights.com/industry-reports/chronic-wound-care-market-100222 (accessed on 26 April 2021).
9. Zou, F.; Sun, X.; Wang, X. Elastic, hydrophilic and biodegradable poly (1, 8-octanediol-co-citric acid)/polylactic acid nano fi brous membranes for potential wound dressing applications. *Polym. Degrad. Stab.* **2019**, *166*, 163–173. [CrossRef]
10. Huang, T.; Wang, G.; Tseng, C.; Su, W. Epidermal cells differentiated from stem cells from human exfoliated deciduous teeth and seeded onto polyvinyl alcohol/silk fi broin nano fiber dressings accelerate wound repair. *Mater. Sci. Eng. C* **2019**, *104*, 109986. [CrossRef]

11. Abid, S.; Hussain, T.; Nazir, A.; Zahir, A.; Ramakhrishna, S.; Hameed, M.; Khenoussi, N. Enhanced antibacterial activity of PEO-chitosan nanofibers with potential application in burn infection management. *Int. J. Biol. Macromol.* **2019**, *135*, 1222–1236. [CrossRef]
12. Hussain, Z.; Thu, H.E.; Shuid, A.N.; Katas, H.; Hussain, F. Recent Advances in Polymer-based Wound Dressings for the Treatment of Diabetic Foot Ulcer: An Overview of State-of-the-art. *Curr. Drug Targets* **2018**, *19*, 527–550. [CrossRef] [PubMed]
13. Dias, J.R.; Baptista-silva, S.; de Oliveira, C.M.T.; Sousa, A.; Oliveira, A.L.; Bartolo, P.J.; Granja, P.L. In situ crosslinked electrospun gelatin nano fi bers for skin regeneration. *Eur. Polym. J.* **2017**, *95*, 161–173. [CrossRef]
14. Wiwatwongwana, F.; Surin, P. In Vitro Degradation of Gelatin/Carboxymethylcellulose Scaffolds for Skin Tissue Regeneretion. *Chem. Eng. Trans.* **2019**, *74*, 1555–1560.
15. Alven, S.; Nqoro, X.; Aderibigbe, B.A. Polymer-Based Materials Loaded with Curcumin for wound healing application. *Polymers* **2020**, *12*, 2286. [CrossRef] [PubMed]
16. Han, G.; Ceilley, R. Chronic Wound Healing: A Review of Current Management and Treatments. *Adv. Ther.* **2017**, *34*, 599–610. [CrossRef] [PubMed]
17. Khan, Z.A.; Jamil, S.; Akhtar, A.; Bashir, M.M.; Yar, M. Chitosan based hybrid materials used for wound healing applications—A short review. *Int. J. Polym. Mater. Polym. Biomater.* **2020**, *69*, 419–436. [CrossRef]
18. Wang, P.; Huang, B.; Horng, H.; Yeh, C.; Chen, Y.-J. Wound healing. *J. Chin. Med. Assoc.* **2018**, *81*, 94–101. [CrossRef] [PubMed]
19. Rieger, K.A.; Birch, N.P.; Schiffman, J.D. Designing electrospun nanofiber mats to promote wound healing—A review. *J. Mater. Chem. B* **2013**, *1*, 4531–4541. [CrossRef]
20. O'Donnell, T.F.; Lau, J. A systematic review of randomized controlled trials of wound dressings for chronic venous ulcer. *J. Vasc. Surg.* **2006**, *44*, 1118–1125. [CrossRef]
21. Stoica, A.E.; Chircov, C.; Grumezescu, A.M. Nanomaterials for Wound Dressings: An Up-to-Date Overview. *Molecules* **2020**, *25*, 2699. [CrossRef]
22. Moeini, A.; Pedram, P.; Makvandi, P.; Malinconico, M.; d'Ayala, G.G. Wound healing and antimicrobial effect of active secondary metabolites in chitosan-based wound dressings: A review. *Carbohydr. Polym.* **2020**, *233*, 115839. [CrossRef]
23. Paul, W.; Sharma, C.P. Chitosan and Alginate Wound Dressings: A Short Review. *Trends Biomater. Artif. Organs* **2004**, *18*, 18–23.
24. Rujitanaroj, P.; Pimpha, N.; Supaphol, P. Wound-dressing materials with antibacterial activity from electrospun gelatin fiber mats containing silver nanoparticles. *Polymers* **2008**, *49*, 4723–4732. [CrossRef]
25. Kang, M.G.; Lee, M.Y.; Cha, J.M.; Lee, J.K.; Lee, S.C.; Kim, J.; Hwang, Y.S.; Bae, H. Nanogels derived from fish gelatin: Application to drug delivery system. *Mar. Drugs.* **2019**, *17*, 246. [CrossRef]
26. Naghibzadeh, M.; Firoozi, S.; Nodoushan, F.S.; Adabi, M.; Khoradmehr, A.; Fesahat, F.; Esnaashari, S.S.; Khosravani, M.; Adabi, M.; Tavakol, S.; et al. Application of eletrospun gelatin in tissue engineering. *Biointerface Res. Appl. Chem.* **2018**, *8*, 3048–3052.
27. Rath, G.; Hussain, T.; Chauhan, G.; Garg, T.; Goyal, A.K. Development and characterization of cefazolin loaded zinc oxide nanoparticles composite gelatin nano fi ber mats for postoperative surgical wounds. *Mater. Sci. Eng. C* **2016**, *58*, 242–253. [CrossRef]
28. Ko, J.H.; Yin, H.; An, J.; Chung, D.J. Characterization of Cross-linked Gelatin Nanofibers through Electrospinning. *Macromol. Biosci.* **2010**, *18*, 137–143. [CrossRef]
29. Agrawal, P.; Soni, A.; Mittal, G.; Bhatnagar, A. Role of polymeric biomaterials as wound healing agents. *Int. J. Low. Extrem. Wounds* **2014**, *13*, 180–190. [CrossRef] [PubMed]
30. Pham-Nguyen, O.-V.; Shin, J.U.; Yoo, H.S. Biomaterials Science mesenchymal stem cells and gelatin nano fi bers for the treatment of full-thickness wounds. *Biomater. Res.* **2020**, *8*, 4535. [CrossRef] [PubMed]
31. Xu, X.; Zhou, M. Antimicrobial Gelatin Nanofibers Containing Silver Nanoparticles. *Fibers Polym.* **2008**, *9*, 685–690. [CrossRef]
32. Schonauer, C.; Tessitore, E.; Barbagallo, G.; Albanese, V.; Moraci, A. The use of local agents: Bone wax, gelatin, collagen, oxidized cellulose. *Eur. Spine J.* **2004**, *13*, 89–96. [CrossRef]
33. Sabel, M.; Stummer, W. The use of local agents: Surgicel and Surgifoam. *Eur. Spin J.* **2004**, *13*, 97–101. [CrossRef] [PubMed]
34. Alven, S.; Aderibigbe, B. Combination Therapy Strategies for the Treatment of Malaria. *Molecules* **2019**, *24*, 3601. [CrossRef]
35. Ajovalasit, A.; Sabatino, M.A.; Todaro, S.; Alessi, S.; Giacomazza, D.; Picone, P.; Carlo, M.D.; Dispenza, C. Xyloglucan-based hydrogel films for wound dressing: Structure-property relationships. *Carbohydr. Polym.* **2018**, *179*, 262–272. [CrossRef] [PubMed]
36. Kamoun, E.A.; Kenawy, E.S.; Chen, X. A review on polymeric hydrogel membranes for wound dressing applications: PVA-based hydrogel dressings. *J. Adv. Res.* **2017**, *98*, 217–233. [CrossRef]
37. Wang, N.; Xiao, W.; Niu, B.; Duan, W.; Zhou, L.; Zheng, Y. Highly efficient adsorption of fluoroquinolone antibiotics using chitosan derived granular hydrogel with 3D structure. *J. Mol. Liq.* **2019**, *281*, 307–314. [CrossRef]
38. Hsu, Y.; Liu, K.; Yeh, H.; Lin, H.; Wu, H.; Tsai, J. Sustained release of recombinant thrombomodulin from cross-linked gelatin/hyaluronic acid hydrogels potentiate wound healing in diabetic mice. *Eur. J. Pharm. Biopharm.* **2019**, *135*, 61–71. [CrossRef]
39. Mao, Q.; Hoffmann, O.; Yu, K.; Lu, F.; Lan, G.; Dai, F.; Shang, S.; Xei, R. Self-contracting oxidized starch/gelatin hydrogel for noninvasive wound closure and wound healing. *Mater. Des.* **2020**, *194*, 108916. [CrossRef]
40. Dang, L.E.H.; Huynh, N.T.; Pham, N.O.; Nguyen, C.T.; Vu, M.T.; Dinh, V.T.; Le, V.T.; Tran, N.Q. Injectable nanocurcumin-dispersed gelatin—Pluronic nanocomposite hydrogel platform for burn wound treatment. *Bull. Mater. Sci.* **2019**, *42*, 71. [CrossRef]

41. Zheng, Y.; Liang, Y.; Zhang, D.; Sun, X.; Liang, L.; Li, J.; Liu, Y.-N. Gelatin-Based Hydrogels Blended with Gellan as an Injectable Wound Dressing. *ACS Omega* **2018**, *3*, 4766–4775. [CrossRef] [PubMed]
42. Dong, Y.; Sigen, A.; Rodrigues, M.; Li, X.; Kwon, S.H.; Kosaric, N.; Khong, S.; Gao, Y.; Wang, W.; Gurther, G.C. Injectable and tunable gelatin hydrogels enhance stem cell retention and improve cutaneous wound healing. *Adv. Funct. Mater.* **2017**, *27*, 1606619. [CrossRef]
43. Khamrai, M.; Banerjee, S.; Paul, S.; Samanta, S.; Kundu, P. Curcumin entrapped gelatin/ionically modified bacterial cellulose based self-healable hydrogel film: An eco-friendly sustainable synthesis method of wound healing patch. *Int. J. Biol. Macromol.* **2019**, *122*, 940–953. [CrossRef]
44. Treesuppharat, W.; Rojanapanthu, P.; Siangsanoh, C.; Manuspiya, H.; Ummartyotin, S. Synthesis and characterization of bacterial cellulose and gelatin-based hydrogel composites for drug-delivery systems. *Biotechnol. Rep.* **2017**, *15*, 84–91. [CrossRef]
45. Li, D.; Ye, Y.; Li, D.; Li, X.; Mu, C. Biological properties of dialdehyde carboxymethyl cellulose crosslinked gelatin-PEG composite hydrogel fibers for wound dressings. *Carbohydr. Polym.* **2016**, *137*, 508–514. [CrossRef] [PubMed]
46. Fan, L.; Yang, H.; Yang, J.; Peng, M.; Hu, J. Preparation and characterization of chitosan/gelatin/PVA hydrogel for wound dressings. *Carbohydr. Polym.* **2016**, *146*, 427–434. [CrossRef] [PubMed]
47. Sood, A.; Granick, M.S.; Tomaselli, N.L. Wound dressings and comparative effectiveness data. *Adv. Wound Care* **2014**, *3*, 511–529. [CrossRef]
48. Gupta, B.; Agarwal, R.; Alam, M. Textile-based smart wound dressings. *Indian J. Fibre Text. Res.* **2010**, *35*, 174–184.
49. Taheri, P.; Jahanmardi, R.; Koosha, M.; Abdi, S. Physical, mechanical and wound healing properties of chitosan/gelatin blend fi lms containing tannic acid and/or bacterial nanocellulose. *Int. J. Biol. Macromol.* **2020**, *154*, 421–432. [CrossRef]
50. Sakthiguru, N.; Sithique, M.A. Fabrication of bioinspired chitosan/gelatin/allantoin biocomposite fi lm for wound dressing application. *Int. J. Biol. Macromol.* **2020**, *152*, 873–883. [CrossRef]
51. Akhavan-kharazian, N.; Izadi-vasa, H. Preparation and characterization of chitosan/gelatin/nanocrystalline cellulose/calcium peroxide fi lms for potential wound dressing applications. *Int. J. Biol. Macromol.* **2019**, *133*, 881–891. [CrossRef]
52. Patel, S.; Srivastava, S.; Singh, M.R.; Singh, D. Preparation and optimization of chitosan-gelatin films for sustained delivery of lupeol for wound healing. *Int. J. Biol. Macromol.* **2018**, *107*, 1888–1897. [CrossRef]
53. Türe, H. Characterization of hydroxyapatite-containing alginate—Gelatin composite fi lms as a potential wound dressing. *Int. J. Biol. Macromol.* **2019**, *123*, 878–888. [CrossRef]
54. Cahú, T.B.; Silva, R.S.; Silva, R.P.F.; Silva, M.M.; Arruda, I.R.S.; Silva, J.F.; Costa, R.M.P.B.; Santos, S.D.; Nader, H.B.; Bezerra, R.S. Evaluation of Chitosan-Based Films Containing Gelatin, Chondroitin 4-Sulfate and ZnO for Wound Healing. *App Biochem.* **2017**, *183*, 765–777. [CrossRef] [PubMed]
55. Evranos, E.; Aycan, D.; Alemdar, N. Production of cipro fl oxacin loaded chitosan/gelatin/bone ash wound dressing with improved mechanical properties. *Carbohydr. Polym.* **2019**, *222*, 115007. [CrossRef] [PubMed]
56. Baek, S.; Park, H.; Kim, M.; Lee, D. Preparation of PCL/(+)-catechin/gelatin film for wound healing using air-jet spinning. *Appl. Surf. Sci.* **2020**, *509*, 145033. [CrossRef]
57. Garcia-orue, I.; Santos-Vizcaino, E.; Etxabide, A.; Uranga, J.; Bayat, A.; Guerrero, P.; Igartua, M.; Caba, K.; Hernandez, R.M. Development of Bioinspired Gelatin and Gelatin/Chitosan Bilayer Hydrofilms for Wound Healing. *Pharmaceutics* **2019**, *11*, 314. [CrossRef]
58. Bhowmik, S.; Islam, J.; Debnath, T.; Miah, M.; Bhattacharjee, S.M.; Khan, M. Reinforcement of gelatin-based nanofilled polymer biocomposite by crystalline cellulose from cotton for advanced wound dressing applications. *Polymers* **2017**, *9*, 222. [CrossRef]
59. Benskin, L.L. Evidence for Polymeric Membrane Dressings as a Unique Dressing Subcategory, Using Pressure Ulcers as an Example. *Adv. Wound Care* **2018**, *7*, 419–426. [CrossRef] [PubMed]
60. Xu, W.; Wang, Z.; Liu, Y.; Wang, L.; Jiang, Z.; Li, T. Carboxymethyl chitosan/gelatin/hyaluronic acid blended-membranes as epithelia transplanting sca ff old for corneal wound healing. *Carbohydr. Polym.* **2018**, *192*, 240–250. [CrossRef] [PubMed]
61. Kenawy, E.; Omer, A.M.; Tamer, T.M.; Elmeligy, M.A.; Eldin, M.S.M. Fabrication of biodegradable gelatin/chitosan/cinnamaldehyde crosslinked membranes for antibacterial wound dressing applications. *Int. J. Biol. Macromol.* **2019**, *139*, 440–448. [CrossRef]
62. Shi, R.; Niu, Y.; Gong, M.; Ye, J.; Tian, W.; Zhang, L. Antimicrobial gelatin-based elastomer nanocomposite membrane loaded with ciprofloxacin and polymyxin B sulfate in halloysite nanotubes for wound dressing. *Mater. Sci. Eng. C* **2018**, *87*, 128–138. [CrossRef]
63. Jayakumar, R.; Prabaharan, M.; Kumar, P.T.S.; Nair, S.V.; Tamura, H. Biomaterials based on chitin and chitosan in wound dressing applications. *Biotechnol. Adv.* **2011**, *29*, 322–337. [CrossRef] [PubMed]
64. Wang, X.; Zhang, D.; Wang, J.; Tang, R.; Wei, W.; Jiang, Q. Succinyl pullulan-crosslinked carboxymethyl chitosan sponges for potential wound dressing. *Int. J. Polym. Mater. Polym. Biomater.* **2017**, *66*, 61–70. [CrossRef]
65. Feng, Y.; Li, X.; Zhang, Q.; Yan, S.; Guo, Y.; Li, M. Mechanically robust and flexible silk protein/polysaccharide composite sponges for wound dressing. *Carbohydr. Polym.* **2019**, *216*, 17–24. [CrossRef]
66. Zou, Y.; Xie, R.; Hu, E.; Qian, P.; Lu, B.; Lan, G.; Lu, F. Protein-reduced gold nanoparticles mixed with gentamicin sulfate and loaded into konjac/gelatin sponge heal wounds and kill drug- resistant bacteria. *Int. J. Biol. Macromol.* **2020**, *148*, 921–931. [CrossRef] [PubMed]
67. Jinno, C.; Morimoto, N.; Ito, R.; Sukamoto, M.; Ogino, S.; Taira, T.; Suzuki, S. A Comparison of Conventional Collagen Sponge and Collagen-Gelatin Sponge in Wound Healing. *BioMed Res. Int.* **2016**, *2016*, 4567146. [CrossRef] [PubMed]

68. Ye, H.; Cheng, J.; Yu, K. In situ reduction of silver nanoparticles by gelatin to obtain porous silver nanoparticle/chitosan composites with enhanced antimicrobial and wound-healing activity. *Int. J. Biol. Macromol.* **2019**, *121*, 633–642. [CrossRef]
69. Naghshineh, N.; Tahvildari, K.; Nozari, M. Preparation of Chitosan, Sodium Alginate, Gelatin and Collagen Biodegradable Sponge Composites and their Application in Wound Healing and Curcumin Delivery. *J. Polym. Environ.* **2019**, *27*, 2819–2830. [CrossRef]
70. Lu, B.; Wang, T.; Li, Z.; Dai, F.; Lv, L.; Tang, F.; Yu, K.; Liu, J.; Lan, G. Healing of skin wounds with a chitosan—Gelatin sponge loaded with tannins and platelet-rich plasma. *Int. J. Biol. Macromol.* **2016**, *82*, 884–891. [CrossRef]
71. Singaravelu, S.; Ramanathan, G.; Raja, M.D.; Nagiah, N.; Padmapriya, P.; Kaveri, K.; Sivagnanam, U.T. Biomimetic interconnected porous keratin—Fibrin—Gelatin 3D sponge for tissue engineering application. *Int. J. Biol. Macromol.* **2016**, *86*, 810–819. [CrossRef]
72. Ye, S.; Jiang, L.; Su, C.; Zhu, Z.; Wen, Y.; Shao, W. Development of gelatin/bacterial cellulose composite sponges as potential natural wound dressings. *Int. J. Biol. Macromol.* **2019**, *133*, 148–155. [CrossRef]
73. Wen, Y. Synthesis of Antibacterial Gelatin/Sodium Alginate Sponges and Their Antibacterial Activity. *Polymers* **2020**, *12*, 1926. [CrossRef] [PubMed]
74. Liu, M.; Duan, X.; Li, Y.; Yang, D.; Long, Y. Electrospun nano fi bers for wound healing. *Mater. Sci. Eng. C* **2017**, *76*, 1413–1423. [CrossRef] [PubMed]
75. Dubsky, M.; Kubinova, S.; Sirc, J.; Voska, L.; Zajicek, R.; Zajicova, A.; Lesny, P.; Jirkovska, A.; Michalek, J.; Munzarova, M.; et al. Nanofibers prepared by needleless electrospinning technology as scaffolds for wound healing. *J. Mater. Sci. Mater. Med.* **2012**, *23*, 931–941. [CrossRef]
76. Dai, X.; Liu, J.; Zheng, H.; Wichmann, J.; Hopfner, U.; Sudhop, P.; Prein, C.; Shen, Y.; Machens, H.-G.; Schilling, A.F. Nano-formulated curcumin accelerates acute wound healing through Dkk-1-mediated fi broblast mobilization and MCP-1-mediated anti-in fl ammation. *NPG Asia Mater.* **2017**, *9*, e368. [CrossRef]
77. Li, H.; Wang, M.; Williams, G.R.; Wu, J.; Sun, X.; Lv, Y.; Zhu, L.-M. Electrospun gelatin nano fi bers loaded with vitamins A and E as antibacterial wound dressing. *RCS Adv.* **2016**, *6*, 50267.
78. Sundaramurthi, D.; Krishnan, U.M.; Sethuraman, S. Electrospun Nanofibers as Scaffolds for Skin Tissue Engineering Electrospun Nanofibers as Scaffolds for Skins. *Polym. Rev.* **2014**, *54*, 348–376. [CrossRef]
79. Ajmal, G.; Bonde, G.V.; Mittal, P.; Khan, G.; Pandey, V.K.; Bakade, B.V.; Mishra, B. Biomimetic PCL-gelatin based nano fi bers loaded with cipro fl oxacin hydrochloride and quercetin: A potential antibacterial and anti-oxidant dressing material for accelerated healing of a full thickness wound. *Int. J. Pharm.* **2019**, *567*, 118480. [CrossRef] [PubMed]
80. Bakhsheshi-rad, H.; Ismail, A.F.; Aziz, M.; Akbari, M.; Hadisi, Z.; Daroonparvar, M.; Chen, X.B. Antibacterial activity and in vivo wound healing evaluation of polycaprolactone-gelatin methacryloyl-cephalexin electrospun nanofibrous. *Mater. Lett.* **2019**, *256*, 126618. [CrossRef]
81. Adeli-sardou, M.; Mehdi, M.; Torkzadeh-mahani, M.; Dodel, M. Controlled release of lawsone from polycaprolactone/gelatin electrospun nano fi bers for skin tissue regeneration. *Int. J. Biol. Macromol.* **2019**, *124*, 478–491. [CrossRef]
82. Murat, I.; Mülaz, G. Production and characterization of bactericidal wound dressing material based on gelatin nanofi ber. *Int. J. Biol. Macromol.* **2019**, *137*, 392–404.
83. Cam, M.E.; Crabbe-Mann, M.; Alehzi, H.; Hazar-Yavuz, A.N.; Ertas, B.; Ekentox, C.; Ozcan, G.S.; Topal, F.; Guler, E.; Yazir, Y.; et al. The comparision of glybenclamide and metformin-loaded bacterial cellulose/gelatin nano fi bres produced by a portable electrohydrodynamic gun for diabetic wound healing. *Eur. Polym. J.* **2020**, *134*, 109844. [CrossRef]
84. Rather, H.A.; Thakore, R.; Singh, R.; Jhala, D.; Singh, S.; Vasita, R. Bioactive Materials Antioxidative study of Cerium Oxide nanoparticle functionalised PCL-Gelatin electrospun fi bers for wound healing application. *Bioact. Mater.* **2018**, *3*, 201–211. [CrossRef]
85. Alishahi, M.; Khorram, M.; Asgari, Q.; Davani, F.; Goudarzi, F.; Emami, A.; Arastehfar, A.; Zomorodian, K. Glucantime-loaded electrospun core-shell nano fi bers composed of poly (ethylene oxide)/gelatin-poly (vinyl alcohol)/chitosan as dressing for cutaneous leishmaniasis. *Int. J. Biol. Macromol.* **2020**, *163*, 288–297. [CrossRef] [PubMed]
86. Zhang, D.; Li, L.; Shan, Y.; Xiong, J.; Hu, Z.; Zhang, Y.; Gao, J. In vivo study of silk fi broin/gelatin electrospun nano fi ber dressing loaded with astragaloside IV on the e ff ect of promoting wound healing and relieving scar. *J. Drug Deliv. Sci. Technol.* **2019**, *52*, 272–281. [CrossRef]
87. Xia, L.; Lu, L.; Liang, Y.; Cheng, B. poly (lactic acid)/gelatin/cipro fl oxacin nano fi bers for antimicrobial wound dressing. *RSC Adv.* **2019**, *9*, 35328. [CrossRef]
88. Fallah, M.; Bahrami, S.H.; Ranjbar-mohammadi, M. Fabrication and characterization of PCL/gelatin/curcumin nanofibers and their antibacterial properties. *J. Ind. Text.* **2016**, *46*, 562–577. [CrossRef]
89. Gharaie, S.S.; Habibi, S.; Nazockdast, H. Fabrication and characterization of chitosan/gelatin/thermoplastic polyurethane blend nanofibers. *J. Text. Fibrous Mater.* **2018**, *1*, 2515221118769324.
90. Pavlinakova, V.; Fohlerová, Z.; Pavlinak, D.; Khunová, V.; Vojtová, L. Effect of halloysite nanotube structure on physical, chemical, structural and biological properties of elastic polycaprolactone/gelatin nano fi bers for wound healing applications. *Mater. Sci. Eng. C* **2018**, *91*, 94–102. [CrossRef] [PubMed]
91. Jiang, Z.; Zhao, L.; He, F.; Tan, H.; Li, Y.; Tang, Y.; Duan, X.; Li, Y. Palmatine-loaded electrospun poly (e-caprolactone)/gelatin nanofibrous scaffolds accelerate wound healing and inhibit hypertrophic scar. *J. Biomater. Appl.* **2021**, *7*, 869–886. [CrossRef]

92. Yang, X.; Yang, J.; Wang, L.; Ran, B.; Jia, Y.; Zhang, L.; Yanga, G.; Shao, H.; Jiang, X. Pharmaceutical Intermediate-Modified Gold Nanoparticles: Against Multidrug-Resistant Bacteria and Wound-Healing Application via an Electrospun Scaffold. *ACS Nano* **2017**, *11*, 5737–5745. [CrossRef] [PubMed]
93. Ong, C.T.; Lim, I.; Kee, I.; Fahamy, M.; Templonuevo, V.; Lim, C.T.; Phan, T.T. Preclinical Evaluation of Tegaderm^{TM} Supported Nanofibrous Wound Matrix Dressing on Porcine Wound Healing Model. *Adv. Wound Care* **2015**, *4*, 110–118. [CrossRef]
94. Hivechi, A.; Bahrami, S.H.; Siegel, R.A.; Milan, P.B.; Amoupour, M. In vitro and in vivo studies of biaxially electrospun poly (caprolactone)/gelatin nanofibers, reinforced with cellulose nanocrystals, for wound healing applications. *Cellulose* **2020**, *27*, 5179–5196. [CrossRef]
95. Jafari, A.; Amirsadeghi, A.; Hassanajili, S.; Azarpira, N. Bioactive antibacterial bilayer PCL/gelatin nanofibrous scaffold promotes full-thickness wound healing. *Int. J. Pharm.* **2020**, *583*, 119413. [CrossRef] [PubMed]
96. Bazmande, A.; Mirzaei, E.; Fadaie, M.; Shirian, S.; Ghasemi, Y. Dual spinneret electrospun nano fi brous/gel structure of chitosan-gelatin/chitosan-hyaluronic acid as a wound dressing: In-vitro and in-vivo studies. *Int. J. Biol. Macromol.* **2020**, *162*, 359–373. [CrossRef]
97. Yao, C.; Chen, K.; Chen, Y.-S.; Li, S.; Huang, C.-H. Lithospermi radix extract-containing bilayer nano fi ber sca ff old for promoting wound healing in a rat model. *Mater. Sci. Eng. C* **2019**, *96*, 850–858. [CrossRef]
98. Hadisi, Z.; Nourmohammadi, J.; Nassiri, S.M. International Journal of Biological Macromolecules The antibacterial and anti-inflammatory investigation of Lawsonia Inermis -gelatin-starch nano-fibrous dressing in burn wound. *Int. J. Biol. Macromol.* **2019**, *107*, 2008–2019. [CrossRef]
99. Ahlawat, J.; Kumar, V.; Gopinath, P. Carica papaya loaded poly (vinyl alcohol)-gelatin nano fi brous sca ff old for potential application in wound dressing. *Mater. Sci. Eng. C* **2019**, *103*, 109834. [CrossRef]
100. Sobhanian, P.; Khorram, M.; Hashemi, S.; Mohammadi, A. Development of nano fi brous collagen-grafted poly (vinyl alcohol)/gelatin/alginate scaffolds as potential skin substitute. *Int. J. Biol. Macromol.* **2019**, *130*, 977–987. [CrossRef] [PubMed]
101. Vázquez, N.; Garnica-Palafox, I.; Ontiveros-Tlachi, R.; Chaires-Rosas, C.; Pinon-Zarate, G.; Herrera-Enriques, M.; Hautefeuillers, M.; Vera-Graziano, R. Influence of the PLGA/gelatin ratio on the physical, chemical and biological properties of electrospun scaffolds for wound dressings In fl uence of the PLGA/gelatin ratio on the physical, chemical and biological properties of electrospun scaffolds f. *Biomed. Mater.* **2019**, *14*, 045006. [CrossRef]
102. Zahedi, P.; Rezaeian, I.; Ranaei-Siadat, S.-O.; Jafari, S.-H.; Supaphol, P. A review on wound dressings with an emphasis on electrospun nanofibrous polymeric bandages. *Polym. Adv. Technol.* **2010**, *21*, 77–95. [CrossRef]
103. Farzamfar, S.; Naseri-Nosar, M.; Samadian, H.; Mahakizadeh, S.; Tajerian, R.; Kahmati, M.; Vaez, A.; Salehi, M. Taurine-loaded poly (ε-caprolactone)/gelatin electrospun mat as a potential wound dressing material: In vitro and in vivo evaluation. *J. Bioact. Compat. Polym.* **2018**, *33*, 282–294. [CrossRef]
104. Unalan, I.; Endlein, S.J.; Slavik, B.; Buettner, A.; Goldmann, W.H.; Detsch, R.; Boccaccini, A.R. Evaluation of Electrospun Poly (ε-Caprolactone)/Gelatin Nanofiber Mats Containing Clove Essential Oil for Antibacterial Wound Dressing. *Pharmaceuticals* **2019**, *11*, 570. [CrossRef]
105. Ramalingam, R.; Dhand, C.; Leung, C.M.; Ezhilarasu, H.; Kamruddin, M.; Lakshminarayanan, R.; Ramakrishna, S.; Verma, N.K.; Arunachalam, K.D. Poly-ε-Caprolactone/Gelatin Hybrid Electrospun Composite Nanofibrous Mats Containing Ultrasound Assisted Herbal Extract: Antimicrobial and Cell Proliferation Study. *Nanomaterials* **2019**, *9*, 462. [CrossRef]
106. Niyakan, M.S.; Ehterami, A.; Haghi-Daredeh, S.; Nazarnezhad, S.; Abbaszadeh-Goudarizi, G.; Vaez, A.; Hashemi, S.F.; Rezaei, N.; Mousavi, S.R. Porous electrospun poly (ε-caprolactone)/gelatin nanofibrous mat containing cinnamon for wound healing application: In vitro and in vivo study. *Biomed. Eng. Lett.* **2020**, *10*, 149–161.
107. Samadian, H.; Salehi, M.; Farzamfar, S.; Vaez, A.; Ehterami, A.; Sahrapeyma, H.; Goodarzi, A.; Ghorbani, S. In vitro and in vivo evaluation of electrospun cellulose acetate/gelatin/hydroxyapatite nanocomposite mats for wound dressing applications. *Artif. Cells Nanomed. Biotechnol.* **2018**, *46*, 964–974. [CrossRef]
108. Zahiri, M.; Khanmohammadi, M.; Goodarzi, A.; Ababzadeh, S.; Farahani, M.S.; Mohandeshezhad, S.; Bahrami, N.; Nabipour, I.; Ai, J. Encapsulation of curcumin loaded chitosan nanoparticle within poly (ε-caprolactone) and gelatin fiber mat for wound healing and layered dermal reconstitution. *Int. J. Biol. Macromol.* **2020**, *153*, 1241–1250. [CrossRef] [PubMed]
109. Yao, C.; Lee, C.; Huang, C.; Chen, Y.; Chen, K. Novel bilayer wound dressing based on electrospun gelatin/keratin nano fi brous mats for skin wound repair. *Mater. Sci. Eng. C* **2017**, *79*, 533–540. [CrossRef] [PubMed]
110. Basar, A.; Castro, S.; Torres-giner, S.; Lagaron, J.M.; Sasmazel, H.T. Materials Science & Engineering C Novel poly (ε-caprolactone)/gelatin wound dressings prepared by emulsion electrospinning with controlled release capacity of Ketoprofen anti- in fl ammatory drug. *Mater. Sci. Eng. C* **2017**, *81*, 459–468.
111. Amer, S.; Attia, N.; Nouh, S.; El-kammar, M.; Korittum, A.; Abu-ahmed, H. Fabrication of sliver nanoparticles/polyvinyl alcohol/gelatin ternary nanofiber mats for wound healing application. *J. Biomater. Appl.* **2020**, *35*, 287–298. [CrossRef] [PubMed]
112. Cai, N.; Li, C.; Han, C.; Luo, X.; Shen, L.; Xue, Y.; Yu, F. Tailoring mechanical and antibacterial properties of chitosan/gelatin nanofiber membranes with Fe3O4 nanoparticles for potential wound dressing application. *Appl. Surf. Sci.* **2016**, *369*, 492–500. [CrossRef]
113. Shi, R.; Geng, H.; Gong, M.; Ye, J.; Wu, C.; Hu, X.; Zhang, L. Long-acting and broad-spectrum antimicrobial electrospun poly (ε-caprolactone)/gelatin micro/for wound dressing. *J. Colloid Interface Sci.* **2018**, *509*, 275–284. [CrossRef] [PubMed]

114. Semnani, D.; Poursharifi, N.; Banitaba, N.; Fakhrali, A. Electrospun polyvinylidene pyrolidone/gelatin membrane impregnated with silver sulfadiazine as wound dressing for burn. *Bull. Mater. Sci.* **2018**, *41*, 72. [CrossRef]
115. Eskandarinia, E.; Kefayat, A.; Agheb, M.; Refienia, M.; Baghbadorani, M.A.; Navid, S.; Ebrahimpour, K.; Khodabakhshi, D.; Ghahremani, F. A Novel Bilayer Wound Dressing Composed of a Dense Polyurethane/Propolis Membrane and a Biodegradable Polycaprolactone/Gelatin Nanofibrous Scaffold. *Sci. Rep.* **2020**, *10*, 3063. [CrossRef]
116. Ogawa, Y.; Azuma, K.; Izawa, H.; Morimoto, M.; Ochi, K.; Osaki, T.; Ito, N.; Okamoto, Y.; Saimoto, H.; Ifuku, S. Preparation and biocompatibility of a chitin nanofiber/gelatin composite film. *Int. J. Biol. Macromol.* **2017**, *104*, 1882–1889. [CrossRef]
117. Naseri-nosar, M.; Farzamfar, S.; Sahrapeyma, H.; Ghorbani, S.; Bastami, F.; Vaez, A.; Salehi, M. Cerium oxide nanoparticle-containing poly (ε-caprolactone)/gelatin electrospun film as a potential wound dressing material: In vitro and in vivo evaluation. *Mater. Sci. Eng. C* **2017**, *81*, 366–372. [CrossRef]
118. Joshi, A.; Xu, Z.; Ikegami, Y.; Yoshida, K.; Sakai, Y.; Joshi, A.; Kaur, T.; Nakao, Y.; Yamashita, Y.; Baba, H.; et al. Exploiting synergistic e ff ect of externally loaded bFGF and endogenous growth factors for accelerated wound healing using heparin functionalized PCL/gelatin co-spun nano fi brous patches. *Chem. Eng. J.* **2021**, *404*, 126518. [CrossRef]
119. Lv, F.; Wang, J.; Xu, P.; Han, Y.; Ma, H.; Xu, H.; Chen, S.; Chang, J.; Ke, Q.; Liu, M.; et al. A conducive bioceramic/polymer composite biomaterial for diabetic wound healing. *Acta Biomater.* **2017**, *60*, 128–143. [CrossRef]
120. Dong, Z.; Meng, X.; Yang, W.; Zhang, J.; Sun, P.; Zhang, H.; Fang, X.; Wang, D.-A.; Fan, C. Progress of gelatin-based microspheres (GMSs) as delivery vehicles of drug and cell. *Mater. Sci. Eng. C* **2021**, *122*, 111949. [CrossRef]
121. Khurshid, M.F.; Hussain, T.; Masood, R.; Hussain, N. Development and evaluation of a controlled drug delivery wound dressing based on polymeric porous microspheres. *J. Ind. Text.* **2016**, *46*, 986–999. [CrossRef]
122. Choudhari, S.J.; Singh, S.R. Microsponge—Novel drug delivery system. *Int. J. Med. Pharm. Sci. Res. Rev.* **2013**, *1*, 26–52.
123. Chen, H.; Xing, X.; Tan, H.; Jia, Y.; Zhou, T.; Chen, Y.; Ling, Z.; Hu, X. Covalently antibacterial alginate-chitosan hydrogel dressing integrated gelatin microspheres containing tetracycline hydrochloride for wound healing. *Mater. Sci. Eng. C* **2017**, *70*, 287–295. [CrossRef] [PubMed]
124. Kozlowska, J.; Stachowiak, N.; Sionkowska, A. Collagen/gelatin/hydroxyethyl cellulose composites containing microspheres based on collagen and gelatin: Design and evaluation. *Polymers* **2018**, *10*, 456. [CrossRef]
125. Fang, Q.; Yao, Z.; Feng, L.; Liu, T.; Wei, S.; Xu, P.; Guo, R.; Cheng, B.; Wang, X. Antibiotic-loaded chitosan-gelatin scaffolds for infected seawater immersion wound healing. *Int. J. Biol. Macromol.* **2020**, *159*, 1140–1155. [CrossRef] [PubMed]
126. Thyagarajan, S.L.; Ramanathan, G.; Singaravelu, S.; Kandhasamy, S.; Perumal, P.T.; Sivagnanam, U.T. Characterization and evaluation of siderophore-loaded gelatin microspheres: A potent tool for wound-dressing material. *Polym. Bull.* **2017**, *74*, 2349–2363. [CrossRef]
127. Yang, J.; Zhou, M.; Li, W.; Lin, F.; Shan, G. Preparation and Evaluation of Sustained Release Platelet-Rich Plasma-Loaded Gelatin Microspheres Using an Emulsion Method. *ACS Omega* **2020**, *5*, 27113–27118. [CrossRef]
128. Li, L.; Du, Y.; Xiong, Y.; Ding, Z.; Lv, G.; Li, H.; Liu, T. Injectable negatively charged gelatin microsphere-based gels as hemostatic agents for intracavitary and deep wound bleeding in surgery. *J. Biomater. Appl.* **2018**, *33*, 647–661. [CrossRef]
129. Zhu, Q.; Teng, J.; Liu, X.; Lan, Y.; Guo, R. Preparation and characterization of gentamycin sulfate-impregnated gelatin microspheres/collagen—Cellulose/nanocrystal scaffolds. *Polym. Bull.* **2018**, *75*, 77–91. [CrossRef]
130. Kirubanandan, S. Ciprofloxacin-Ioaded Gelatin Microspheres Impregnated Collagen Scaffold for Augmentation of Infected Soft Tissue. *Asian J. Pharm.* **2017**, *11*, 12. [CrossRef]
131. Nešović, K.; Janković, A.; Radetić, T.; Vukašinović-Sekulić, M.; Kojić, V.; Živković, L.; Perić-Grujić, A.; Rhee, K.Y.; Mišković-Stanković, V. Chitosan-based hydrogel wound dressings with electrochemically incorporated silver nanoparticles—In vitro study. *Eur. Polym. J.* **2019**, *121*, 109257. [CrossRef]
132. Alven, S.; Aderibigbe, B.A. Hyaluronic Acid-Based Scaffolds as Potential Bioactive Wound Dressings. *Polymers* **2021**, *13*, 2102. [CrossRef] [PubMed]
133. Koehler, J.; Brandl, F.P.; Goepferich, A.M. Hydrogel wound dressings for bioactive treatment of acute and chronic wounds. *Eur. Polym. J.* **2018**, *100*, 1–10. [CrossRef]
134. Sezer, A.D.; Cevher, E. Biopolymers as wound healing materials: Challenges and new strategies. In *Biomaterials Applications for Nanomedicine*; Pignatello, R., Ed.; InTech: Rijeka, Croatia, 2011; pp. 383–414.

polymers

MDPI

Review

Silver Micro-Nanoparticle-Based Nanoarchitectures: Synthesis Routes, Biomedical Applications, and Mechanisms of Action

Md Abdul Wahab [1,2,*,†], Li Luming [1,†], Md Abdul Matin [3], Mohammad Rezaul Karim [4,5], Mohammad Omer Aijaz [4], Hamad Fahad Alharbi [4,6], Ahmed Abdala [7] and Rezwanul Haque [2]

1 Institute for Advanced Study, Chengdu University, Chengdu 610106, China; liluming@cdu.edu.cn
2 School of Science, Technology and Engineering, University of the Sunshine Coast, Sippy Downs, QLD 4556, Australia; rhaque@usc.edu.au
3 Department of Pharmacy, NUB School of Health Sciences, Northern University Bangladesh, Globe Center, 24 Mirpur Road, Dhaka 1205, Bangladesh; mamatin76@yahoo.com
4 Center of Excellence for Research in Engineering Materials (CEREM), Deanship of Scientific Research (DSR), King Saud University, Riyadh 11421, Saudi Arabia; mkarim@ksu.edu.sa (M.R.K.); maijaz@ksu.edu.sa (M.O.A.); harbihf@ksu.edu.sa (H.F.A.)
5 K.A. CARE Energy Research and Innovation Center, Riyadh 11451, Saudi Arabia
6 Mechanical Engineering Department, College of Engineering, King Saud University, Riyadh 11421, Saudi Arabia
7 Chemical Engineering Program, Texas A&M University at Qatar, Doha POB 23874, Qatar; ahmed.abdalla@qatar.tamu.edu
* Correspondence: mawahab@cdu.edu.cn or mawahab@gmail.com
† Equally contributed to this paper.

Citation: Wahab, M.A.; Luming, L.; Matin, M.A.; Karim, M.R.; Aijaz, M.O.; Alharbi, H.F.; Abdala, A.; Haque, R. Silver Micro-Nanoparticle-Based Nanoarchitectures: Synthesis Routes, Biomedical Applications, and Mechanisms of Action. *Polymers* **2021**, *13*, 2870. https://doi.org/10.3390/polym13172870

Academic Editors: Bramasta Nugraha and Faisal Raza

Received: 8 July 2021
Accepted: 23 August 2021
Published: 26 August 2021

Abstract: Silver has become a potent agent that can be effectively applied in nanostructured nanomaterials with various shapes and sizes against antibacterial applications. Silver nanoparticle (Ag NP) based-antimicrobial agents play a major role in different applications, including biomedical applications, as surface treatment and coatings, in chemical and food industries, and for agricultural productivity. Due to advancements in nanoscience and nanotechnology, different methods have been used to prepare Ag NPs with sizes and shapes reducing toxicity for antibacterial applications. Studies have shown that Ag NPs are largely dependent on basic structural parameters, such as size, shape, and chemical composition, which play a significant role in preparing the appropriate formulation for the desired applications. Therefore, this review focuses on the important parameters that affect the surface interaction/state of Ag NPs and their influence on antimicrobial activities, which are essential for designing future applications. The mode of action of Ag NPs as antibacterial agents will also be discussed.

Keywords: antibacterial; pathogens; infectious diseases; silver nanoparticles

1. Introduction

With the emergence of various infectious pathogens that show resistance toward one or more antibiotics, the treatment of patients becomes very difficult, eventually leading to deaths [1–6]. These various microorganisms include bacteria, protozoans, infectious agents, fungi, viruses, and prions. More critical is that foodborne, waterborne, and airborne pathogens can also enter the body via different modes of infection [4,6,7]. Over a million deaths per annum worldwide are reported due to these harmful infectious pathogens [6]. Pathogens such as *Escherichia coli* (*E. coli*) and *Staphylococcus aureus* (*S. aureus*) and viruses, including norovirus and influenza virus, are the most reported. Such infectious pathogens can vary in virulence, contagiousness, mode of transmission, and degree of severity of the infection [5–7]. To get rid of the infections associated with pathogens, antibiotics are successfully used to treat infected patients. Still, unfortunately, the excess use of antibiotics has increased antibiotic resistance and, broadly, antimicrobial resistance [8].

Meanwhile, combined treatments, such as the use and overuse of antibiotics and other associated antimicrobial agents, have shown a higher level of multi-drug antibiotic microbial resistance (known as MDR), resulting in low treatment efficacy [9]. Therefore, the rise of resistance to harmful pathogenic microorganisms has received huge attention globally from researchers, pharmaceutical manufacturers, and medical professionals [10]. For example, a person already shown MDR will be treated with a spectrum of antibiotics even if recovery is slow. Therefore, the additional antimicrobial resistance characteristics of different pathogens will bring a severe threat to the world [11–13]. Based on the pandemic and epidemic diseases report made by the World Health Organization (WHO), the death rate for the infection with drug-resistant pathogens was high [12]. Under these circumstances, health science requires new types of disinfection systems [1–3].

In this context, with the development of nanoscience and nanotechnology, particularly, Ag NPs have become one of the most prominent disinfection systems as a disinfectant in biomedical science for several decades [1–5]. Therefore, recently, the design and development of Ag NP-based antimicrobial agents with better efficacy have received huge attention [1–3]. Ag NPs with unique characteristics including excellent control of size and shape, loading, and antibacterial activities have emerged. Some studies have even shown that the size and shape can control antibacterial activities better [14–19]. Therefore, the modifications of Ag NPs from bulky to micro-size and then to nano-size scale along with designed shapes, sizes, and targeted compositions have been found to extend the bactericidal activities of Ag NPs [20–35]. Furthermore, the surface chemistry of Ag NPs has a crucial role in their potency because of the influence exerted from physical and chemical phenomena [36–46].

A Scopus survey [47] with the keyword *'silver nanoparticle'* revealed 55,309 documents. The authors added a keyword, 'synthesis', with the Logic operator 'AND' to narrow this down. After this, 18,182 documents were revealed. To narrow down the literature further, the authors added another keyword, *'biocompatible'*, with the *'AND'* logic operator. This ultimately revealed 549 documents from the year range of 2003–2021. The analysis of the search results is shown in Figure 1 and Table 1. More and more researchers are involved in this topic, and the research interest is increasing every day. As a result, an exponential trend is observed in the published document (Figure 1).

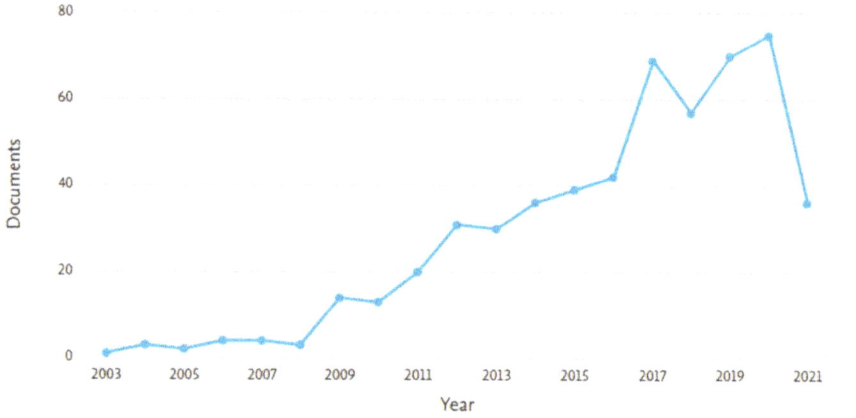

Figure 1. The number of annual publications on the topic of interest showing exponential growth (created using Scopus database [47]).

It is also evident from Table 1 that a significant number of review articles have been published on this topic (44 out of 549). However, only a handful of reviews were on silver nanoparticles [48–52]. Although various aspects were reviewed, a review article focused on the formation with different shapes and sizes, and the on-demand release of silver nanoparticles is highly demanded.

Table 1. The analysis of the search results is shown in Figure 1.

Documents Type	No. of Documents
Article	472
Review	44
Conference paper	19
Book chapter	9
Short survey	2
Conference review	1
Erratum	1
Note	1

This review focuses on the synthesis of Ag NPs by considering some individual potential factors: synthesis routes and their impact on the particle size, shape, aggregation, and composition and their antimicrobial activities will also be discussed. The mode of action and side effects of Ag NPs will be demonstrated in this review.

2. Synthesis of Ag NPs

Several synthesis methods were reported for preparing nanoengineered Ag NP-based antimicrobial agents. Significantly, the types of particles will directly affect the final properties, which are highly associated with applications [53–59]. For example, Ag NPs capped with galactose and mannose have lower toxicity against hepatocytes and neuronal-like cell lines than NPs stabilized with citrate [60]. It is expected that nanoparticles (NPs) with better biocompatibility are more suitable for biomedical fields [61–65]. Therefore, the judicious choice of the Ag NP synthesis method is crucial to produce Ag NPs with special features for desired applications, particularly biomedical applications. However, the following existing methods will be briefly discussed in the following sections as they are predominantly used to prepare Ag NPs.

2.1. Wet Chemical Synthesis Route

The conventional wet chemical routes allow the preparation of Ag NPs with different sizes and shapes through chemical transformations of the Ag precursor by varying the experimental conditions. This route consists mainly of a few materials such as a Ag metal source, solvent, stabilizing/capping agent, and reducing agent [66,67]. The reduction is usually carried out with some reducing agents such as hydrazine, citrate of sodium, and sodium dodecyl sulfate. The reduction of Ag NPs also consists of two steps: nucleation and the growth of particles.

The chemicals used to synthesize Ag NPs such as citrate, borohydride, thioglycerol, 2-mercaptoethanol, solvents, and substrates are toxic and hazardous [68–70]. Additionally, the reaction will form byproducts. Some of them are toxic and harmful to the living system. Based on the reported literature, the preparation methods of Ag NPs could be broadly classified into (i) "Top-down" and (ii) "Bottom-up" methods [68–70] as shown in Scheme 1. "Top-down" processes use mechanical force to grind the bulk of the Ag source; then, the particle stabilization is carried out via some colloidal protecting agents [68–70]. The "Bottom-up" processes include chemical reduction, electrochemical routes, and sonolytic decomposition, also known as the wet chemical process. The advantage of these chemical routes is the high yield of Ag NPs [71–75]. These routes produce particles on which surfaces are sedimented with chemicals, which require further steps to remove them. On the other hand, it is hard to prepare Ag NPs with a well-controlled size and nonaggregated morphology. Therefore, an additional step is needed to prevent the aggregation of particles [76–80].

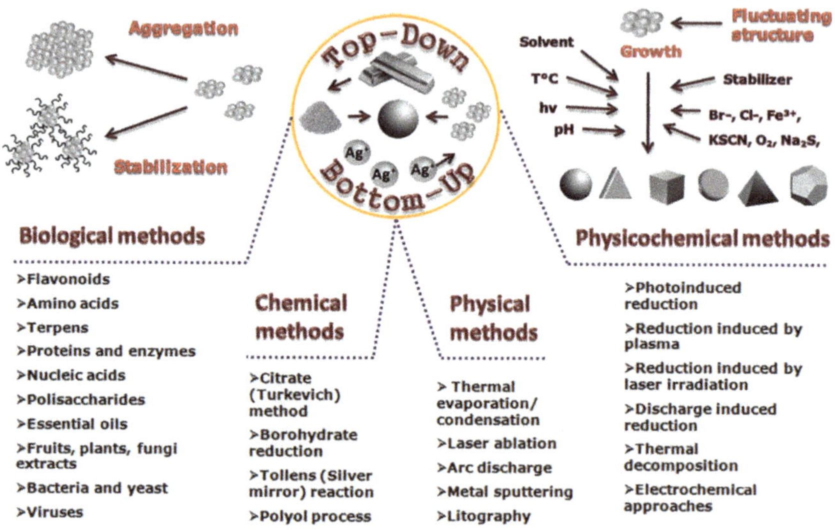

Scheme 1. The synthesis scheme of Ag NPs via various methods GO (adapted with permission from reference [67]).

2.2. Physical Synthesis Routes

The physical synthesis routes mainly use force/pressure (mechanical grinding), temperature, electromagnetic radiation, and energy [67,81–88]. The advantages of physical routes are speed, minimal chemical consumption, and no hazardous agents involved. Still, they require high energy for the process and produce an extensive range of particles with low yield [67,68]. The "Top-down" approach is usually based on physical synthesis routes, which are less expensive, fast, and simple techniques than wet chemical routes. For example, the arc discharge is often employed for pure Ag atomization for forming Ag NPs [81]. Based on various studies, the shape and size of Ag NPs can easily be controlled by employing different synthetic conditions and media [84]. The synthesis medium has a significant impact on the shape, size, distribution, and aggregation of Ag NPs. Additionally, oxygen might help form the unexpected Ag_2O instead of metallic Ag NPs, even by using an Ar jet at the interaction zone. Other methods, including sputtering, plasma during gas-phase synthesis, and lithography, are also used to prepare Ag NPs. Among these methods, lithography offers better control over the shape and size [82]. It should also be noted that lithography is a highly labor-intensive process that will provide rather expensive products.

2.3. Green/Biological Synthesis Route

Recently, the bioinspired method for the preparation of Ag NPs has become an alternative process to other reported methods because it is cost-effective, facile and straightforward, reliable, and more environmentally friendly. Therefore, tremendous attention has been devoted to preparing Ag NPs with various sizes and shapes using different biological approaches [89–95]. For example, Ganaie et al. [80] have reported the green synthesis of Ag NPs with controlled shape and size using weed mimosa. The process is more economical and could improve the economics of the production of Ag NPs. In the meantime, various kinds of Ag NPs were reported via green and biocompatible approaches without chemicals, including toxic agents [58,88,96–102]. These studies have suggested alternative preparing methods for the synthesis of Ag NPs, which largely depend on the following factors: the solvent, the reducing agent, and the non-toxic material. The great benefit of these biological approaches is the availability of various functional groups, including amino acids, proteins, or secondary metabolites, and a vast array of biological resources.

In contrast, the disadvantage of these methods is the additional steps needed to prevent the formation of nanoparticle aggregation. Overall, the preparation of Ag NPs was found to be very eco-friendly, cost-effective, and pollution-free in comparison to chemical-dependent processes. These methods produce NPs with a controlled size and shape [88,97–102], which are critical factors that should be considered for different biomedical-based applications.

2.4. *Size and Shape That Contribute to the Inhibition of Bacterial Growth*

Many studies have shown that the type of Ag NPs, including in terms of their size, shape, and concentration, has a significant impact on the inhibition process of the growth of bacteria [1–3,67–69,88,97–102]. For example, those Ag NPs having a similar active surface area will display how the shape of the particle can inhibit the growth of bacteria. Additionally, the active facets of the employed nanoparticles show different interactions with microorganisms. The wet chemical method mediated two Ag NPs that were prepared: (i) spherical of 15–90 nm and (ii) triangular of a ~150 nm size. Spherical particles of 15–90 nm have better antibacterial performance than triangular particles of a ~150 nm size against *Pseudomonas aeruginosa* and *Escherichia coli* [55]. Therefore, results have suggested that size does matter to penetrate bacterial cells [53,55,57] effectively. The spherical Ag NPs dominated by the (111) facets have effectively killed bacteria compared to the triangular-shaped Ag NPs [55,102], suggesting that each facet interacts differently with the bacterial surface [53,57]. Additionally, the highly reactive facets (111) with Ag NPs of <10 nm in size can effectively kill the bacteria cells via tagging Ag NPs into the sulfur-containing membrane [53], which is consistent with the previously reported antibacterial studies that focused on three sizes of stable Ag NPs (5, 15, and 55 nm mean values) tested against various bacteria [16,57,59].

2.5. *Role of Support and Stabilizer*

Ag NPs with different shapes and sizes have already displayed strong antibacterial activity against infectious pathogens, but particle instability in different media remains challenging. The size and aggregation of Ag NPs show dependency on the type of employed media. The stability of NPs is enhanced by using suitable stabilizing agents, which can prevent the agglomeration and precipitation of NPs during synthesis [60,103–108]. Among the stabilizers, polyvinyl pyrrolidone (PVP) is more effectively employed for controlling the size and agglomeration of NPs [109–114]. Therefore, its presence as the stabilizing agent can enhance their final functional activities because of structural advantages. The homogeneous dispersion of Ag NPs can enhance the antibacterial activity of pure supports such as carbon nitride against infectious pathogens [115]. Roman et al. [116] have reported Ag NPs under different polymeric stabilizers. The study suggested that 0.01% of sodium carboxymethylcellulose (CMC) can form better nanoparticles. Another study was conducted by Jung et al. [117] on the effects of polymeric stabilizers for the formation of various Ag NPs. Based on the coordination of Ag^+ ions with PVP and poly(4-styrene sulfonic acid-co-maleic acid) sodium salt (PSSMA), it is suggested that PSSMA has better controllability over the final morphology of nanoparticles [117].

2.6. *The Functional Properties of Ag NPs*

Physical and chemical properties of Ag NPs are highly dependent on size and shape, distribution, type of morphology/facet, surface chemistry, surface area, composition, aggregation, and Ag^0/Ag^+, and all these factors will play a role in antibacterial activities. Additionally, the type of employed reducing agent and synthesis methods for preparing Ag NPS will have a significant role in determining cytotoxicity and inhibiting bacterial growth [61,63,118–131]. Various kinds of Ag NPs can easily be manipulated by different synthesis routes that will control the shape and sizes and impact the final materials' toxicity, particularly for biomedical applications [132–138]. Studies have shown that particles with smaller dimensions can produce more toxicity than those larger particles employed because they have a larger surface area and due to their ability to penetrate the cell/membrane of bacteria [1–3,17–19,26,132–135,138]. The role of types of shapes and facets cannot be ruled out for controlling the toxicity of Ag NPs [26,133–135]. Suresh et al. [134] reported the comparative analysis on the effects of different surface coatings to prepare various Ag NPs via chemical and or biological coating methods. Results suggested that either method on the NPs surface can significantly affect the toxicity [134]. Ag NP surface charges also determine the toxicity effect in cells. More prominently, Tabata et al. [135] have reported that positive charges of NPs can stay for a long time in the bloodstream compared to negatively charged NPs [66,135], which is a major route for the administration of anticancer agents reported by other groups of authors [26,135].

3. Applications

Ag NPs have already become known as broad-spectrum antimicrobial agents, and their antibacterial activities depend on the nature and type of Ag NPs. However, Ag has been used by humankind for many years [1–3]. For example, Ag plays a significant role against some infections developed by infectious pathogens.

3.1. Burn and Wound Healing

The applications of Ag NPs are not limited to these: medical, antiseptic sprays, wound dressings, and thin antibacterial coatings on the surface of medical devices for preventing infection against infectious pathogens [1–3,8,9,56]. For example, Zhou et al. [63] have reported graphene-supported Ag/AgCl nanoparticles under various conditions in Figures 2 and 3 against antimicrobial activity, and burn wound healing was assessed. Figure 2 also shows how to control the size and shape of Ag/AgCl NPs using the poly(diallyl dimethylammonium chloride) (PDDA) surfactant and graphene oxide (GO) sheets. Both PDDA and GO are also included in Figure 2. In this study, the presence of oxygen in GO functions as a site for coating the Ag NPs and prohibited the formation of the agglomeration of Ag NPs. The attached PDDA surfactant molecules on GO further enhanced the prevention of the aggregation of Ag NPs, which was confirmed by an image in Figure 3f. Therefore, the synergistic ability from both PDDA and GO has enabled the ultrafine-sized Ag/AgCl NPs in Figure 3. Among the images in Figure 3, Figure 3a shows that particles with less than 10 nm are uniformly distributed over the surface of GO sheets. In contrast, Figure 3b,c confirm the homogenous distribution of 4 nm Ag NPs on the rGO sheets facilitated by ultrasonication, which is well-consistent with previous reports on how the employed method impacts the formation of metal nanoparticles on the support [115]. These NPs were tested for antibacterial performance and suggested for the burn wound healing process, as displayed in Figures 4 and 5 against Gram-negative and Gram-positive pathogens.

The antibacterial performance of the Ag/AgCl/rGO against *Escherichia Coli* (*E. coli*) and *Staphylococcus aureus* (*S. aureus*) was evaluated qualitatively in Figure 4. The Ag/AgCl/rGO-based agent has shown antibacterial activity against both bacteria based on the presence of inhibition zones. The growth kinetics profile of the employed pathogens in the Luria–Bertani (LB) medium in Figure 5 has confirmed the dose-dependent antibacterial effect of the Ag/AgCl/rGO. The minimum inhibitory concentrations (MICs) for Ag/AgCl/rGO in Figure 5 against *E. coli* and *S. aureus* were found to be 2 and 4 mg L^{-1}, respectively, and the complete inhibition was reported at 10 mg L^{-1} for *E. coli* and *S. aureus* 10 mg L^{-1}. The result from the biocompatibility is at <5 mg L^{-1}, while antibacterial activity against both bacteria performed well. On the other hand, the burn wounds of healthy mice were treated with the Ag/AgCl/rGO sample for two weeks. A negligible scab was noted for Ag/AgCl/rGO-treated mice, while the control showed a big scab, indicating that the Ag/AgCl/rGO-treated burn wound had a fast-healing rate and epidermis regeneration.

Recently, Wahab et al. [115] used an in situ ultrasonication process to incorporate Ag NPs along with a single C-N precursor into the pore size (PS) (9.17 nm) of SBA15 silica to prepare highly nanoporous carbon nitride (NCN)-supported Ag NPs (NCN-Ag NPs).

The resulting Ag NPs with less than 8 nm in NCN were tested against both wild type and multidrug-resistant *E. coli* pathogens, as shown in Figure 6.

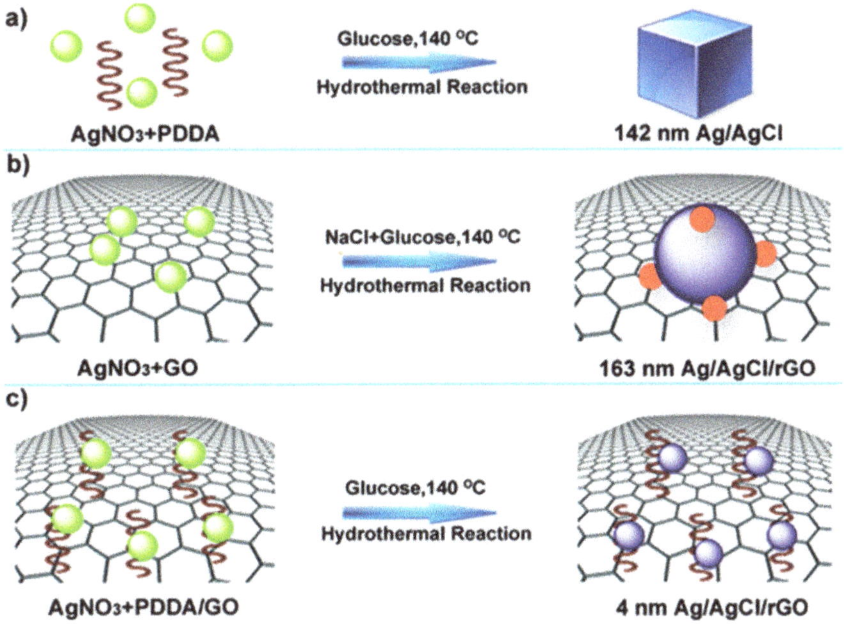

Figure 2. Schematic illustration of the size and shape of Ag/AgCl NPs controlled by (**a**) the PDDA surfactant, (**b**) GO sheets, and (**c**) both PDDA and GO (adapted with permission from reference [63]).

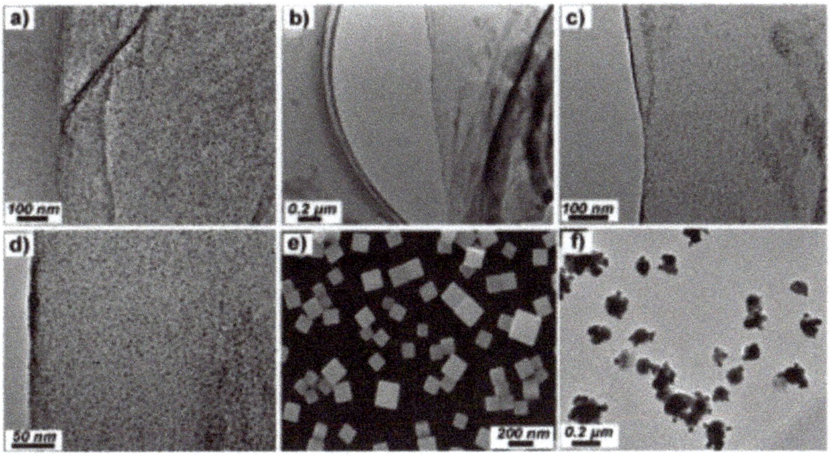

Figure 3. TEM images of Ag NPs: (**a**) Ag/AgCl/GO and (**b**–**d**) Ag/AgCl/rGO synthesized in the presence of GO and PDDA, (**e**) scanning electron microscope (SEM) images of Ag/AgCl synthesized in the presence of the PDDA surfactant, and (**f**) TEM image of Ag/AgCl/rGO synthesized without PDDA (adapted with permission from reference [63]).

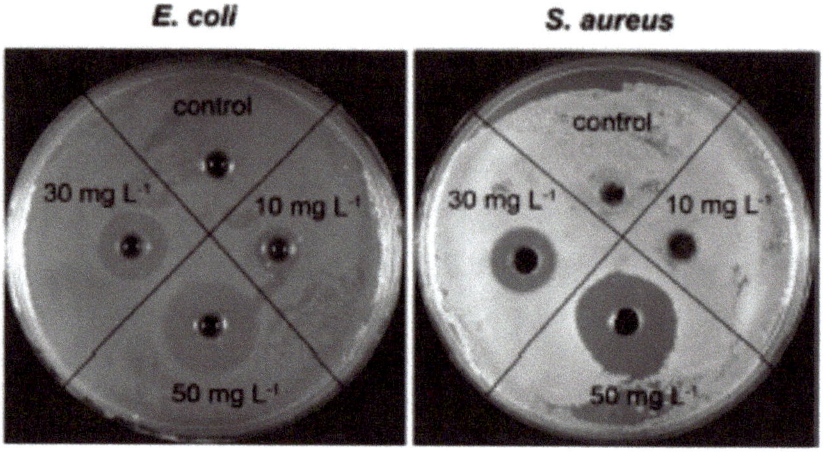

Figure 4. Photographs of *E. coli* and *S. aureus* grown around a series of concentrations of Ag/AgCl/rGO nanomaterials on the plates (adapted with permission from reference [63]).

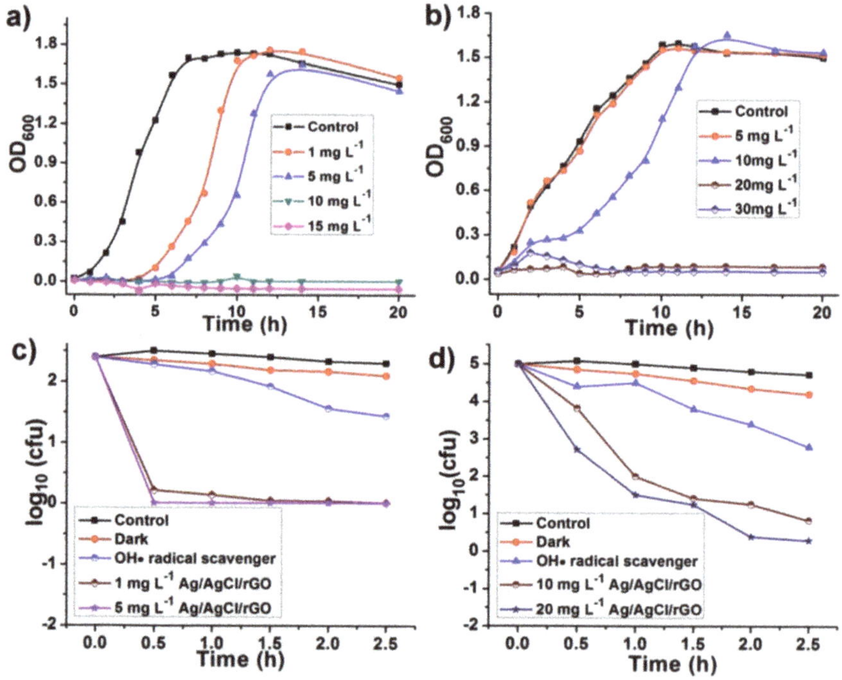

Figure 5. Growth profile in LB medium with serial concentrations of Ag/AgCl/rGO nanomaterial added to the culture of (**a**) *E. coli* and (**b**) *S. aureus*. Bacteria time–kill profiles within 2.5 h for (**c**) *E. coli* in the presence of 1 or 5 mg L^{-1} Ag/AgCl/rGO nanomaterial and (**d**) *S. aureus* in the presence of 10 or 20 mg L^{-1} Ag/AgCl/rGO nanomaterial. The bacteria time−kill profiles of *E. coli* (**c**) and *S. aureus* (**d**) treated with Ag/AgCl/rGO were also performed in a dark environment or with the OH* radical scavenger (adapted with permission from reference [63]).

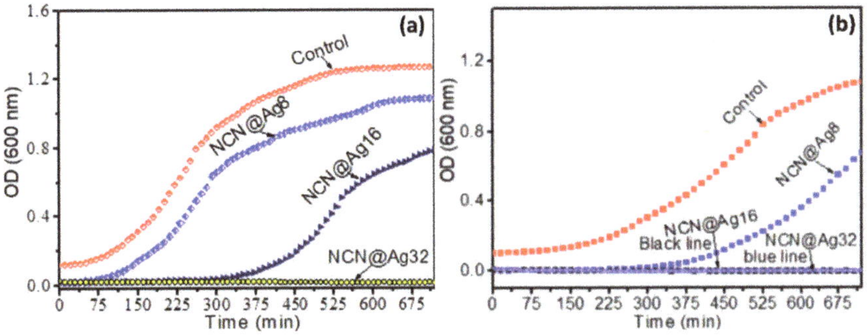

Figure 6. (**a**) Growth profiles of wild-type *E. coli* and (**b**) of MDR *E. coli* strains in the presence of control and various concentration of NCN@Ag NPs (adapted with permission from reference [115]).

Pure NCN was less effective against both pathogens, but NCN-supported Ag NPs have shown excellent antibacterial performance against both pathogens tested. It was reported that the complete inhibition at 32 μg/mL for the wild type and 16 μg/mL for the multidrug-resistant strain was achieved, indicating that MDR *E. coli* was found to be more susceptible in the presence of NCN@Ag NPs than wild-type *E. coli*. It should be noted that NCN alone could not show such antibacterial performance, but the presence of homogeneously dispersed Ag NPs in the NCN support efficiently inhibited the growth of both bacteria.

Microbial infection becomes a serious complication when it occurs in burn and wound sites [139–143]. In this context, Ag NPs/Ag NP-based composites play an essential role in wound healing/dressing applications [139–143]. Pat et al. [140] have reported Ag NPs (5–12 nm)/bacterial cellulose (BC) composites (Ag/BC) by the photochemical reduction process using UV radiation against *E. coli* for wound-healing [140]. The minimum amount of Ag NPs incorporated in BC showed the maximum ability to kill bacteria, even for a longer amount of time. The specific amount of Ag released after a specific time indicated the stability of the Ag NPs within BC and reduced the risk of toxicity if applied in wound healing [140]. Recently, Jin et al. [141] investigated the possible applications of the synergistic and on-demand release of Ag NPs-AMPs (antimicrobial peptide) incorporated into porous silicon for antibacterial and wound healing processes. In this study, the wound site was loaded with a Ag NPs-AMP@PSiMPs composite. The results have shown outstanding in vivo bacteria-killing activity, accelerated wound-healing, and low biotoxicity in an *S. aureus*-infected rat wound model [141]. Based on the results, the authors have suggested that this research could be useful as an on-demand release to fight wound infection and promote wound healing. More studies on Ag-NPs-based composites were reported [139–143].

3.2. Eco-Friendly and Biocompatible Application

Recently, green synthesis-mediated Ag NPs have been more preferred for biomedical applications than physical and chemical route-mediated Ag NPs because NPs from green synthesis are more eco-friendly, safe, biocompatible, and effective. For example, Azizi et al. [61] synthesized Ag NPs using hydrogel beads based on k-Carrageenan. Briefly, the Ag NPs were synthesized in aqueous *Citrullus colocynthis* seed extract. *Citrullus colocynthis* was used as both a reducing and capping agent, and cross-linked k-Carrageenan/Ag NPs hydrogel beads were also fabricated with the assistance of KCl. Green synthesis-mediated Ag NPs were effective as an antibacterial agent against *S. aureus*, Methicilin Resistant *S. aureus*, *P. aeruginosa*, and *E. coli*, with maximum zones of inhibition of 11 ± 2 mm.

Figure 7 shows how Ag NP concentration affected color, which changed from dark yellow to dark brown [61]. FESEM studies confirmed the formation of spherical Ag NPs of less than 25 nm. This study also conducted cytotoxicity as shown in Figure 8. The values of growth of inhibition at 1000 μg/mL were found to be much lower than 50%, indicating that the employed bio-nano composites do not have any toxicity effect, damaging elements for living cells. This could be a new avenue where hydrogels with the reported level of toxicity should impact pharmacological potential.

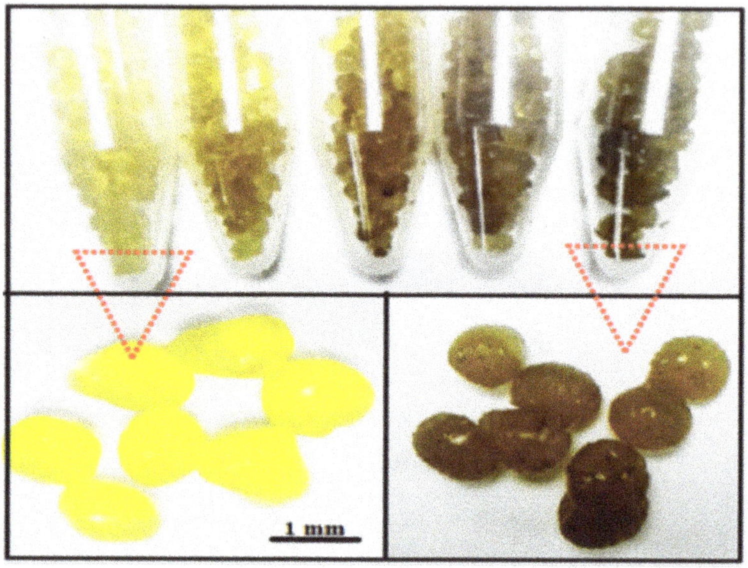

Figure 7. Digital image of Kappa-Carrageenan/Ag bio-nano composite with the various ratios of Ag-NPs (adapted with permission from reference [61]).

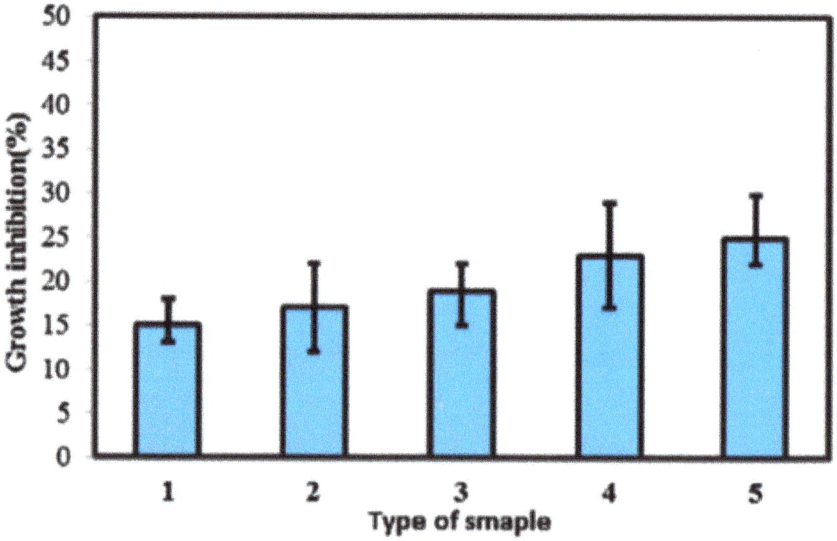

Figure 8. Cytotoxic effect of hydrogel Kappa-Carrageenan/Ag nanocomposites on the growth inhibition of VERO cells (adapted with permission from reference [61]).

Among the studied pathogens, the antibacterial activity of PP-Ag NPs has shown the highest inhibition against *E. coli* (16.33 ± 0.14 mm) at a 40 μL concentration. In addition to the antibacterial application, free radical scavenging, anticancer, larvicidal, anti-acetylcholinesterase, reusability, and durability have also been assessed, and an associated discussion is available in [61].

3.3. Enhancing Tribological Properties

Recently, alloy nanoparticles of metals have become popular in biomaterial applications since combining two metals can provide enhanced functional activities, including stability, chemical, and tribological properties [65,120]. Vijayalakshmi et al. [119] have used various stabilizing agents to form a Ag@SnO_2 core–shell. The antibacterial activity of chalcone dendrimer stabilized Ag@SnO_2 core–shell NPs was tested against multiple pathogens, including *Bacillus subtilis*, *Proteus mirabilis*, *Candida albicans*, and *Aspergillus niger*. Interestingly, antibacterial activity against the Bacillus subtilis was more effective among the tested pathogens, whereas it did not show any activity against *Aspergillus niger*. In contrast, it acted mildly as an antibacterial agent against *Proteus mirabilis* and *Candida albicans*.

Torres et al. [120] demonstrated Ag NP-coated Ti porous substrates and dense particles against *S. aureus*, as shown in Figure 9, using a substrate of 40% of porosity [120]. Based on the inhibition experiment, particles with porosity are more effective toward antibacterial activity because more Ag NPs can be embedded into the wall of large pores of the porous Ti substrate.

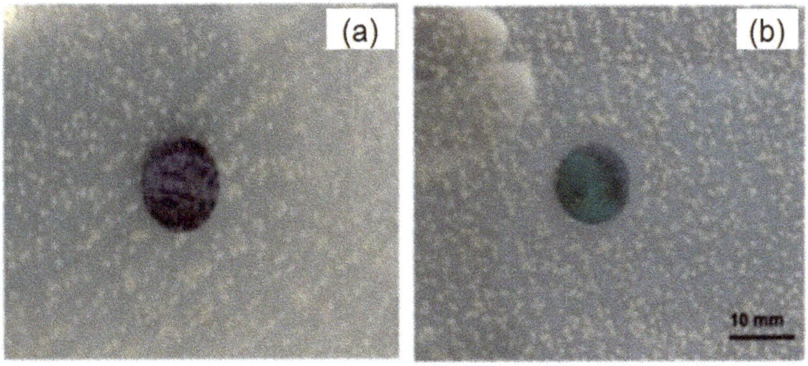

Figure 9. Inhibition experiments: images for 355–500 um after silanization and before Ag NP coating (**a**) and after Ag NP coating (**b**). Ten millimeter scale bar for both images (adapted with permission from reference [120]).

Iqbal et al. [64] demonstrated Ag_2O NPs with a dominated crystallite size of 64.3 nm from the plane (111) via the wet chemical route. To support their use as an anticancer agent, cellular adsorption, phototoxicity analysis, and reactive oxygen species (ROS) analysis were systematically carried out. Figure 10 shows how the concentration of Ag_2O NPs has impacted the percentage loss in cell viability.

The significant loss in cell viability occurred when the concentration of Ag_2O NPs was 60 mg/mL. Afterward, no change in the loss in cell viability is found, indicating that the optimal concentration of Ag_2O NPs is (60 mg/mL) [64]. Figure 11 displays the ROS study results using the fluorescence which was found to depend on the employed concentration of Ag_2O NPs [64]. The obtained results suggested that after a certain concentration, Ag_2O NPs are found to be very toxic, which might be helpful for biomedical and clinical applications, as indicated by the authors. Based on the various analysis, Ag_2O NPs have bio-interaction characteristics and physicochemical properties as an anticancer agent. This study was limited to spherical particles of 64.3 nm, but any analysis that can be carried out on less than 64.3 nm along with different particle facets might have more interesting results.

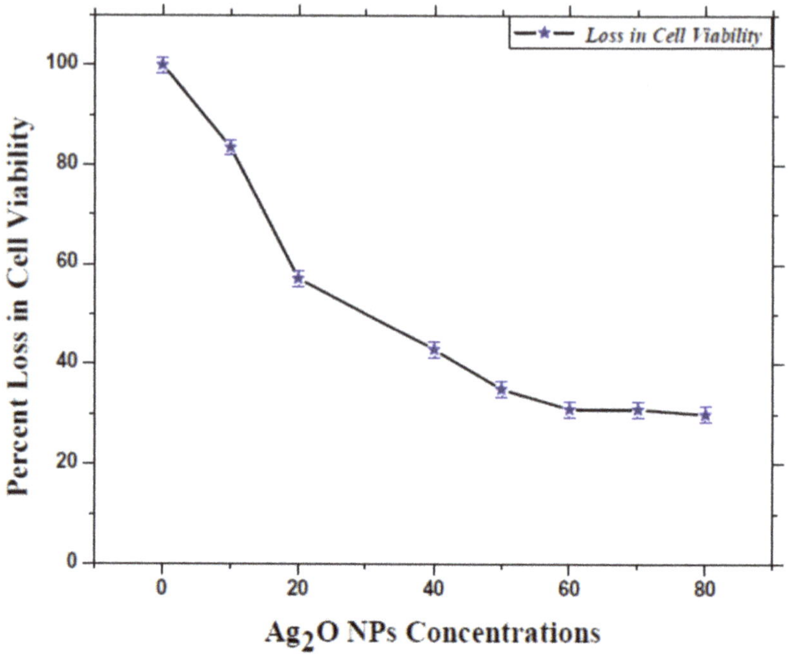

Figure 10. Percent cell viability loss in HepG2 cell viability (adapted with permission from reference [64]).

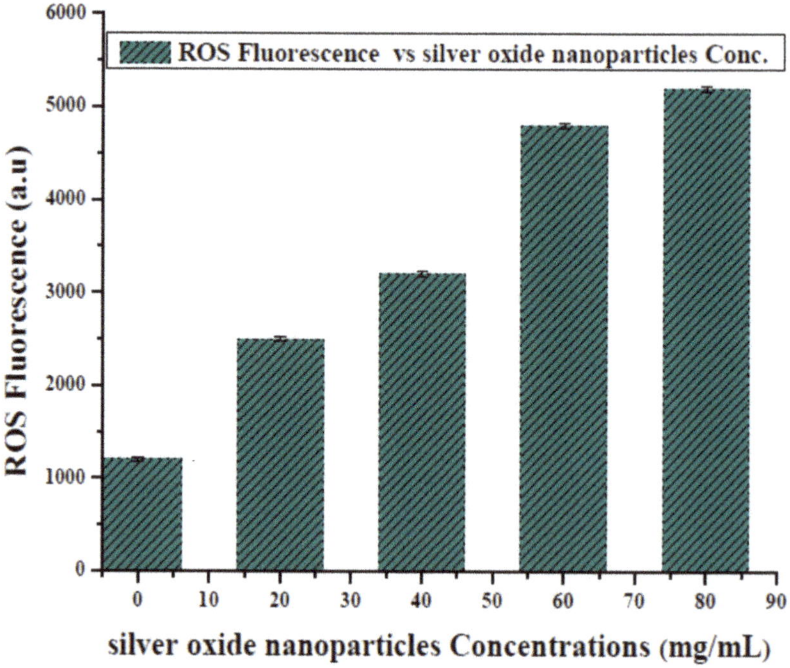

Figure 11. ROS fluorescence (a.u) for silver oxide nanoparticles exposed in in vitro HepG2 model (adapted with permission from reference [64]).

3.4. Aerobic and Anaerobic Environmental Activities

Interestingly, Park et al. [118] have reported ROS generation by Ag ions in the presence or absence of oxygen. Their anti-bactericidal activity was well-compared against *E. coli* and *S. aureus* in Figure 12. For the aerobic environment, 0.5 mg/L Ag ions required 2.2 log inactivation of *E. coli* in 60 min. In contrast, the same dose of Ag ions affected ~0.5 log inactivation for the anaerobic environment. As seen in Figure 12b, aerobic conditions have inactivated more efficiently than anaerobic conditions, suggesting that in the presence of O_2, Ag ions killed bacteria effectively due to the production of superoxide radicals. This study has suggested that superoxide-radical-independent antibacterial activity is due to the thiol-interaction mechanism of Ag ions. Under the same conditions, a similar antibacterial activity was demonstrated against *S. aureus* in Figure 12c,d and suggested that Ag ions' superoxide-radical-facilitated extra inactivation ability towards killing bacteria could be a general phenomenon [118].

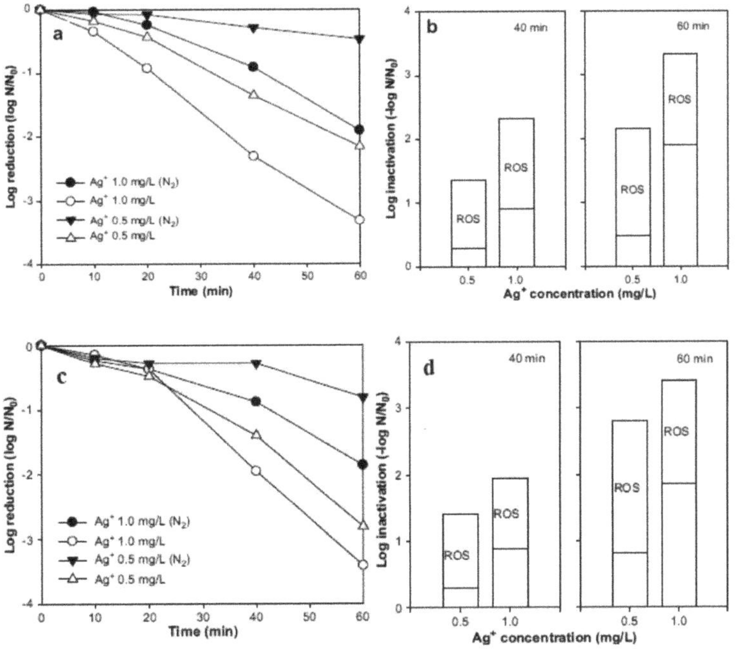

Figure 12. (**a**) The effect of Ag ions on the inactivation of *E. coli* ATCC8739 in the absence or presence of oxygen. (**c**) The effect of silver ions on the inactivation of *S. aureus* ATCC6538. (**b**,**d**) The proportion of ROS-mediated inactivation by silver ions at 40 and 60 min (N_0 = 10^6 CFU/mL, pH 7.1) (adapted with permission from reference [118]).

Xiu et al. [121] systematically demonstrated the antibacterial activity of Ag NPs through manipulation of oxygen availability, particle size, shape, and/or type of coating. As depicted in Figure 13, it is evident that the presence of oxygen indeed has a significant impact on the killing of *E. coli*, which is consistent with other reported works [118].

According to the toxicity assay, aerobic conditions enhanced the toxicity of the system. Therefore, Ag^+ ions released during the toxicity assay showed a significant antimicrobial effect, and even prolonged air exposure showed more impact on antibacterial toxicity of Ag NPs of 5 nm. These results evidenced that the toxicity of Ag NPs is quite sensitive to oxygen availability, and oxidative dissolution of the crystalline cores can result under an aerobic environment and increase the concentration of soluble Ag^+ ions, which are needed to have a significant impact on the antibacterial activity [118,121].

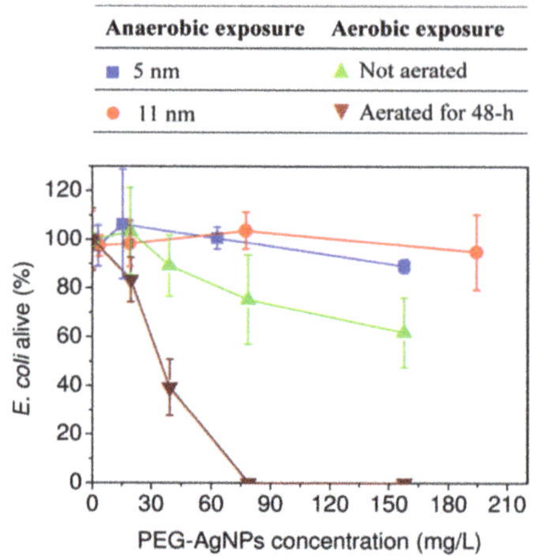

Figure 13. Antibacterial action of Ag NPs under aerobic and anaerobic atmosphere (adapted with permission from reference [121]).

3.5. *Important Parameters That Control the Mechanism of Action*

Based on the available literature [1–5,122,123,125–128], since the 1800s, Ag NPs have been used for food handling, currency, and preventing wound infections. Recently, the applications of Ag NPs have been tremendously expanded into various emerging advanced biomedical areas. Most of the reported studies have described the antimicrobial activity of Ag NPs due to the presence of Ag in the system. The addition of Ag NPs into the growth media of pathogens/bacteria will push Ag NPs towards the membrane of bacteria and possibly form the aggregation of Ag NPs that will slowly deteriorate the integrity of the bacterial membrane. Finally, cell death will occur [8,58,59].

Additionally, the overall mechanism of the antibacterial activity largely depends on the interaction between pathogens employed by Ag NPs. The particle size controls the interaction since small particles have a different interaction with the bacterial membrane than larger particles [8,58,59,121]. Figure 14 shows several phenomena affecting Ag NP dissolution, which will inhibit the growth of bacteria [5].

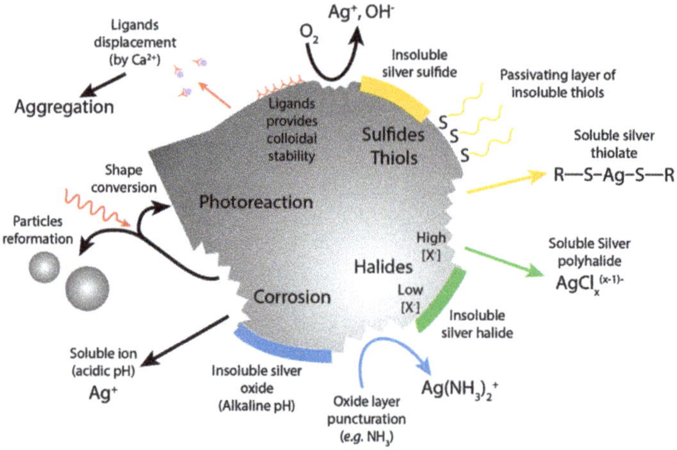

Figure 14. Summary of the factors affecting Ag NP dissolution and inhibition of growth of bacteria (adapted with permission from reference [5]).

Since the first few reports of Ag particles, most of the studies have used the following factors that helped to develop the mode of action against antibacterial activity, which are highly related to each other [1–3,8,9,56]. Based on the above discussion, we can summarize the following factors already discussed for the mechanism of action.

(i) One of the main components is the design of the effective and potent antibacterial system that influences the overall mode of action since the mode of action of Ag NPs against pathogens is highly dependent on some factors such as modification, aggregation, size, shape, dissolution, ROS production, the release of adsorbed silver species, adsorption or desorption of ions, and the nature of polymers/supports/surfaces of supports [1–3,8,9,56].

(ii) The type of silver species (Ag^0/Ag^+) can be produced when a Ag source is added into the growth media of bacteria because the production of Ag particles in the media will first penetrate the cell wall of bacteria and react with peptidoglycans [125,127]. It is also noted here that the degree of interaction between the cell wall of bacteria and Ag NPs will be primarily controlled by previously mentioned parameters such as size, shape, aggregation, and type of Ag species already existing in the media.

(iii) The binding of Ag NPs to the cell wall of bacteria will release Ag^+ ions that will show toxicity to kill the bacteria. Ag NPs can easily bind to membrane proteins, which can significantly affect the membrane's permeability and lead to the breakage of cells [130]. Additionally, Ag NPs that bind to membrane proteins can significantly affect the uptake and release of phosphate ions, thus disrupting the respiratory chain and energy production [130].

(iv) Smaller particles can bind more effectively to the membrane and penetrate the cell wall of bacteria, and final inhibition of transcription occurs. The penetration of Ag NPs into the cell is also associated with intracellular structural components such as lipids, proteins, and DNA [130]. More clearly, they can damage DNA and act on protein synthesis [129].

(v) The produced ROS will affect cell membrane disruption and DNA modification. As the process goes on, the continuous release of Ag NPs' Ag+ ions is more and more considered to be the mechanism of destroying infectious pathogens [128]. Thus, the result of cell death is a consequence of their action from this process [129].

3.6. Side Effects of Ag NPs

Since the 1800s, the applications of Ag NPs have been expanded in different areas, including environmental, biomedical, and domestic appliances. Moreover, recently, the development of nanomedicines using NPs is one of the promising strategies to combat various diseases, including infectious pathogen-caused diseases. Therefore, research on Ag NPs is carried out with different shapes and sizes, and how they impact users should be investigated thoroughly since each type of Ag NP particle shows not only a different level of toxicity but also antibacterial activity, which is highly related to size, shape, and concentration [1–3,10,67]. It is found that a smaller size of particles has shown better penetration ability. For example, if higher doses release more Ag NPs in aqueous media, this might lead to severe health complications [1–3,8,9,56]. Thus, it could be fairly suggested that caution in their use and further investigation of the mechanism of action based on available employed Ag NPs are necessary for avoiding long-term consequences. Based on the literature, it could be fairly suggested that Ag NPs could reach the body's vital organs (such as lungs, intestine, liver, and so on) through the skin as nanosilver may penetrate more easily than micro/macro-silver particles. Eventually, the availability of such small nanoparticles might sometimes create some toxicity around the organs, leading to serious complications [128,144–146].

4. Conclusions and Outlook

Bacterial infections have become one of the main health concerns because more than a million deaths worldwide per annum are the result of these highly infectious pathogens. It is found that the absence of effective treatments will lead to various types of serious health complications. In addition, MDR is becoming another key problem in clinical scenarios. In this context, the use of Ag NPs at the nanoscale could provide an opportunity for antibacterial treatments because the nanosized effects and exotic behavior of Ag NPs have produced some outstanding characteristics including biological properties related to biomedical applications.

The research reviewed in this article has comprehensively demonstrated synthesis routes and their impacts on the formation of particles, shapes, and biomedical applications of Ag NPs, particularly focusing on the antibacterial activity of various infectious pathogens and their mechanisms. As discussed, because of multi-drug resistance, both researchers from academia and industry have explored Ag NPs as a possible alternative broad-spectrum antibacterial agent for reducing the risk of microbial infections. Hence, the design and development of Ag NP antibacterial agents over the last several years has been found to be one of the promising approaches to combatting diseases caused by various microorganisms. It is noteworthy to mention that Ag NPs of less than 10 nm are found to be more effective in inhibiting the growth of bacteria.

If this becomes true, it will help nanoscience and nanotechnology researchers to develop safer, biocompatible, and efficient antibacterials based on Ag NPs. Nonetheless, studies dealing with Ag NPs' biocompatibility of interaction with cells and tissues are inevitable to avoid risks to human health as well as the environment since the overdose of Ag NP-based agents could have long-term adverse effects on both humans and the environment. Such detailed studies will provide sound ground to treat various infectious and harmful pathogen-based diseases cautiously. Biomolecules including peptides and proteins are well-known for their self-assembling capability to prepare nanostructures via non-covalent interactions (e.g., H-bonding, electrostatic, Π-Π stacking, and hydrophobic interactions) and are functioned as capping, stabilizing, and reducing agents for metal ions. Therefore, the biomolecule-based approach could be a good technique to prepare Ag nanoparticles that might be able to overcome the toxicity and stability highly associated with being used in healthcare systems. More intensive research is required to prepare Ag incorporating peptide and protein nanomaterials, with precise control over their formation, stability, biocompatibility, and other biophysical properties being needed for clinical studies.

Author Contributions: M.A.W.: conceptualization, figure analysis and collection, writing, and revision. L.L.: conceptualization, figure analysis and collection, writing, and revision. M.A.M.: revision and correction. M.R.K., M.O.A. and H.F.A.: writing, discussion, and revision. A.A.: writing original draft, revision, and editing. R.H.: writing, revision, figure analysis, and resource collection. All authors have read and agreed to the published version of the manuscript.

Funding: This work was supported by Chengdu University, China.

Institutional Review Board Statement: Not applicable.

Informed Consent Statement: Not applicable.

Data Availability Statement: The data presented in this study are available in this study with copyright permissions.

Acknowledgments: M.A.W. gratefully thanks Chengdu University for supporting this work. The authors extend their appreciation to the Deanship of Scientific Research at King Saud University, Riyadh, for funding this work through Research Group "RGP-1438-025".

Conflicts of Interest: The authors declare no conflict of interest.

References

1. McDonnell, G.; Russell, A.D. Antiseptics and Disinfectants: Activity, Action, and Resistance. *Clin. Microbiol. Rev.* **1999**, *12*, 147–179. [CrossRef] [PubMed]
2. Jiang, W.; Kim, B.Y.S.; Rutka, J.T.; Chan, W.C.W. Nanoparticle-mediated cellular response is size-dependent. *Nat. Nanotechnol.* **2008**, *3*, 145–150. [CrossRef] [PubMed]
3. Lemire, J.A.; Harrison, J.J.; Turner, R.J. Antimicrobial activity of metals: Mechanisms, molecular targets and applications. *Nat. Rev. Microbiol.* **2013**, *11*, 371–384. [CrossRef] [PubMed]

4. You, C.; Han, C.; Wang, X.; Zheng, Y.; Li, Q.; Hu, X.; Sun, H. The progress of silver nanoparticles in the antibacterial mechanism, clinical application and cytotoxicity. *Mol. Biol. Rep.* **2012**, *39*, 9193–9201. [CrossRef] [PubMed]
5. Le Ouay, B.; Stellacci, F. Antibacterial activity of silver nanoparticles: A surface science insight. *Nano Today* **2015**, *10*, 339–354. [CrossRef]
6. Dye, C. After 2015: Infectious diseases in a new era of health and development. *Philos. Trans. R. Soc. B Biol. Sci.* **2014**, *369*. [CrossRef]
7. Li, Y.; Wang, Z.; Sun, L.; Liu, L.; Xu, C.; Kuang, H. Nanoparticle-based sensors for food contaminants. *TrAC—Trends Anal. Chem.* **2019**, *113*, 74–83. [CrossRef]
8. Bresee, J.; Bond, C.M.; Worthington, R.J.; Smith, C.A.; Gifford, J.C.; Simpson, C.A.; Carter, C.J.; Wang, G.; Hartman, J.; Osbaugh, N.A.; et al. Nanoscale structure-activity relationships, mode of action, and biocompatibility of gold nanoparticle antibiotics. *J. Am. Chem. Soc.* **2014**, *136*, 5295–5300. [CrossRef]
9. Fan, W.; Yung, B.; Huang, P.; Chen, X. Nanotechnology for Multimodal Synergistic Cancer Therapy. *Chem. Rev.* **2017**, *117*, 13566–13638. [CrossRef]
10. Brigger, I.; Dubernet, C.; Couvreur, P. Nanoparticles in cancer therapy and diagnosis. *Adv. Drug Deliv. Rev.* **2012**, *64*, 24–36. [CrossRef]
11. Supraja, N.; Dhivya, J.; Prasad, T.N.V.K.V.; David, E. Synthesis, characterization and dose dependent antimicrobial and anti-cancerous efficacy of phycogenic (Sargassum muticum) silver nanoparticles against Breast Cancer Cells (MCF 7) cell line. *Adv. Nano Res.* **2018**, *6*, 183–200. [CrossRef]
12. Baptista, P.V.; McCusker, M.P.; Carvalho, A.; Ferreira, D.A.; Mohan, N.M.; Martins, M.; Fernandes, A.R. Nano-strategies to fight multidrug resistant bacteria–"A Battle of the Titans". *Front. Microbiol.* **2018**, *9*, 1441. [CrossRef] [PubMed]
13. Kailasa, S.K.; Park, T.-J.; Rohit, J.V.; Koduru, J.R. Chapter 14—Antimicrobial activity of silver nanoparticles. In *Nanoparticles in Pharmacotherapy*; Grumezescu, A.M., Ed.; William Andrew Publishing: Norwich, NY, USA, 2019; pp. 461–484.
14. Wang, T.; Ma, B.; Jin, A.; Li, X.; Zhang, X.; Wang, W.; Cai, Y. Facile loading of Ag nanoparticles onto magnetic microsphere by the aid of a tannic acid—Metal polymer layer to synthesize magnetic disinfectant with high antibacterial activity. *J. Hazard. Mater.* **2018**, *342*, 392–400. [CrossRef] [PubMed]
15. Agnihotri, S.; Mukherji, S.; Mukherji, S. Size-controlled silver nanoparticles synthesized over the range 5-100 nm using the same protocol and their antibacterial efficacy. *RSC Adv.* **2014**, *4*, 3974–3983. [CrossRef]
16. Bragg, P.D.; Rainnie, D.J. The effect of silver ions on the respiratory chain of *Escherichia coli*. *Can. J. Microbiol.* **1974**, *20*, 883–889. [CrossRef] [PubMed]
17. Carlson, C.; Hussein, S.M.; Schrand, A.M.; Braydich-Stolle, L.K.; Hess, K.L.; Jones, R.L.; Schlager, J.J. Unique cellular interaction of silver nanoparticles: Size-dependent generation of reactive oxygen species. *J. Phys. Chem. B* **2008**, *112*, 13608–13619. [CrossRef]
18. Wahab, M.A.; Islam, N.; Hoque, M.E.; Young, D.J. Recent advances in silver nanoparticle containing biopolymer nanocomposites for infectious disease control—A mini review. *Curr. Anal. Chem.* **2018**, *14*, 198–202. [CrossRef]
19. Wahab, M.A.; Li, L.; Li, H.; Abdala, A. Silver nanoparticle-based nanocomposites for combating infectious pathogens: Recent advances and future prospects. *Nanomaterials* **2021**, *11*, 581. [CrossRef]
20. Potara, M.; Jakab, E.; Damert, A.; Popescu, O.; Canpean, V.; Astilean, S. Synergistic antibacterial activity of chitosan-silver nanocomposites on *Staphylococcus aureus*. *Nanotechnology* **2011**, *22*, 135101. [CrossRef]
21. Magaña, S.M.; Quintana, P.; Aguilar, D.H.; Toledo, J.A.; Ángeles-Chávez, C.; Cortés, M.A.; León, L.; Freile-Pelegrín, Y.; López, T.; Sánchez, R.M.T. Antibacterial activity of montmorillonites modified with silver. *J. Mol. Catal. A Chem.* **2008**, *281*, 192–199. [CrossRef]
22. An, J.; Luo, Q.; Li, M.; Wang, D.; Li, X.; Yin, R. A facile synthesis of high antibacterial polymer nanocomposite containing uniformly dispersed silver nanoparticles. *Colloid Polym. Sci.* **2015**, *293*, 1997–2008. [CrossRef]
23. Długosz, M.; Bulwan, M.; Kania, G.; Nowakowska, M.; Zapotoczny, S. Hybrid calcium carbonate/polymer microparticles containing silver nanoparticles as antibacterial agents. *J. Nanoparticle Res.* **2012**, *14*, 1313. [CrossRef] [PubMed]
24. Taglietti, A.; Arciola, C.R.; D'Agostino, A.; Dacarro, G.; Montanaro, L.; Campoccia, D.; Cucca, L.; Vercellino, M.; Poggi, A.; Pallavicini, P.; et al. Antibiofilm activity of a monolayer of silver nanoparticles anchored to an amino-silanized glass surface. *Biomaterials* **2014**, *35*, 1779–1788. [CrossRef] [PubMed]
25. Munteanu, B.S.; Aytac, Z.; Pricope, G.M.; Uyar, T.; Vasile, C. Polylactic acid (PLA)/Silver-NP/VitaminE bionanocomposite electrospun nanofibers with antibacterial and antioxidant activity. *J. Nanoparticle Res.* **2014**, *16*. [CrossRef]
26. Kumar-Krishnan, S.; Prokhorov, E.; Hernández-Iturriaga, M.; Mota-Morales, J.D.; Vázquez-Lepe, M.; Kovalenko, Y.; Sanchez, I.C.; Luna-Bárcenas, G. Chitosan/silver nanocomposites: Synergistic antibacterial action of silver nanoparticles and silver ions. *Eur. Polym. J.* **2015**, *67*, 242–251. [CrossRef]
27. Pishbin, F.; Mouriño, V.; Gilchrist, J.B.; McComb, D.W.; Kreppel, S.; Salih, V.; Ryan, M.P.; Boccaccini, A.R. Single-step electrochemical deposition of antimicrobial orthopaedic coatings based on a bioactive glass/chitosan/nano-silver composite system. *Acta Biomater.* **2013**, *9*, 7469–7479. [CrossRef] [PubMed]
28. Dubey, P.; Bhushan, B.; Sachdev, A.; Matai, I.; Uday Kumar, S.; Gopinath, P. Silver-nanoparticle-Incorporated composite nanofibers for potential wound-dressing applications. *J. Appl. Polym. Sci.* **2015**, *132*. [CrossRef]

29. Kiriyama, T.; Kuroki, K.; Sasaki, K.; Tomino, M.; Asakura, M.; Kominami, Y.; Takahashi, Y.; Kawai, T. Antibacterial properties of a self-cured acrylic resin composed of a polymer coated with a silver-containing organic composite antibacterial agent. *Dent. Mater. J.* **2013**, *32*, 679–687. [CrossRef] [PubMed]
30. Macocinschi, D.; Filip, D.; Paslaru, E.; Munteanu, B.S.; Dumitriu, R.P.; Pricope, G.M.; Aflori, M.; Dobromir, M.; Nica, V.; Vasile, C. Polyurethane-extracellular matrix/silver bionanocomposites for urinary catheters. *J. Bioact. Compat. Polym.* **2015**, *30*, 99–113. [CrossRef]
31. Thomas, R.; Soumya, K.R.; Mathew, J.; Radhakrishnan, E.K. Electrospun Polycaprolactone Membrane Incorporated with Biosynthesized Silver Nanoparticles as Effective Wound Dressing Material. *Appl. Biochem. Biotechnol.* **2015**, *176*, 2213–2224. [CrossRef]
32. Vigneshwaran, N.; Ashtaputre, N.M.; Varadarajan, P.V.; Nachane, R.P.; Paralikar, K.M.; Balasubramanya, R.H. Biological synthesis of silver nanoparticles using the fungus *Aspergillus flavus*. *Mater. Lett.* **2007**, *61*, 1413–1418. [CrossRef]
33. Lee, H.Y.; Park, H.K.; Lee, Y.M.; Kim, K.; Park, S.B. A practical procedure for producing silver nanocoated fabric and its antibacterial evaluation for biomedical applications. *Chem. Commun.* **2007**, 2959–2961. [CrossRef]
34. Ghilini, F.; Rodríguez González, M.C.; Miñán, A.G.; Pissinis, D.; Creus, A.H.; Salvarezza, R.C.; Schilardi, P.L. Highly Stabilized Nanoparticles on Poly-L-Lysine-Coated Oxidized Metals: A Versatile Platform with Enhanced Antimicrobial Activity. *ACS Appl. Mater. Interfaces* **2018**, *10*, 23657–23666. [CrossRef] [PubMed]
35. Pissinis, D.E.; Benítez, G.A.; Schilardi, P.L. Two-step biocompatible surface functionalization for two-pathway antimicrobial action against Gram-positive bacteria. *Colloids Surf. B Biointerfaces* **2018**, *164*, 262–271. [CrossRef] [PubMed]
36. Lichter, J.A.; Van Vlietpa, K.J.; Rubner, M.F. Design of antibacterial surfaces and interfaces: Polyelectrolyte multilayers as a multifunctional platform. *Macromolecules* **2009**, *42*, 8573–8586. [CrossRef]
37. D'Agostino, A.; Taglietti, A.; Desando, R.; Bini, M.; Patrini, M.; Dacarro, G.; Cucca, L.; Pallavicini, P.; Grisoli, P. Bulk surfaces coated with triangular silver nanoplates: Antibacterial action based on silver release and photo-thermal effect. *Nanomaterials* **2017**, *7*, 7. [CrossRef]
38. Pallavicini, P.; Arciola, C.R.; Bertoglio, F.; Curtosi, S.; Dacarro, G.; D'Agostino, A.; Ferrari, F.; Merli, D.; Milanese, C.; Rossi, S.; et al. Silver nanoparticles synthesized and coated with pectin: An ideal compromise for antibacterial and anti-biofilm action combined with wound-healing properties. *J. Colloid Interface Sci.* **2017**, *498*, 271–281. [CrossRef]
39. Liu, J.; Hurt, R.H. Ion release kinetics and particle persistence in aqueous nano-silver colloids. *Environ. Sci. Technol.* **2010**, *44*, 2169–2175. [CrossRef]
40. Pallavicini, P.; Preti, L.; Vita, L.D.; Dacarro, G.; Diaz Fernandez, Y.A.; Merli, D.; Rossi, S.; Taglietti, A.; Vigani, B. Fast dissolution of silver nanoparticles at physiological pH. *J. Colloid Interface Sci.* **2020**, *563*, 177–188. [CrossRef]
41. Grunlan, J.C.; Choi, J.K.; Lin, A. Antimicrobial behavior of polyelectrolyte multilayer films containing cetrimide and silver. *Biomacromolecules* **2005**, *6*, 1149–1153. [CrossRef]
42. Konop, M.; Damps, T.; Misicka, A.; Rudnicka, L. Certain Aspects of Silver and Silver Nanoparticles in Wound Care: A Minireview. *J. Nanomater.* **2016**, *2016*, 47. [CrossRef]
43. Kumar, S.S.D.; Rajendran, N.K.; Houreld, N.N.; Abrahamse, H. Recent advances on silver nanoparticle and biopolymer-based biomaterials for wound healing applications. *Int. J. Biol. Macromol.* **2018**, *115*, 165–175. [CrossRef]
44. Duan, K.; Wang, R. Surface modifications of bone implants through wet chemistry. *J. Mater. Chem.* **2006**, *16*, 2309–2321. [CrossRef]
45. Abdelhalim, A.O.E.; Galal, A.; Hussein, M.Z.; El Sayed, I.E.T. Graphene Functionalization by 1,6-Diaminohexane and Silver Nanoparticles for Water Disinfection. *J. Nanomater.* **2016**, *2016*, 1485280. [CrossRef]
46. Deshmukh, S.P.; Patil, S.M.; Mullani, S.B.; Delekar, S.D. Silver nanoparticles as an effective disinfectant: A review. *Mater. Sci. Eng. C* **2019**, *97*, 954–965. [CrossRef]
47. Scopus. Available online: www.scopus.com/results/results.uri?sid=adb0e4cff6baeefdf9d96511c97c4cd5&src=s&sot=b&sdt=b&origin=searchbasic&rr=&sl=98&s= (accessed on 18 June 2021).
48. Ratan, Z.A.; Haidere, M.F.; Nurunnabi, M.; Shahriar, S.M.; Ahammad, A.J.S.; Shim, Y.Y.; Reaney, M.J.T.; Cho, J.Y. Green chemistry synthesis of silver nanoparticles and their potential anticancer effects. *Cancers* **2020**, *12*, 855. [CrossRef]
49. Ahmad, S.; Munir, S.; Zeb, N.; Ullah, A.; Khan, B.; Ali, J.; Bilal, M.; Omer, M.; Alamzeb, M.; Salman, S.M.; et al. Green nanotechnology: A review on green synthesis of silver nanoparticles—An ecofriendly approach. *Int. J. Nanomed.* **2019**, *14*, 5087–5107. [CrossRef] [PubMed]
50. Mousavi, S.M.; Hashemi, S.A.; Ghasemi, Y.; Atapour, A.; Amani, A.M.; Savar Dashtaki, A.; Babapoor, A.; Arjmand, O. Green synthesis of silver nanoparticles toward bio and medical applications: Review study. *Artif. Cells Nanomed. Biotechnol.* **2018**, *46*, S855–S872. [CrossRef] [PubMed]
51. Daniel, S.C.G.K.; Joseph, P.; Sivakumar, M. Biosynthesized silver nanoparticle based hybrid materials. *Nanosci. Nanotechnol.-Asia* **2018**, *8*, 4–12. [CrossRef]
52. Rafique, M.; Sadaf, I.; Rafique, M.S.; Tahir, M.B. A review on green synthesis of silver nanoparticles and their applications. *Artif. Cells Nanomed. Biotechnol.* **2017**, *45*, 1272–1291. [CrossRef]
53. Morones, J.R.; Elechiguerra, J.L.; Camacho, A.; Holt, K.; Kouri, J.B.; Ramírez, J.T.; Yacaman, M.J. The bactericidal effect of silver nanoparticles. *Nanotechnology* **2005**, *16*, 2346–2353. [CrossRef] [PubMed]
54. Sondi, I.; Salopek-Sondi, B. Silver nanoparticles as antimicrobial agent: A case study on *E. coli* as a model for Gram-negative bacteria. *J. Colloid Interface Sci.* **2004**, *275*, 177–182. [CrossRef] [PubMed]

55. Raza, M.A.; Kanwal, Z.; Rauf, A.; Sabri, A.N.; Riaz, S.; Naseem, S. Size- and shape-dependent antibacterial studies of silver nanoparticles synthesized by wet chemical routes. *Nanomaterials* **2016**, *6*, 74. [CrossRef] [PubMed]
56. Alshareef, A.; Laird, K.; Cross, R.B.M. Shape-dependent antibacterial activity of silver nanoparticles on *Escherichia coli* and *Enterococcus faecium* bacterium. *Appl. Surf. Sci.* **2017**, *424*, 310–315. [CrossRef]
57. Lu, Z.; Rong, K.; Li, J.; Yang, H.; Chen, R. Size-dependent antibacterial activities of silver nanoparticles against oral anaerobic pathogenic bacteria. *J. Mater. Sci. Mater. Med.* **2013**, *24*, 1465–1471. [CrossRef] [PubMed]
58. Pal, S.; Tak, Y.K.; Song, J.M. Does the antibacterial activity of silver nanoparticles depend on the shape of the nanoparticle? A study of the gram-negative bacterium *Escherichia coli*. *Appl. Environ. Microbiol.* **2007**, *73*, 1712–1720. [CrossRef] [PubMed]
59. Feng, Q.L.; Wu, J.; Chen, G.Q.; Cui, F.Z.; Kim, T.N.; Kim, J.O. A mechanistic study of the antibacterial effect of silver ions on *Escherichia coli* and *Staphylococcus aureus*. *J. Biomed. Mater. Res.* **2000**, *52*, 662–668. [CrossRef]
60. Kennedy, D.C.; Orts-Gil, G.; Lai, C.H.; Müller, L.; Haase, A.; Luch, A.; Seeberger, P.H. Carbohydrate functionalization of silver nanoparticles modulates cytotoxicity and cellular uptake. *J. Nanobiotechnol.* **2014**, *12*. [CrossRef]
61. Azizi, S.; Mohamad, R.; Abdul Rahim, R.; Mohammadinejad, R.; Bin Ariff, A. Hydrogel beads bio-nanocomposite based on Kappa-Carrageenan and green synthesized silver nanoparticles for biomedical applications. *Int. J. Biol. Macromol.* **2017**, *104*, 423–431. [CrossRef]
62. Schauermann, S.; Nilius, N.; Shaikhutdinov, S.; Freund, H.J. Nanoparticles for heterogeneous catalysis: New mechanistic insights. *Acc. Chem. Res.* **2013**, *46*, 1673–1681. [CrossRef]
63. Zhou, Y.; Chen, R.; He, T.; Xu, K.; Du, D.; Zhao, N.; Cheng, X.; Yang, J.; Shi, H.; Lin, Y. Biomedical Potential of Ultrafine Ag/AgCl Nanoparticles Coated on Graphene with Special Reference to Antimicrobial Performances and Burn Wound Healing. *ACS Appl. Mater. Interfaces* **2016**, *8*, 15067–15075. [CrossRef] [PubMed]
64. Iqbal, S.; Fakhar-e-Alam, M.; Akbar, F.; Shafiq, M.; Atif, M.; Amin, N.; Ismail, M.; Hanif, A.; Farooq, W.A. Application of silver oxide nanoparticles for the treatment of cancer. *J. Mol. Struct.* **2019**, *1189*, 203–209. [CrossRef]
65. Calderon, V.S.; Galindo, R.E.; Oliveira, J.C.; Cavaleiro, A.; Carvalho, S. Ag^+ release and corrosion behavior of zirconium carbonitride coatings with silver nanoparticles for biomedical devices. *Surf. Coat. Technol.* **2013**, *222*, 104–111. [CrossRef]
66. Zhang, X.F.; Liu, Z.G.; Shen, W.; Gurunathan, S. Silver nanoparticles: Synthesis, characterization, properties, applications, and therapeutic approaches. *Int. J. Mol. Sci.* **2016**, *17*, 1534. [CrossRef] [PubMed]
67. Pryshchepa, O.; Pomastowski, P.; Buszewski, B. Silver nanoparticles: Synthesis, investigation techniques, and properties. *Adv. Colloid Interface Sci.* **2020**, *284*. [CrossRef] [PubMed]
68. Deepak, V.; Umamaheshwaran, P.S.; Guhan, K.; Nanthini, R.A.; Krithiga, B.; Jaithoon, N.M.H.; Gurunathan, S. Synthesis of gold and silver nanoparticles using purified URAK. *Colloids Surf. B Biointerfaces* **2011**, *86*, 353–358. [CrossRef]
69. Amulyavichus, A.; Daugvila, A.; Davidonis, R.; Sipavichus, C. Study of chemical composition of nanostructural materials prepared by laser cutting of metals. *Fiz. Met. I Metalloved.* **1998**, *85*, 111–117.
70. Mahmoudi, M.; Serpooshan, V. Silver-coated engineered magnetic nanoparticles are promising for the success in the fight against antibacterial resistance threat. *ACS Nano* **2012**, *6*, 2656–2664. [CrossRef]
71. Malik, M.A.; O'Brien, P.; Revaprasadu, N. A simple route to the synthesis of core/shell nanoparticles of chalcogenides. *Chem. Mater.* **2002**, *14*, 2004–2010. [CrossRef]
72. Sergeev, B.M.; Kasaikin, V.A.; Litmanovich, E.A.; Sergeev, G.B.; Prusov, A.N. Cryochemical synthesis and properties of silver nanoparticle dispersions stabilised by poly(2-dimethylaminoethyl methacrylate). *Mendeleev Commun.* **1999**, *9*, 130–131. [CrossRef]
73. Mafuné, F.; Kohno, J.Y.; Takeda, Y.; Kondow, T.; Sawabe, H. Formation and size control of silver nanoparticles by laser ablation in aqueous solution. *J. Phys. Chem. B* **2000**, *104*, 9111–9117. [CrossRef]
74. Hulteen, J.C.; Treichel, D.A.; Smith, M.T.; Duval, M.L.; Jensen, T.R.; Van Duyne, R.P. Nanosphere lithography: Size-tunable silver nanoparticle and surface cluster arrays. *J. Phys. Chem. B* **1999**, *103*, 3854–3863. [CrossRef]
75. Zhu, J.J.; Liao, X.H.; Zhao, X.N.; Chen, H.Y. Preparation of silver nanorods by electrochemical methods. *Mater. Lett.* **2001**, *49*, 91–95. [CrossRef]
76. Abid, J.P.; Wark, A.W.; Brevet, P.F.; Girault, H.H. Preparation of silver nanoparticles in solution from a silver salt by laser irradiation. *Chem. Commun.* **2002**, *7*, 792–793. [CrossRef] [PubMed]
77. Talebi, J.; Halladj, R.; Askari, S. Sonochemical synthesis of silver nanoparticles in Y-zeolite substrate. *J. Mater. Sci.* **2010**, *45*, 3318–3324. [CrossRef]
78. Hosseinpour-Mashkani, S.M.; Ramezani, M. Silver and silver oxide nanoparticles: Synthesis and characterization by thermal decomposition. *Mater. Lett.* **2014**, *130*, 259–262. [CrossRef]
79. Zhang, Q.; Li, N.; Goebl, J.; Lu, Z.; Yin, Y. A systematic study of the synthesis of silver nanoplates: Is citrate a "magic" reagent? *J. Am. Chem. Soc.* **2011**, *133*, 18931–18939. [CrossRef]
80. Ganaie, S.U.; Abbasi, T.P.; Abbasi, S.A. Green synthesis of silver nanoparticles using an otherwise worthless weed mimosa (*Mimosa pudica*): Feasibility and process development toward shape/size control. *Part. Sci. Technol.* **2015**, *33*, 638–644. [CrossRef]
81. Kang, W.J.; Cheng, C.Q.; Li, Z.; Feng, Y.; Shen, G.R.; Du, X.W. Ultrafine Ag Nanoparticles as Active Catalyst for Electrocatalytic Hydrogen Production. *ChemCatChem* **2019**, *11*, 5976–5981. [CrossRef]
82. Biswas, A.; Bayer, I.S.; Biris, A.S.; Wang, T.; Dervishi, E.; Faupel, F. Advances in top-down and bottom-up surface nanofabrication: Techniques, applications & future prospects. *Adv. Colloid Interface Sci.* **2012**, *170*, 2–27. [CrossRef]

83. Kibis, L.S.; Stadnichenko, A.I.; Pajetnov, E.M.; Koscheev, S.V.; Zaykovskii, V.I.; Boronin, A.I. The investigation of oxidized silver nanoparticles prepared by thermal evaporation and radio-frequency sputtering of metallic silver under oxygen. *Appl. Surf. Sci.* **2010**, *257*, 404–413. [CrossRef]
84. Miranzadeh, M.; Kassaee, M.Z. Solvent effects on arc discharge fabrication of durable silver nanopowder and its application as a recyclable catalyst for elimination of toxic p-nitrophenol. *Chem. Eng. J.* **2014**, *257*, 105–111. [CrossRef]
85. Kylián, O.; Kuzminova, A.; Štefaníková, R.; Hanuš, J.; Solař, P.; Kúš, P.; Cieslar, M.; Choukourov, A.; Biederman, H. Silver/plasma polymer strawberry-like nanoparticles produced by gas-phase synthesis. *Mater. Lett.* **2019**, *253*, 238–241. [CrossRef]
86. Tien, D.C.; Tseng, K.H.; Liao, C.Y.; Huang, J.C.; Tsung, T.T. Discovery of ionic silver in silver nanoparticle suspension fabricated by arc discharge method. *J. Alloy. Compd.* **2008**, *463*, 408–411. [CrossRef]
87. Khan, I.; Bahuguna, A.; Krishnan, M.; Shukla, S.; Lee, H.; Min, S.H.; Choi, D.K.; Cho, Y.; Bajpai, V.K.; Huh, Y.S.; et al. The effect of biogenic manufactured silver nanoparticles on human endothelial cells and zebrafish model. *Sci. Total Environ.* **2019**, *679*, 365–377. [CrossRef]
88. Thakkar, K.N.; Mhatre, S.S.; Parikh, R.Y. Biological synthesis of metallic nanoparticles. *Nanomed. Nanotechnol. Biol. Med.* **2010**, *6*, 257–262. [CrossRef]
89. Gurunathan, S.; Kalishwaralal, K.; Vaidyanathan, R.; Venkataraman, D.; Pandian, S.R.K.; Muniyandi, J.; Hariharan, N.; Eom, S.H. Biosynthesis, purification and characterization of silver nanoparticles using Escherichia coli. *Colloids Surf. B Biointerfaces* **2009**, *74*, 328–335. [CrossRef] [PubMed]
90. Gurunathan, S.; Han, J.W.; Kim, J.H. Green chemistry approach for the synthesis of biocompatible graphene. *Int. J. Nanomed.* **2013**, *8*, 2719–2732. [CrossRef] [PubMed]
91. Gurunathan, S.; Han, J.W.; Park, J.H.; Kim, E.; Choi, Y.J.; Kwon, D.N.; Kim, J.H. Reduced graphene oxide-silver nanoparticle nanocomposite: A potential anticancer nanotherapy. *Int. J. Nanomed.* **2015**, *10*, 6257–6276. [CrossRef] [PubMed]
92. Kalimuthu, K.; Suresh Babu, R.; Venkataraman, D.; Bilal, M.; Gurunathan, S. Biosynthesis of silver nanocrystals by Bacillus licheniformis. *Colloids Surf. B Biointerfaces* **2008**, *65*, 150–153. [CrossRef]
93. Kalishwaralal, K.; Deepak, V.; Ramkumarpandian, S.; Nellaiah, H.; Sangiliyandi, G. Extracellular biosynthesis of silver nanoparticles by the culture supernatant of Bacillus licheniformis. *Mater. Lett.* **2008**, *62*, 4411–4413. [CrossRef]
94. Nair, B.; Pradeep, T. Coalescence of Nanoclusters and Formation of Submicron Crystallites Assisted by Lactobacillus Strains. *Cryst. Growth Des.* **2002**, *2*, 293–298. [CrossRef]
95. Kalishwaralal, K.; Deepak, V.; Ram Kumar Pandian, S.; Kottaisamy, M.; BarathManiKanth, S.; Kartikeyan, B.; Gurunathan, S. Biosynthesis of silver and gold nanoparticles using *Brevibacterium casei*. *Colloids Surf. B Biointerfaces* **2010**, *77*, 257–262. [CrossRef]
96. Shankar, S.S.; Ahmad, A.; Sastry, M. Geranium Leaf Assisted Biosynthesis of Silver Nanoparticles. *Biotechnol. Prog.* **2003**, *19*, 1627–1631. [CrossRef]
97. Gurunathan, S.; Han, J.W.; Dayem, A.A.; Eppakayala, V.; Park, J.H.; Cho, S.G.; Lee, K.J.; Kim, J.H. Green synthesis of anisotropic silver nanoparticles and its potential cytotoxicity in human breast cancer cells (MCF-7). *J. Ind. Eng. Chem.* **2013**, *19*, 1600–1605. [CrossRef]
98. Leung, T.C.Y.; Wong, C.K.; Xie, Y. Green synthesis of silver nanoparticles using biopolymers, carboxymethylated-curdlan and fucoidan. *Mater. Chem. Phys.* **2010**, *121*, 402–405. [CrossRef]
99. Kumar, B.; Smita, K.; Cumbal, L.; Debut, A.; Pathak, R.N. Sonochemical synthesis of silver nanoparticles using starch: A comparison. *Bioinorg. Chem. Appl.* **2014**, *2014*, 784268. [CrossRef] [PubMed]
100. Shankar, S.; Rhim, J.W. Amino acid mediated synthesis of silver nanoparticles and preparation of antimicrobial agar/silver nanoparticles composite films. *Carbohydr. Polym.* **2015**, *130*, 353–363. [CrossRef] [PubMed]
101. Pyatenko, A.; Yamaguchi, M.; Suzuki, M. Synthesis of spherical silver nanoparticles with controllable sizes in aqueous solutions. *J. Phys. Chem. C* **2007**, *111*, 7910–7917. [CrossRef]
102. Khodashenas, B.; Ghorbani, H.R. Synthesis of silver nanoparticles with different shapes. *Arab. J. Chem.* **2019**, *12*, 1823–1838. [CrossRef]
103. Silva, T.; Pokhrel, L.R.; Dubey, B.; Tolaymat, T.M.; Maier, K.J.; Liu, X. Particle size, surface charge and concentration dependent ecotoxicity of three organo-coated silver nanoparticles: Comparison between general linear model-predicted and observed toxicity. *Sci. Total Environ.* **2014**, *468–469*, 968–976. [CrossRef]
104. Yasin, H.M.; Ahmed, W.; Ali, A.; Bhatti, A.S.; Rehman, N.U. Micro-plasma assisted synthesis of multifunctional D-fructose coated silver nanoparticles. *Mater. Res. Express* **2019**, *6*. [CrossRef]
105. Hsiao, I.L.; Bierkandt, F.S.; Reichardt, P.; Luch, A.; Huang, Y.J.; Jakubowski, N.; Tentschert, J.; Haase, A. Quantification and visualization of cellular uptake of TiO2 and Ag nanoparticles: Comparison of different ICP-MS techniques. *J. Nanobiotechnology* **2016**, *14*. [CrossRef] [PubMed]
106. Alarcon, E.I.; Udekwu, K.; Skog, M.; Pacioni, N.L.; Stamplecoskie, K.G.; González-Béjar, M.; Polisetti, N.; Wickham, A.; Richter-Dahlfors, A.; Griffith, M.; et al. The biocompatibility and antibacterial properties of collagen-stabilized, photochemically prepared silver nanoparticles. *Biomaterials* **2012**, *33*, 4947–4956. [CrossRef] [PubMed]
107. Xing, L.; Xiahou, Y.; Zhang, P.; Du, W.; Xia, H. Size Control Synthesis of Monodisperse, Quasi-Spherical Silver Nanoparticles to Realize Surface-Enhanced Raman Scattering Uniformity and Reproducibility. *ACS Appl. Mater. Interfaces* **2019**, *11*, 17637–17646. [CrossRef]

108. Blommaerts, N.; Vanrompay, H.; Nuti, S.; Lenaerts, S.; Bals, S.; Verbruggen, S.W. Unraveling Structural Information of Turkevich Synthesized Plasmonic Gold–Silver Bimetallic Nanoparticles. *Small* **2019**, *15*. [CrossRef]
109. Hegde, H.; Santhosh, C.; Sinha, R.K. Seed mediated synthesis of highly stable CTAB capped triangular silver nanoplates for LSPR sensing. *Mater. Res. Express* **2019**, *6*. [CrossRef]
110. Huang, T.; Xu, X.H.N. Synthesis and characterization of tunable rainbow colored colloidal silver nanoparticles using single-nanoparticle plasmonic microscopy and spectroscopy. *J. Mater. Chem.* **2010**, *20*, 9867–9876. [CrossRef] [PubMed]
111. Ashkarran, A.A. A novel method for synthesis of colloidal silver nanoparticles by arc discharge in liquid. *Curr. Appl. Phys.* **2010**, *10*, 1442–1447. [CrossRef]
112. Da Silva, R.R.; Yang, M.; Choi, S.I.; Chi, M.; Luo, M.; Zhang, C.; Li, Z.Y.; Camargo, P.H.C.; Ribeiro, S.J.L.; Xia, Y. Facile Synthesis of Sub-20 nm Silver Nanowires through a Bromide-Mediated Polyol Method. *ACS Nano* **2016**, *10*, 7892–7900. [CrossRef]
113. Chen, Z.; Balankura, T.; Fichthorn, K.A.; Rioux, R.M. Revisiting the Polyol Synthesis of Silver Nanostructures: Role of Chloride in Nanocube Formation. *ACS Nano* **2019**, *13*, 1849–1860. [CrossRef]
114. Monteiro, D.R.; Silva, S.; Negri, M.; Gorup, L.F.; De Camargo, E.R.; Oliveira, R.; Barbosa, D.B.; Henriques, M. Silver nanoparticles: Influence of stabilizing agent and diameter on antifungal activity against Candida albicans and Candida glabrata biofilms. *Lett. Appl. Microbiol.* **2012**, *54*, 383–391. [CrossRef] [PubMed]
115. Wahab, M.A.; Hasan, C.M.; Alothman, Z.A.; Hossain, M.S.A. In-situ incorporation of highly dispersed silver nanoparticles in nanoporous carbon nitride for the enhancement of antibacterial activities. *J. Hazard. Mater.* **2021**, *408*. [CrossRef]
116. Verkhovskii, R.; Kozlova, A.; Atkin, V.; Kamyshinsky, R.; Shulgina, T.; Nechaeva, O. Physical properties and cytotoxicity of silver nanoparticles under different polymeric stabilizers. *Heliyon* **2019**, *5*. [CrossRef]
117. Jung, Y.J.; Govindaiah, P.; Choi, S.W.; Cheong, I.W.; Kim, J.H. Morphology and conducting property of Ag/poly(pyrrole) composite nanoparticles: Effect of polymeric stabilizers. *Synth. Met.* **2011**, *161*, 1991–1995. [CrossRef]
118. Park, H.J.; Kim, J.Y.; Kim, J.; Lee, J.H.; Hahn, J.S.; Gu, M.B.; Yoon, J. Silver-ion-mediated reactive oxygen species generation affecting bactericidal activity. *Water Res.* **2009**, *43*, 1027–1032. [CrossRef] [PubMed]
119. Vijayalakshmi, R.V.; Kuppan, R.; Kumar, P.P. Investigation on the impact of different stabilizing agents on structural, optical properties of Ag@SnO_2 core-shell nanoparticles and its biological applications. *J. Mol. Liq.* **2020**, *307*. [CrossRef]
120. Gaviria, J.; Alcudia, A.; Begines, B.; Beltrán, A.M.; Villarraga, J.; Moriche, R.; Rodríguez-Ortiz, J.A.; Torres, Y. Synthesis and deposition of silver nanoparticles on porous titanium substrates for biomedical applications. *Surf. Coat. Technol.* **2021**, *406*. [CrossRef]
121. Xiu, Z.M.; Zhang, Q.B.; Puppala, H.L.; Colvin, V.L.; Alvarez, P.J.J. Negligible particle-specific antibacterial activity of silver nanoparticles. *Nano Lett.* **2012**, *12*, 4271–4275. [CrossRef] [PubMed]
122. Ahmed, S.; Ahmad, M.; Swami, B.L.; Ikram, S. A review on plants extract mediated synthesis of silver nanoparticles for antimicrobial applications: A green expertise. *J. Adv. Res.* **2016**, *7*, 17–28. [CrossRef]
123. Barillo, D.J.; Marx, D.E. Silver in medicine: A brief history BC 335 to present. *Burns* **2014**, *40*, S3–S8. [CrossRef]
124. Gao, S.S.; Zhao, I.S.; Duffin, S.; Duangthip, D.; Lo, E.C.M.; Chu, C.H. Revitalising silver nitrate for caries management. *Int. J. Environ. Res. Public Health* **2018**, *15*, 80. [CrossRef] [PubMed]
125. Talapko, J.; Matijević, T.; Juzbašić, M.; Antolović-Požgain, A.; Škrlec, I. Antibacterial activity of silver and its application in dentistry, cardiology and dermatology. *Microorganisms* **2020**, *8*, 1400. [CrossRef] [PubMed]
126. Logaranjan, K.; Raiza, A.J.; Gopinath, S.C.B.; Chen, Y.; Pandian, K. Shape- and Size-Controlled Synthesis of Silver Nanoparticles Using Aloe vera Plant Extract and Their Antimicrobial Activity. *Nanoscale Res. Lett.* **2016**, *11*, 520. [CrossRef] [PubMed]
127. Sim, W.; Barnard, R.T.; Blaskovich, M.A.T.; Ziora, Z.M. Antimicrobial silver in medicinal and consumer applications: A patent review of the past decade (2007–2017). *Antibiotics* **2018**, *7*, 93. [CrossRef] [PubMed]
128. Yin, I.X.; Zhang, J.; Zhao, I.S.; Mei, M.L.; Li, Q.; Chu, C.H. The antibacterial mechanism of silver nanoparticles and its application in dentistry. *Int. J. Nanomed.* **2020**, *15*, 2555–2562. [CrossRef]
129. Mathur, P.; Jha, S.; Ramteke, S.; Jain, N.K. Pharmaceutical aspects of silver nanoparticles. *Artif. Cells Nanomed. Biotechnol.* **2018**, *46*, 115–126. [CrossRef] [PubMed]
130. Tang, S.; Zheng, J. Antibacterial Activity of Silver Nanoparticles: Structural Effects. *Adv. Healthc. Mater.* **2018**, *7*. [CrossRef]
131. Möhler, J.S.; Sim, W.; Blaskovich, M.A.T.; Cooper, M.A.; Ziora, Z.M. Silver bullets: A new lustre on an old antimicrobial agent. *Biotechnol. Adv.* **2018**, *36*, 1391–1411. [CrossRef]
132. Stoehr, L.C.; Gonzalez, E.; Stampfl, A.; Casals, E.; Duschl, A.; Puntes, V.; Oostingh, G.J. Shape matters: Effects of silver nanospheres and wires on human alveolar epithelial cells. *Part. Fibre Toxicol.* **2011**, *8*. [CrossRef]
133. Rycenga, M.; Cobley, C.M.; Zeng, J.; Li, W.; Moran, C.H.; Zhang, Q.; Qin, D.; Xia, Y. Controlling the synthesis and assembly of silver nanostructures for plasmonic applications. *Chem. Rev.* **2011**, *111*, 3669–3712. [CrossRef]
134. Suresh, A.K.; Pelletier, D.A.; Wang, W.; Morrell-Falvey, J.L.; Gu, B.; Doktycz, M.J. Cytotoxicity induced by engineered silver nanocrystallites is dependent on surface coatings and cell types. *Langmuir* **2012**, *28*, 2727–2735. [CrossRef]
135. Tabata, Y.; Ikada, Y. Macrophage phagocytosis of biodegradable microspheres composed of L-lactic acid/glycolic acid homo- and copolymers. *J. Biomed. Mater. Res.* **1988**, *22*, 837–858. [CrossRef] [PubMed]
136. Schlinkert, P.; Casals, E.; Boyles, M.; Tischler, U.; Hornig, E.; Tran, N.; Zhao, J.; Himly, M.; Riediker, M.; Oostingh, G.J.; et al. The oxidative potential of differently charged silver and gold nanoparticles on three human lung epithelial cell types. *J. Nanobiotechnol.* **2015**, *13*. [CrossRef] [PubMed]

137. Lallemand, F.; Felt-Baeyens, O.; Besseghir, K.; Behar-Cohen, F.; Gurny, R. Cyclosporine A delivery to the eye: A pharmaceutical challenge. *Eur. J. Pharm. Biopharm.* **2003**, *56*, 307–318. [CrossRef]
138. Wei, L.; Lu, J.; Xu, H.; Patel, A.; Chen, Z.S.; Chen, G. Silver nanoparticles: Synthesis, properties, and therapeutic applications. *Drug Discov. Today* **2015**, *20*, 595–601. [CrossRef]
139. Neacsu, I.A.; Leau, S.A.; Marin, S.; Holban, A.M.; Vasile, B.S.; Nicoara, A.I.; Ene, V.L.; Bleotu, C.; Albu Kaya, M.G.; Ficai, A. Collagen-carboxymethylcellulose biocomposite wound-dressings with antimicrobial activity. *Materials* **2021**, *14*, 1153. [CrossRef]
140. Pal, S.; Nisi, R.; Stoppa, M.; Licciulli, A. Silver-Functionalized Bacterial Cellulose as Antibacterial Membrane for Wound-Healing Applications. *ACS Omega* **2017**, *2*, 3632–3639. [CrossRef]
141. Jin, Y.; Yang, Y.; Duan, W.; Qu, X.; Wu, J. Synergistic and On-Demand Release of Ag-AMPs Loaded on Porous Silicon Nanocarriers for Antibacteria and Wound Healing. *ACS Appl. Mater. Interfaces* **2021**, *13*, 16127–16141. [CrossRef]
142. Wang, Y.; Shi, L.; Wu, H.; Li, Q.; Hu, W.; Zhang, Z.; Huang, L.; Zhang, J.; Chen, D.; Deng, S.; et al. Graphene Oxide-IPDI-Ag/ZnO@Hydroxypropyl Cellulose Nanocomposite Films for Biological Wound-Dressing Applications. *ACS Omega* **2019**, *4*, 15373–15381. [CrossRef]
143. Wang, S.; Yuan, L.; Xu, Z.; Lin, X.; Ge, L.; Li, D.; Mu, C. Functionalization of an Electroactive Self-Healing Polypyrrole-Grafted Gelatin-Based Hydrogel by Incorporating a Polydopamine@AgNP Nanocomposite. *ACS Appl. Bio Mater.* **2021**, *4*, 5797–5808. [CrossRef]
144. Ferdous, Z.; Nemmar, A. Health impact of silver nanoparticles: A review of the biodistribution and toxicity following various routes of exposure. *Int. J. Mol. Sci.* **2020**, *21*, 2375. [CrossRef]
145. Mao, B.H.; Chen, Z.Y.; Wang, Y.J.; Yan, S.J. Silver nanoparticles have lethal and sublethal adverse effects on development and longevity by inducing ROS-mediated stress responses. *Sci. Rep.* **2018**, *8*. [CrossRef] [PubMed]
146. Manzar, A.; Atia, A.; Ruirui, X.; Xuehai, Y. Silver-incorporating peptide and protein supramolecular nanomaterials for biomedical applications. *J. Mater. Chem. B* **2021**, *9*, 4444–4458.

polymers

MDPI

Review

Articular and Artificial Cartilage, Characteristics, Properties and Testing Approaches—A Review

Mohammad Mostakhdemin [1,*], Ashveen Nand [2,3] and Maziar Ramezani [1,*]

1 Department of Mechanical Engineering, Auckland University of Technology, Auckland 1142, New Zealand
2 School of Environmental and Animal Sciences, Unitec Institute of Technology, Auckland 1025, New Zealand; anand2@unitec.ac.nz
3 School of Healthcare and Social Practice, Unitec Institute of Technology, Auckland 1025, New Zealand
* Correspondence: demin.mostakhdemin@aut.ac.nz (M.M.); maziar.ramezani@aut.ac.nz (M.R.)

Abstract: The design and manufacture of artificial tissue for knee joints have been highlighted recently among researchers which necessitates an apt approach for its assessment. Even though most re-searches have focused on specific mechanical or tribological tests, other aspects have remained underexplored. In this review, elemental keys for design and testing artificial cartilage are dis-cussed and advanced methods addressed. Articular cartilage structure, its compositions in load-bearing and tribological properties of hydrogels, mechanical properties, test approaches and wear mechanisms are discussed. Bilayer hydrogels as a niche in tissue artificialization are presented, and recent gaps are assessed.

Keywords: articular cartilage; hydrogels; mechanical properties; tribological properties

Citation: Mostakhdemin, M.; Nand, A.; Ramezani, M. Articular and Artificial Cartilage, Characteristics, Properties and Testing Approaches—A Review. *Polymers* **2021**, *13*, 2000. https://doi.org/10.3390/polym13122000

Academic Editor: Bramasta Nugraha

Received: 19 May 2021
Accepted: 14 June 2021
Published: 18 June 2021

1. Introduction

The complex structure of healthy articular cartilage facilitates the joint withstanding the imposed pressures and retaining interstitial fluid to lessen stresses on its soft tissue while easing the locomotion and minimizing friction between cartilage mates. Avascular nature of this tissue results in unrecoverable damaged lesions and severe pain over time. Polymeric hydrogels are promising candidate materials for the replacement of the damaged cartilage. Moreover, polymeric scaffolds have been applied in interface tissue engineering and their uses have extended to bone to tendon and muscle to tendon interface reconstruction [1]. Recently, bilayer hydrogels have been developed with distinct techniques as promising artificial cartilage due to their resemblance to the native cartilage structure. Bilayer hydrogels contain bulk and lubricious layers that enhance water retention in their lubricious layer and advance tribological properties such as wear-resistance and coefficient of friction (CoF). The absence of optimum mechanical and tribological properties has been highlighted as a research gap in recent years because promoting mechanical properties results in a reduction in the tribological properties or vice versa.

In this study, summaries of recent research are covered, also essential elements in designing of artificial cartilage, common materials, required tests according to standard regulations and strengthening method are discussed broadly. Recent research has been highlighted and gaps addressed adequately. This review further discusses the fundamental resources that are considered in design of wide ranges of hydrogels specially bilayer hydrogels which have gained researchers' attention due to their promising mechanical and tribological properties.

2. Synovial Joints

Synovial joints, being the most common joints in mammals, are characterized by allowing movement in multiple planes. They allow for the articulation of long bones, ends of which are covered with articular cartilage (AC), within a fluid-filled cavity. AC, incorporated with a viscous synovial fluid, is a biphasic tissue that provides extremely low friction [2]. It mitigates overstressing on the tissue's solid phase, while dissipating energy and enabling smooth joints movements. The synovial fluid consists of hyaluronic acid (HA), glycosaminoglycans (GAGs) containing chondroitin-4-sulfate, chondroitin-6-sulfate, keratan sulfate and mobile ions and is a dialysate of blood plasma without hemoglobin [3]. The synovial fluid is contained mainly within the molecular pore spaces of the cartilage cells [4]. AC incorporates the viscous synovial fluid to mitigate shock-loadings initiated by physiological activities and body weight [5]. Hence, AC supports smooth joint movements at an extremely low coefficient of friction (CoF) [6].

3. The Structure of Articular Cartilage

The AC structure is complex, as the compositions of GAGs, chondrocytes and collagen are in random orientations and densities; with the main components of this composition contains water (60–85%), collagen type II (15–22%) and Proteoglycan (PG) (4–7%) [7]. Its deep zone includes hydroxyapatite (Hap) combined with collagen and chondrocyte in the vertical orientation [8], as illustrated in Figure 1. AC is a biphasic substrate categorized as a nonlinear, anisotropic, viscoelastic and inhomogeneous material [7,9].

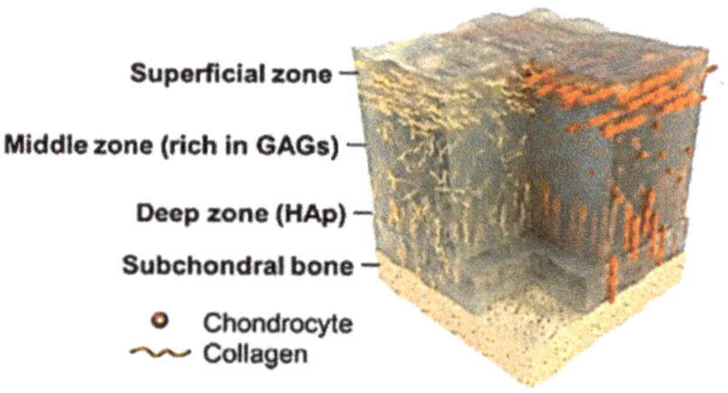

Figure 1. Illustration of the AC structure: superficial, transition and deep zones. Reproduced from [10].

Zonal Categories of Articular Cartilage

AC is a soft avascular tissue with a 3–4 mm thickness and integrates three depth-dependent layers of superficial, transition and deep zones. Each layer is responsible for minimizing either the imposing load or friction of the sliding movement, as described in the following sections.

The top layer (superficial zone) contains collagen fibrils cells in the horizontal orientation, which confers high tensile stiffness and strength. This layer is just 10–20% of the tissue's thickness [11]; both fibrils and chondrocytes are stretched along their length and surrounded at the surface with the finest size compared to the other layers' chondrocytes [12]. This feature also custodies the tissue against high tensile stresses and prevents interstitial fluid permeation, which plays a vital role in sliding on cartilage surface mates [13]. While this layer has high water content, it has the lowest PG [14]. The superficial zone is also called the surface amorphous layer (SAL) that is acellular with no fibril content [7]. Its thickness is a few micrometers, containing proteins, glycoproteins, PGs, hyaluronic acid-protein complexes, chondroitin/keratin sulfates and lipids [15]. In summary, the superficial zone is shear resistant because of the low content of PGs and low permeability [16,17]. This layer plays a crucial role in attaining smooth sliding contact, while controlling synovial fluid diffusion rate. The transition zone is the thickest part of the tissue, contributing to 40–60% of the total thickness of the AC [18]. Collagen fibrils and chondrocytes are both ringed by an extracellular matrix (ECM) that includes GAGs [19]. Moreover, compared to the superficial zone, the transition zone has a higher PG content. The deep zone consists of orthogonally oriented collagen fibers in hydroxyapatite content and has the lowest water content. Its collagen structure is bundled together with fibers in the perpendicular direction to the articular surface. The deep zone forms an interface with the subchondral bone. The stiffness of the whole structure varies gradually through the thickness. The PG, water content and cell density are the lowest in the deep zone [18].

4. Osteoarthritis

Osteoarthritis (OA) is the result of AC degeneration. The recovery process of the damaged lesions is prolonged because of tissue avascularity [7]. Therefore, degenerated tissue experiences high-pressure upon sliding of bones at the joints, which results in severe pain as well as movement disorders [20]. Factors that lead to OA are aging, musculoskeletal disordering and over-pressuring due to either physiological activities or obesity [21]. It is worth mentioning that joint immobilization yields to PG loss, contributing to AC thinning [22,23].

OA is categorized into two types, namely primary and secondary. Primary OA occurs in healthy AC without any abnormality of ligaments and menisci. The reason for primary OA in the elderly is repetitive loadings on thinned AC [20]. Secondary OA, however, is due to injury, trauma or inflammatory factors [24]. In the last decade, studies showed that OA does not result only from AC disease, but also from defects in the ligament, menisci, periarticular muscles and bone [25]. AC engrossed with any of the mentioned factors instigate knee instability and alteration in joint kinematics and consequently nonuniformly distributed stresses, which initiate OA [2].

Treatment Methods for the Cartilage Subjected to OA

The gold standard treatment for patients with OA are total knee/hip replacement (TKR/THR) or hemiarthroplasty. In hemiarthroplasty, only half of the joint in which cartilage deteriorated would be reamed, and either metallic or ceramic components are implanted. In case of hip joint damage, the acetabular cup is left intact, and damaged lesions of the femoral head cartilage would be reamed, and a metallic or ceramic cup is replaced. However, TKR or THR is not the practical solution at mid-adulthood ages due to the limitation of arthroplasty prostheses' life span [26]. Due to the short implant service life (15–20 years), THR/TKR procedures are only suitable for elderly patients [27].

Moreover, any failure after primary surgery yields to a revision surgery. The revision surgery can be implemented for patients just once in their treatment life, since the second revision may result in the implant's loosening [28]. Other procedures that have been developed for damaged cartilage are microfracture [29], autologous-matrix induced chondrogenesis [30], autologous chondrocyte implantation, autologous cultured chondrocytes on porcine collagen membrane (MACI) [31]. However, long-term clinical follow-ups have revealed durability issues with all the above-mentioned procedures [32]. Therapeutically, nonsteroidal drugs, corticosteroids and hyaluronic acid just relieve the pain in short-term and are pushed out of the joint within a few days [32].

Therefore, TKR/THR is the only clinical solution for older patients. However, there is not much attention for developing procedures and treatments suitable for younger patients suffering from dysfunctional cartilage, to eliminate or at least postpone the need for TKR/THR. Young patients between the age of 20–25 years old have reported the highest incidence of joint injury [3]. It turns into OA by 35–40 years old and implementing TKR/THR is high-risk at this age. If TKR, for instance, is performed at the age of 35–40 years, then based on 15–20 years' service life of prosthesis, patients may need revision surgery at the age of 55–60 years. Revision surgery could potentially lead to disability at this age due to the loosening of the prosthesis. In this case, a novel orthopedics implant with minimally invasive surgery that could mimic the mechanical and biological behavior of the native cartilage has been highlighted among researchers as a better alternative to TKR surgery for younger patients [33].

5. Mechanical Characteristics of Articular Cartilage

AC can withstand imposed load under its lifetime which is estimated at 100–200 million loading cycles [34]. AC is categorized as viscoelastic due to variations of its deformation under various strain-rates [35]. It is anisotropic, since the tensile stiffness varies with the direction of loadings [36]. Furthermore, AC is inhomogeneous and performs diverged mechanical functions of tension and compression through the thickness from the superficial to the deep zone [37]. AC incorporation with the synovial fluid, which is incompressible and pressurizes noticeably, supports the significant portion of joint contact pressure [5]. These mentioned properties provide a unique cartilage structure to withstand cyclic loading from the body and transfer those loads smoothly to the bones.

AC tolerates contact pressures in the range of 3–5 MPa during the walking state in hip and knee joints [38]. Moreover, cartilage compressive and shear modulus are reported to be less than 1.5 MPa and 0.5 MPa, respectively. Its Poissons's ratio also ranges from 0.34 to 0.48 [7,39]. AC is also classified as a poroelastic material as its stiffness is highly dependent on strain-rate [40]. Oloyede et al. [41] have reported that at low strain-rates ($0.01 > \varepsilon$ (t)) AC response is consolidation-type deformation, which is stiffness-dependent. In contrast, at higher strain-rates ($0.01 \leq \varepsilon$ (t)) hyperelastic deformation mechanism is dominant that results in high stiffness according to the classical elastic deformation process [41]. Eric et al. [42] studied correlation of cartilage stiffness and strain rate and reported that strain rate increases from 2.7×10^{-3} s^{-1} to 3.5×10^{-2} s^{-1} by increasing stiffness. Their studies employing a wide range of strain rates, showed two primary mechanical responses for AC. At low strain rates, stiffness increases considerably by a minimum increase in strain rate. In contrast, at the upper strain rates regime, stiffness does not vary significantly when the strain-rate increases. Moreover, there is a critical point beyond which the stiffness does not change much by high-strain rate loading [41]. It indicates that the compressive response of AC is strain-rate dependent at low strain-rate regime.

ECM significantly affects the mechanical properties of AC. AC exhibits time-dependent responses with viscoelasticity, poroelasticity or the combination of both phenomena [43]. Research studies demonstrate that AC responds to the loads based on PGs and chondrocyte arrangement [12,44]. However, cartilage's viscoelastic properties support the continuity of the inner tissue interactions by solid and fluid phase incorporation and fluid migration rates through the solid architecture [45]. Therefore, categorizing AC as viscoelastic or poroelastic material is highly dependent on several test factors, such as the size of the indenter, indentation depth and strain rates. Joseph et al. [43] demonstrated that the AC neither follows the classical poroelastic nor the viscoelastic model; In fact, the best model characterizing AC is a nonlinear biphasic material.

As AC is a heterogeneous, anisotropic and multiphasic biomaterial, the mechanical properties depend on its different zones. AC with three main zones and variation of collagen fibrils, PG and water contents in different layers show different responses based on the structure depth or thickness. AC with its relative strength through its thickness is in accordance with its non-homogeneity [46]. Therefore, to analyze the AC responses under loadings, the non-homogeneous poroelastic model has been recommended [47]. This model presented that the collagen fibril reinforces the cartilage through its thickness resulting in stress-strain ranges. This range is not limited just to the axial-loading direction, but also to the radial direction due to the pressurized pores by the interstitial fluid.

Hydration and dehydration are factors that affect the dissipation of pressure energy [48]. AC dissipation response is analyzed by uncoupling poroelastic and intrinsic viscoelastic mechanisms. In the dehydration state, energy dissipation reduction presents the essence of hydration in both poroelastic and viscoelastic functionality [48]. Several elements affect the mechanical properties of AC; however, researchers have circumnavigated through the complexities using customized techniques. For example, the sample-specific tissue composition has been used to predict the compressive mechanical behavior [49].

Depth-dependent mechanical properties of cartilage were also attained with optical imaging techniques such as relaxometry by MRI, which has demonstrated that under similar loading, different deformation patterns at different anatomical sites [50]. Cartilage degeneration is associated with deformation and its mechanics patterns before morphological symptoms. This finding complies with the depth-dependent mechanical properties under contact loading [50].

The cyclic loading effect on cartilage compaction was highlighted when its relaxation time was altered [40]. Moreover, static and dynamic loadings are other factors that significantly affect stress distribution over the cartilage. By dynamic loading, more uniform deformation across cartilage depth occurs, and this is because of substantial synovial fluid pressure in dynamic loading imposed on the cartilage compared to static loading. Thus, it exemplifies cartilage characteristics in reducing local strains in daily high intense physiological activities [51].

A novel method, known as Principle Component Analysis (PCA), has been developed to characterize cartilage mechanical properties with more abilities than conventional methods. This method is based on the surrounding tissue of the loaded area (L) and the transient strain (TS) of the AC during loading and unloading. L would be a benchmark to differentiate healthy and PG-depleted cartilage under loadings (deformation) and unloading (recovery) modes [52]. This framework is proving how PGs play a significant role in mechanical functioning.

6. Tribological Properties of Articular Cartilage

6.1. *Wear and CoF of Articular Cartilage Components*

Human knee or hip joints are subjected to up to one million cycles of loading per year during daily activities [53]. The rupture of the anterior cruciate ligament (ACL), or meniscal tears, is attributed to joints' misalignment, consequently affecting the joint kinematics, which increases the OA risk [54]. ACL and meniscus deficiency also cause excess tribological contact stresses due to instability of the joint and immediate fibrillation on the tibial plateau [55]. Several studies have presented that cartilage properties vary as the function of local contact stresses and mechanical environment; however, tribological properties have been reported to be location-independent [56,57]. Moore et al. [58] have shown that cartilage properties are location-independent and claimed that tribological properties also vary with respect to the local mechanics of the healthy joint. They found four primary tribological responses of the healthy cartilage: first, different regions have different damage tolerances. Secondly, material properties vary remarkably due to OA diseases. Third, different properties are the results of the healthy tibial plateau and OA cartilage. Fourth, OA tissues demonstrate different tribological performances that increase the shear stresses due to mechanical failure or biomechanical degradation [58]. Since cartilage is avascular, degenerated cartilage initiated from the superficial zone and propagated to the deep zone causes destruction of the layers through the thickness, resulting in gradual material loss. Cyclic loading induces stress through the entire cartilage structure yielding microscopic damage [59]. The superficial zone in AC experiences shear stresses and cracks within its collagen fibers. Therefore, AC damage occurs when the fibers crack rate exceeds the cell repair rate [60], and this phenomenon is called AC wear-off. AC presents a rubbery surface with a meager wear rate and CoF [6] but can be escalated by the absence of lubrication, abnormal loading due to varus or valgus knee alignment, aging and excess physiological activities [61].

Wear is the amount of material loss from the surfaces due to contacting asperities and friction. In AC, the wear mechanism is categorized as adhesive, abrasive and fatigue wear [62]. Cartilage wear is because of PGs loss and alterations in the collagen network [63]. Cartilage wear could be initiated due to biochemical degradation and biomechanical factors such as knee misalignment, which induces higher pressure on either the medial or lateral side of the knee joint [64]. Most of the studies have fallen short of quantifying wear mechanism due to its complex nature; hence only frictional properties have been investigated. Several studies used metal abrader against AC to quantify wear depth, and their results demonstrated that synovial fluid incorporation with trypsin effectively protects the cartilage surface against wear [65,66]. Other studies showed that the wear rate increases with increased contact pressure, area of contact, and sliding speed [67,68]. Wear rate can be quantified by biochemical characterization of collagen and GAGs content [69]. Another method to capture wear depth and wear scar is surface topography, using scanning electron microscopy (SEM), transmission electron microscopy (TEM), atomic force microscopy (AFM), contact and non-contact profilometric methods [70,71]. Quantifying wear in AC is complex because of the deficient wear volume of soft tissues. An experiment was conducted to assess wear in AC and cartilage specimens loaded against stainless steel ball by steady sliding motion with 4.62 MPa contact pressure. Collagen loss was monitored as the wear rate indicator, and the results showed a low wear rate (0.5 μg/h at 4.62 MPa) in AC [7].

McCutchen [72] worked on the interstitial fluid and hypothesized that this fluid is the most load-bearing element in AC functioning. The author highlighted that since AC has deformable architecture, the interstitial fluid withstood most of the compressive state load. After this theory, Mow et al. [73] studied the biphasic structure and categorized it as incompressible and immiscible tissue. Katta et al. [56] then assessed that fluid could migrate through the porous AC architecture with tiny pore sizes in the range of 2.0–6.5 nm. In addition, Lai et al. [74] presented the triphasic theory, which considers monovalent ions in the interstitial fluid as the third phase. It showed three elements of fluid, solid and ion concentration are vital in identifying compressive stiffness of cartilage. Joint under compressive loading pressurize the interstitial fluid in the tissue. Such a pressure gradient in the tissue supports a significant contribution of the applied loads until the fluid is exuded away at the very beginning of the unloading period [75]. By the fluid pressurizing phase, the applied load is gradually transferred to the soft cartilage tissue, while the imposed load on the fluid is also gradually dissipated. At the equilibrium state, however, the load is tolerated by the soft cartilage tissue. Therefore, the solid phase of cartilage incorporated with interstitial fluid deprives CoF between cartilage mates. It can be maintained at a very low level as long as sufficient interstitial fluid is lubricating superficial layers of the cartilage [57].

Rehydration, contact stress, sliding contact materials and speeds are proportionally related to AC lubrication [76]. The sliding speed and stroke length are primary factors for controlling CoF and rehydration time. These factors control the wear in the cartilage surface as fluid carries the maximum load and results in a very low CoF in AC [77]. Contact stress was also reported to impact CoF significantly; increasing contact stress resulted in the reduction of CoF [78]. On the other hand, it has been shown that experimental parameters and rehydration would change the trend of decreasing CoF by increasing contact stress [57]. Consequently, Katta et al. [78] demonstrated that with increased contact stresses from 0.2 to 0.5 MPa, CoF decreased upon regular rehydration. Most of the cartilage frictional studies conducted have been based on the linear relationship between the applied load and CoF; however, further study is needed to investigate this relationship by a nonlinear trend.

Krishnan et al. [79] investigated friction in AC under cyclic compressive loading with various frequencies (0.05, 0.5 and 1 Hz). They reported that cyclic loading does not decrease CoF by increasing the interstitial fluid's pressurization compared to the static loading. Their study showed that relocation of contact areas effectively lowered CoF rather than the cyclic loading. On the other hand, another study showed that contact stress and stroke length (for rehydration process time) affect CoF detrimentally [80].

While fluid lubrication has been highlighted as a critical element of CoF variations in experimental studies [58,81], boundary lubrication shows a remarkable improvement since cartilage is biphasic and retains fluid in its superficial layer [82]. By lubricant depletion, the CoF is mostly altered as a function of surface chemistry [56]. Boundary lubrication has been recognized for its usefulness in tissue engineering purposes, joint lubrication, cartilage substitution therapies and several other applications [75].

Biological factors also have a significant impact on CoF in cartilage. GAGs/PGs formation and existence result in fluid pressurization and consequently variation in tribological properties [83]. These materials exhibit resistance against the interstitial fluid flow, leading to a low permeability rate (~10–15 to 10–16 m^4/Ns) [84]. Aging or joint disease leads to a reduction of GAG [85], which effectively increases the CoF rate [86]. Chondroitin sulfate is recommended in case of GAGs depletion; however, lubrication conditions must be considered [87]. Diffusing chondroitin sulfate into the cartilage reported results in a deficiency of ECM integration with chondroitin sulfate, and after imposing load, it is exuded out [56]. Collagen, another major component of cartilage, has also been reported to be effective in reducing CoF, and the lower level of collagen could exacerbate friction [88] and reduce water contents [89]. The SAL contains sulfated sugars, glycoproteins and lipids, which can be removed by wiping, resulting in higher friction than the unwiped surface [84].

6.2. Boundary Lubrication

Transition time in joint is shifting of dynamic to static loading or vice versa. When dynamic loading is gradually transformed to static loading, dissipating energy is mitigated by the interstitial fluid, and it permeates into the cartilage. At this stage, cartilage components absorb the synovial fluids, which initiate the boundary lubrication process [90]. Therefore, it yields to cartilage-on-cartilage contact that increases CoF.

Several studies have demonstrated the role of synovial fluid in minimizing CoF drastically under boundary lubrication regime [91,92]. Radin et al. [93] demonstrated that the proteinaceous layer has a load-bearing duty and not hyaluronic acid (HA) in the synovial fluid. In contrast, other researchers have shown that HA significantly supports the interstitial fluid in withstanding load [88,94,95]. Tests using HA on healthy and dysfunctional cartilage for both humans and bovine showed a remarkable decrease in CoF [88]. This effect is limited to lowering CoF in dynamic loading, even under static pressure, while boundary lubrication occurs. HA penetrates into the cartilage structure and surrounds the chondrocytes, which preserves the CoF levels [95].

Lubricin, a mucinous glycoprotein, is another component of synovial fluid has been reported that lack of lubricin in synovial fluid resulted in inadequate boundary lubrication and increases wear in cartilage [70]. This research showed that in the presence of lubricin, adhesion between contacting cartilage is minimized, and this process yields to decreased friction upon boundary lubrication [70].

As another component of synovial fluid, phospholipids contributed significantly to boundary lubrication due to the hydrophobic nature of its fatty acid [96]. Hills and Crawford [97] reported that phospholipids are a component of lubricin in the boundary lubrication, whereas lubricin and HA only supported the phospholipids. Furthermore, Pickard et al. [98] demonstrated that elimination of phospholipid from the cartilage increases the CoF of cartilage minimally. Their study was just limited to the short time; however, no remarkable effect was reported at a prolonged time regarding the cartilage friction properties.

According to the literature, all mentioned components of synovial fluid effects boundary lubrication, and isolating any component can compromise the boundary lubrication process. Moreover, the biomechanical and biochemical synergies may also be insufficiently controlled, as it is in a synovial joint. Nevertheless, all these findings are the expedient benchmark to characterize wear and CoF in AC.

7. Tissue Engineering of Articular Cartilage

Cartilage tissue engineering has been investigated extensively by researchers since this tissue is avascular, and confined migration of chondrocyte reduces its self-recovery considerably. Therefore, the essence of artificial cartilage motivates researchers to design and manufacture materials mimicking mechanical and tribological responses of the native cartilage. Polymeric hydrogels have been highlighted as candidates for this application as they resemble the biomechanical, biochemical and architectural properties of native cartilage [99]. Hydrogels have also appealed to researchers due to their biocompatibility [100], nontoxicity effects and no stimuli on the immune system [101]. Hydrogels are categorized as natural and synthetic and can be modulated with cell-free or cell-laden scaffolds. Some of the cell-free scaffolds have been presented with the use of bacterial nano-cellulose [102], polyethylene glycol (PEG) in combination with HA [103], collagen-hydroxyapatite hybrids [104], aragonite-hyaluronate membranes [105], acrylamide (AAm) hydrogels [106], alginate (Alg)/chitosan compounds, agarose/polyglycolic acids (PGA) [107], and porous polycaprolactone (PCL) [108]. The mentioned scaffolds were used clinically; however, after clinical follow-up in the longer term, they were rejected due to the lack of strength and durability. The following sections describe some of the common materials used in the manufacture of hydrogels.

7.1. Hydrogel Materials

7.1.1. Hydrogel Classifications

Hydrogels are classified based on raw materials, chemical composition, physical structure, type of crosslinking, physical appearances and electrical charge, presented in Table 1.

Table 1. Classification of hydrogels.

Classification of Hydrogels Based on	Ref.	Subdomains	Features
Source		Natural origin Synthetic origin	—
Polymeric composition	[32,109]	Homopolymeric hydrogels	Network formation by single species of monomer.
		Copolymeric hydrogels	Network formation by various monomer species with at least one hydrophilic monomer.
		Multipolymer hydrogels	Synthesized by two independent crosslinked natural or synthetic polymer.
Physical structure and chemical composition	[110]	Amorphous	- Non crystallized polymer chains contain an abundant amount of water. - Mechanically weak. - Very soft and homogenously heparinized.
	[111]	Semi-crystalline	- Moderately water-swollen hydrogels. - Mechanically stable and performing melt-processability, and self-healing function.
	[112]	Crystalline	- Structurally unique and hierarchical. - Morphologies depend on their molecular architectures.
Type of crosslinking	[113]	Chemically crosslinked (permanent joints)	Covalent bonding between polymer chains.
		Physical crosslinked (transient junctions)	Physical interactions between chains result in chain entanglement, hydrogen bonding, hydrophobic interactions and crystallite formation.
Physical appearances post-polymerization		Matrix, film and Microsphere	—
Network electrical charge	[114]	Non-ionic (neutral)	Less toxic to the cells in vitro.
	[115]	Ionic (including anionic or cationic)	High strain sensitivity and many superior mechanical properties.
		Amphoteric electrolyte	—
	[116]	Zwitterionic (polybetaines)	Anti-polyelectrolyte" behavior, unusual pH sensitivity and temperature sensitivity.

7.1.2. Polymer Materials Used for Articular Cartilage Synthesis

Table 2 presents comparative advantages and applications of wide ranges of materials in synthesizing polymeric hydrogels for articular applications.

Table 2. Commonly used polymers in articular cartilage synthesis.

Polymers	Ref.	Advantages	Applications
Acrylamide	[117]	- High level of toughness and stretch ratio - Similar elastic properties to that of native cartilage	The base of the most polymeric hydrogels.
Acrylic Acid	[118]	- Great impact on tensile strength and elastic modulus - Usage amounts effects on more crosslinking and shorter polymer chains, yields higher toughness - Usage results in nonlinearity in mechanical response - High capacity in water retention for swelling applications	Used in synthesizing hydrogels.
METAC *	[119]	- Deprive wear loss rate - Retain water in the hydrogel matrix and decrease CoF	Utilized in hydrogels that must be riched of water in prolonged time in biomedical and pharmaceutical applications.
Hyaluronic acid	[120]	- Tissue healing, expansion of cell proliferation and migration - Angiogenesis - Inflammatory response control	For treatment purpose of osteochondral diffusion, enhancing chondrogenesis within the damaged tissues.
Cellulose	[121]	- Special fibrous nanostructure, with excellent mechanical and physical characteristics	Methylcellulose includes producing thermosensitive hydrogels applicable in drug delivery systems.
Dextran	[122]	- Biodegradable - Biocompatible - Bioadhesive	Wound healing, Relief patient pain, Hard for installation and removal.
Alginate	[123]	- Biocompatible - Availability and reproducibility - Low cost	Wound healing, Encapsulation of therapeutic agents, Tissue engineering applications.
Chitosan	[124]	- Biocompatibility - Biodegradability - Non-toxicity - Biological characteristics	Hydrogel synthesized by Chitosan and beads applicable to embedding drugs for transport bioactive substances. Drug delivery applications.
Gelatin	[125]	- Biopolymer's biotoxicity - Biodegradability - Potential to induce cell migration	The optimal candidate for applications for extracellular matrix (ECM), 3D structure, Cell transplantation.
Polyvinyl alcohol (PVA)	[126]	Biocompatibility Biodegradability	An ideal option for tissue engineering applications, appropriate for mimicking tissue, vascular cell culture, nontoxicity and mechanical strength.

* METAC: 2-(methacryloyloxy)ethyltrimethlammonium chloride.

7.2. Synthesis of Hydrogels

7.2.1. Crosslinking Hydrogels

Various crosslinking approaches have been reported to synthesize hydrogel, such as chemically modified process, crystallization process, free-radical polymerization and ionic polymerization [127,128]. Table 3 presents four prevalent approaches that are used to synthesize hydrogels for medical applications.

Table 3. Crosslinking methods to design hydrogels.

Methods	Ref.	Category	Advantages
1. Chemically crosslinked gels	[129,130]	Crosslinking by radical polymerization	Water-soluble polymers can be achieved with an initiator and catalyst. Such a system is very efficient, and at ambient temperature, gel forms quickly. Water solubility, short-chain and solubility activity.
		Crosslinking by chemical reaction of interdependent groups	A group of polymer chains can be connected with covalent linkages due to their interdependent reactivity.
		Crosslinking by high energy irradiation	-
	[131]	Crosslinking using enzymes	In an equilibrium state (more than 90% water content), gelatin is formed.
2. Physically crosslinked gels	[128]	Crosslinking ionically	Very effective on the self-healing properties of hydrogels.
	[126]	Crosslinking by crystallization	By the process of freeze-thawing, a very elastic gel is formed.
	[132]	Physically crosslinked hydrogels from by graft copolymers	The uniform structure is formed in water.
3. Crosslinking by hydrogen bonds	[133]	-	Swelling is a function of pH.
4. Crosslinking by protein interactions	[134]	Use of genetically designed proteins	By manipulating genetic DNA code, physical and chemical properties are controllable parameters (More related to Genetic Engineering).
		Crosslinking by antigen-antibody interactions	Good for drug delivery to target specific antigens.

The major limitations for the biomedical application of hydrogels are the non-biocompatibility of some hydrogels and potential toxicity of residual unreacted small cross-linkers in chemically crosslinked hydrogels [135]. However, among methods mentioned above, free-radical polymerization is a prevalent method used to synthesize hydrogels for biomedical applications [136].

7.2.2. Free Radical Polymerization

Free radical polymerization (FRP) is a capable technique to produce about 50% of monomers to polymers [137]. The major advantage of FRP is its insensitivity to monomer and impurities compared to ionic polymerization [138]. It can be applied in normal room conditions, which minimize the cost of production. A broad range of monomers can be utilized in FRP to turn to polymers which is the great advantage of this technique [139].

Free radical polymerization involves the conversion of monomers into polymers through the initiation, propagation and termination steps. The ''initiation'' process involves the production of radicals that start the reaction with monomer. An existing free-radical interacts with the monomer resulting in a new radical, which in turn opens another molecule monomer. This process repeats to result in a polymer, and this step is called "propagation". The polymerization reaction stops when the last radical of one polymer chain meets another chain with the free radical, and when they combine, the polymerization process is completed, hence the "termination" step [140].

7.3. Bilayer Hydrogels

Bilayer hydrogel consists of a porous architecture layer integrated with a bulk layer covalently. The porous architecture is the result of the interruption in the polymerization process. The porous layer benefits hydrogel in water retention, impact on diffusion rate, minimizing CoF and wear rate [104,119]. Gong et al. [141] developed a bilayer hydrogel with varying crosslinking degrees in the top layer. A lower degree of crosslinking resulted in high porosity and the hydrogel had a higher fluid retention capacity, which consequently minimized the CoF. The bilayer architecture formation in hydrogels is due to branch dangling chemical phenomenon [141]. A branched dangling polymer chain is achieved by polymerizing the monomers, while in contact with a hydrophobic surface. Hydrogen-rich moieties are located within close vicinity of the hydrophobic surfaces yielding a low density highly porous structure. This is attributed to the high concentration of hydrogen affecting the propagation step of polymerization. The bulk area, which is far from the hydrophobic surface, could accomplish the polymerization process due to hydrogen deficiency in this zone. Consequently, a very dense structure is formed, and the bulk area's strength enhances compared to its porous counterpart [142,143]. The SEM image of a bilayer hydrogel cross-section is presented in Figure 2.

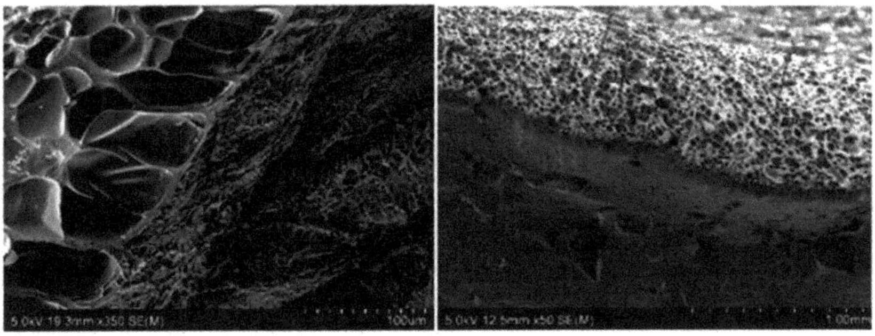

Figure 2. PAAm-Alg bilayer hydrogels: cross-section view.

7.4. Mechanical Testing of Articular Cartilage and Hydrogels

AC as a soft tissue articulates the full range of motions and experiences complex loading scenario, which is compression, tension, shear and friction [144]. Most studies focused on assessing recovered tissue based on biochemical, gene expression, or histological aspects [145]. Comprehensive protocols for mechanical evaluations showed a lack of standardization for their unit reference. Therefore, remarkable tolerances in the reported data are inevitable. The compression testing is categorized as unconfined, confined and in situ. For the confined compression test, a porous plate or indenter is used to let fluid flow out of the tissue.

Four test configurations are commonly used to characterize cartilage mechanical responses: ramp, stress relaxation, creep and indentation tests. Jay et al. [70] reported that the most utilized test configuration in studies from 2009 to 2018 were: ramp, stress relaxation and creep. Thus, the ramp test has been configured to simulate the load-bearing properties of the tissue. After recording the stress-strain response by the ramp test, the first-order differential equation of the curve, which is the slope of the stress-strain curve, results in the tangent modulus of the tissue. Tangent modulus quantifies softening and hardening of the material and plastic deformation beyond yield stress [132]. Softened materials endure a higher load before ultimate failure compared to hardened materials and are suitable for replacing tissues that undergo large deformations [146]. Two factors that considerably affect the tangent modulus are strain rate and strain point. Healthy knee cartilage typically experiences average strains under 10% [36] and a maximum of 17% [147]. The tangent modulus is estimated by laying on the curve less than 10% strain at different strain points, hence, tangent modulus data would not be clinically helpful. However, it shows at each strain point how hard or soft tissue responses are. This is relative to the micro-architecture of the tissue matrix, porosity and fluid flow rate within the matrix [148].

It has been highlighted that compression tests are essential with modeling of viscoelasticity responses according to required tests of the United States Food and Drug Administration (FDA) and International Cartilage Repair Society (ICRS) [149,150]. Moreover, the American Society for Testing and Materials (ASTM) standard is focused on confined creep testing as a requirement for mechanical evaluation of designed tissues [151]. Alternatively, creep or stress relaxation is needed to quantify material properties recommended by ASTM. A systematic review of literature from 2009 to 2018 [152] showed only 11.4% of studies had performed stress relaxation or creep tests, which demonstrates that most studies did not meet the requirements of the FDA and ICRS guidance documents.

7.5. *Tribological Testing of Articular Cartilage and Hydrogels*

In the tribology testing of both native and engineered cartilage, there are two methods of testing the lubrication properties; the first method is sliding mate with a specified stroke length, which yields to matrix deformation. The CoF would be very low as the fluid resistance is against imposed load in the active deformation region. It is reported that the load support can be analyzed by Peclet number, where low friction occurs by the condition of $Pe >> 1$ and connective fluid velocity surpasses diffusive fluid velocity [5,75]. The second method of lubrication analysis is aimed more at boundary lubrication which is a stationary contact area. In this method, a sample is compressed to a solid mate, and CoF is recorded as the fluid pressure drops to the ambient pressure [81]. Therefore, interstitial fluid pressure lessens, and only contact pressure between two solid mates determines the CoF associated with the biochemical and articular surface. Thus, this method is suitable to analyze boundary lubrication and its biomolecular interactions. It is worth mentioning that a correct interpretation of using the two methods is necessary and depends on the surface and pressuring mechanism. If a tissue provides excellent permeability, which increases the localization of lubricants, it will have a relatively low CoF in stationary and high CoF in migrating contact areas. In contrast, a tissue with a remarkable pressurizing fluid mechanism but poor in boundary lubricants would have a relatively low CoF in migrating contact area and high CoF in stationary contact area [152].

8. Mechanical Properties of Hydrogels

Crosslinking process within polymer chains improves the compressive strength, stretchability and toughness of the hydrogels to withstand shear or compressive stresses [141]. There are two conventional crosslinking approaches. Covalent crosslinking enhances materials' strength and dissipates mechanical energy against deformation, whereas ionically crosslinked augments self-healing properties and controls degradation of the polymeric network [26]. Furthermore, it was reported that ionically crosslinked hydrogels using Fe^{3+} or Al^{3+} also exhibited enhanced mechanical strength [153]. Crosslinking density affects the polymer chain length, and consequently, different properties can be achieved [154]. The dangling chains phenomenon exploits the hydrophobicity and hydrophilicity interaction to form a low-crosslinked density that improves lubricious fluid retention. The high-crosslinked density, however, results in a bulk layer that enhances structure load-bearing [153]. Furthermore, interpenetrating polymer networks (IPNs) are formed by interpenetrating entanglement of two or more crosslinked polymers. A semi-IPN results when only one polymer in the system is crosslinked, whereas, crosslinking of all polymers in the system results in full-IPN. Hence, the mechanical strengths of hydrogels in the form of full-IPN structure is superior compared to semi-IPN structures [155].

An improvement in the mechanical properties mitigates the lubrication properties of hydrogels. Subsequently, research on having a load-bearing structure with a sufficient lubricational threshold has not yielded the desired success; therefore, this subject warrants further research attention. It has been proven that monomers molar ratio, initiator and crosslinking degree determine the mechanical properties of hydrogels [156]. Zhang et al. [119] reported that the mechanical properties of bilayer hydrogels improved notably by meticulously increasing monomer (acrylic acid, AAc) content. Increasing the amount of AAc, resulted in ultimate tensile strength and elastic modulus increase. However, when AAc was more than 50%, hydrogels become very brittle and stiff, resulting in inferior tensile properties [132], and were not suitable for practical applications. Xu et al. [157] found that the titanium nanocomposite hydrogels having 10% AAc had significant tensile strength and enhanced water stability (low swelling ratio) compared to the higher molar percentage of AAc. Optimum AAc amount improves the mechanical strength and affects the nonlinearity of the hydrogels, which is a premium consideration in tissue engineering applications [158]. Arjmandi et al. [26] reported that their hydrogel's mechanical properties improved by increasing crosslinking concentration up to 21% and 32% for elastic modulus and hardness, respectively. Trivalent cations (Al^{3+} or Fe^{3+}) also presented a momentous factor in increasing the strength and stiffness when hydrogels were synthesized using alginate monomer [159].

Among polymers, alginate and polyacrylamide (Alg/PAAm) have been reported to provide a high level of toughness and stretch ratio [160]. The elastic properties, furthermore, were reported to be similar to that of AC. Alg/PAAm also proved a 3-fold decrease in CoF compared to either Alg or PAAm as single network hydrogels [161]. Alg, however, has some disadvantages such as low tensile properties and difficulty in sterilization and controlling the hygiene process during synthesis. Its impurities may also affect material properties [162]. To sum up, optimum amounts of AAc, AAm, Alg and relevant crosslinking ratios would significantly improve both the mechanical and tribological properties of hydrogels.

Viscoelastic and Poroelastic Relaxation

Viscoelastic and poroelastic are associated with the rate of fluid migration within the networks, and their interaction with polymer chains results in dissipating energy [163]. Therefore, the assessment of hydrogel materials and their viscoelastic or poroelastic relaxation response is essential in designing tissues where they are subjected to high-impact loads. Hydrogels are formed by fiber networks similar to fibrin and collagen in AC and can be categorized as viscoelastic due to the exhibition of stress relaxation [164]. A nanoporous hydrogel structure, such as acrylamide hydrogels, performs minor viscoelasticity and is nearly elastic [46]. It was reported that stress relaxes promptly when the hydrogel is crosslinked ionically compared with covalently crosslinked [165]. More details were reported by Zhao et al. [165] and showed that binding and unbinding of alginate hydrogels that are crosslinked ionically show quicker stress relaxation compared to the covalently crosslinked. By exerting a force that results in unbinding of ionically crosslinked fibers, divalent cations detach from the anions of alginate chains and re-bond with another anion. In contrast, the covalently crosslinked network does not detach and re-attach fibers. Thus, instead of detaching, it yields to a longer time to relax the stress [166]. The covalently crosslinked hydrogels exhibited time-dependent mechanical properties.

It is highlighted that an abundant amount of water in hydrogels also affects viscoelastic responses. Fluid motion within the network would significantly impact dissipating energy from external loadings [165]. Hong et al. [167] formulated a coupled mass transport theory and large deformation within the hydrogel network. The motion of fluid inside the network and the resistance of the porous structure against the fluid migration yield to macroscopic mechanical relaxation, which is different from relaxation resulting from structural deformation in the network. This phenomenon is called poroelasticity and is characterized by diffusion coefficient D of the fluid in the network [168] and can be obtained by the following equation:

$$D \sim Er2/\eta \quad (1)$$

where E is the elastic modulus, r is the pore radius of the polymer network and η is the fluid viscosity in the hydrogel. According to the equation, the rate of relaxation depends on poroelasticity. As mentioned above, regarding the fluid migration, the smaller pore size results in slower fluid migration and thus slower stress relaxation. Therefore, diffusion rate D, and geometric scale L of the sample are inversely proportional to the time of stress relaxation. A smaller L yields to a faster stress relaxation due to the fluid migration at a shorter distance. However, the rate of deformations of a hydrogel is independent of the geometric scale [165]. In addition, viscoelastic responses are always attributed to fluid flow and network deformation. Therefore, when L >> $\sqrt{(D\tau\_v)}$ which was obtained for hydrogels when the sample scale is large enough to prevent the fluid from migrating to the end, viscoelastic relaxation occurs before poroelastic relaxation [169]. If we consider two states of time required for hydrogel to reach viscoelastic and poroelastic relaxation, therefore, $t \sim \tau\_v$ is the time of viscoelastic relaxation from deformation and $t \sim \tau\_p$ is the time of poroelastic relaxation resulting from fluid flow. τ_v is the time of viscoelastic relaxation and τ_p is the time of poroelastic relaxation. Therefore, it is essential in the design of artificial cartilage to assess the viscoelastic and poroelastic time of relaxation based on material properties.

9. Tribological Properties of Hydrogels

Wear is the loss of material, a continuous damage process due to the sliding of contact mates throughout cycles. Wear, V, is defined as the total volume of material loss. Wear rate (w) reported by Archard et al. [170] is defined as volume loss per unit sliding distance. Archard's equation predicts that the wear rate is proportional to the normal contact pressure and inversely proportional to the hardness of the material surface:

$$w = V/s = K\,P/H \quad (2)$$

where V is the total volume loss in [mm^3], P is the normal load in [N], H is the hardness of the material, s is the sliding distance and K is the so-called wear coefficient, a constant that is usually determined by experiment for two specific contact partners under certain environmental conditions.

A conventional system for analyzing tribological parameters is the pin-on-disk tribometer, where a small pin slides on a larger circular disk. The sliding motion is between the specimen and the rotating disk. Several types of motions and sliding between solids have been introduced (i.e., sliding wear, rolling wear, impact wear and oscillation wear) [171]. The dominant wear mechanisms are abrasion, adhesion, surface fatigue and tribochemical reactions. Abrasive wear is the subtraction of a soft material by a hard adjacent surface [172]. The most substantial part of the abrasive wear is caused by tangential sliding motions and removal of the microscopic asperities. Adhesive wear is associated with an increase in the CoF, μ between the interfaces [172]. Up to $\mu = 1.0$, the presence of friction can be explained by adhesion itself, which means that frictional resistance is caused by asperities coming into contact and adhering to one another. Corrosive wear is a mechanism of materials and environment interface; development of worn surface may yield to different scenarios as relative motions of the bodies. Finally, wear due to fracture is a description of removal of chunks of material due to microcrack occurs within material either due to surface cracks or subsurface cracks [57].

Bilayer hydrogels that consist of a bulk layer for bearing load, and a thin porous layer to retain fluid and minimize the CoF have been developed recently [119,153]. In these bilayer hydrogels, the bulk layer exhibited significant compressive strength up to 0.35 MPa. The reciprocating sliding test reported a 0.038 CoF associated with its lubricious layer. However, the lubricious layer was worn after a few thousand cycles due to its low network density. Surface network density is inversely proportional to water retention, which in turn influences the CoF reported by Zhang et al. [119]. Crosslinking density is proportionally related to the mesh size and showed a remarkable correlation at the transition of low to high frictions [173].

In an earlier study, the lateral and normal friction forces were not directly correlated to the stiffness but varied with the hydrogel architecture and composition [174]. The contact pressure and pore pressurization within interconnected channels are the key factors that control hydration levels in tribological assessments [168]. The contact pressure experienced by AC was reported in the range of 0.1–2.0 MPa in the hip and knee joints [76,175]. By increasing contact stress on AC, the CoF decreases [78]. However, research showed that experimental parameters and rehydration would change the trend of decreasing CoF by increasing contact stress [176].

Beyond CoF values, the determination of lubrication mechanisms in hydrogel has rarely been addressed. The effects of load and speed on lubrication regimes have been studied with the aid of the classical engineering Stribeck curve [177]. They found that hydrogels are not covered the engineering Stribeck curve regimes, and the main regimes were developed: mesh-confined, elastoviscous transition and fluid film.

In the engineering system, a prompt transition occurs over narrow ranges of the Hersey number, which is also the dimensionless fluid thickness. It is worth mentioning that stiff engineering materials have elastic moduli in the scale of GPa; therefore, the hydrodynamic fluid film would form by increasing speed or decreasing load. However, hydrogels with conformational surfaces with respect to contacting mate and a much lower range of elastic modulus (kPa) do not fall into this lubrication regime. Therefore, hydrogels are viscoelastic materials, and their wear behavior is similar to that of rubbers; thus, fatigue and adhesion wear mechanisms are dominant [178].

Furthermore, effects of applied load and sliding speed on shifting wear mechanisms have been investigated recently, and it was shown that unlike applied load, sliding speed has a minor influence on the wear mechanism [179]. Addressing these tribological properties is essential to ensure hydrogels under various contact pressures and sliding speeds can perform similar to AC [177].

A knee joint represents a situation of soft elastohydrodynamic lubrication (EHL). Artificial implants are examples of hard EHL. Hard EHL can be very successful in tribological situations, but only when the lubricating fluid has superior high-pressure rheology. This is not the case for synovial fluid, [180]; thus, the soft EHL results in thicker lubricant films than hard EHL in vivo. To this end, a porous architecture of polymer would mimic natural cartilage in terms of EHL lubrication and yields significant performance to conventional fully dense polymers. The CoF associated with different polymeric materials are presented in Table 4.

Table 4. Effects of monomers and polymers materials on hydrogels' CoF.

Author	Ref.	Year	Materials	CoF	Findings
Gong et al.	[142]	2001	PAMPS	0.001	Polymers with dangling chains reduce CoF substantially.
Covert et al.	[77]	2003	PVA-c	*Stc.: 0.285 Dyn.: 0.143	Friction significantly depends on material stiffness and toughness.
Yasuda et al.	[117]	2005	PAMPS	0.040	Excellent wear properties compared to UHMWPE.

Table 4. *Cont.*

Author	Ref.	Year	Materials	CoF	Findings
Lin et al.	[181]	2009	PAAm-Alg-SNPs	0.00026	The incorporation of nano-silica significantly increased the compressive strength and fracture toughness but lowered the cross-linking density and CoF.
Arkaki et al.	[182]	2010	PAMPS/PDMAAm	0.029	Low CoF on normal cartilage, no significant detrimental effects on counterface cartilage.
Liao et al.	[161]	2013	PAAm-Alg-caprolactone	0.150	Tough material and potential for cell-based artificial cartilage.
Li et al.	[183]	2016	PVA on cartilage	0.114	The CoF significantly depends on load and speed.
Zhang et al.	[119]	2017	PAAm-AAc-METAC	<0.07	Salt leaching method was used to modulate porosity on the surface of the hydrogel, and it reduced CoF.
Arjmandi et al.	[26]	2018	PAAm-Alg	0.01	Less material was removed under higher sliding speed in their tribology tests.
Li et al.	[184]	2020	PAAm and different crosslinking concentrations	0.008–0.04	In the low normal force regime, friction is mainly adhesion-controlled and increases with polymer volume fraction. In the high normal force regime, friction is predominantly load-controlled and shows a slow increase with normal force.

*Stc: Static; *Dyn: Dynamics; *PAMPS: Poly 2-acrylamido−2-methyl−1-propanesulfonic acid; *PVA-c: Poly vinyl-alcohol cryogel; *PAMPS: Poly (2-acrylamide−2-metyl-propane sulfonic acid) and polyacrylamide; *PAMPS/PDMAAm: Poly-(2-Acrylamido−2-methylpropane sulfonic acid)/poly-(N,N′-dimetyl acrylamide).

10. Strengthening of Hydrogels with Nanoparticles

TiO_2 nanoparticles (TiO_2 NPs), due to their low toxicity, excellent biocompatibility, low cost and high-level stability, have been explored for the synthesis of polymeric hydrogels for medical applications [185]. However, due to the hydrophobic nature of these nanoparticles, having a homogenous solution that affects mechanical and tribological properties would be challenging. These challenges are because of TiO_2 NPs surface and electrostatic attraction among particle molecules [186]. TiO_2 nanoparticles tend to agglomeration or aggregation due to solution ionic strength (IS), pH level, surface charge or coating [187]. Using different techniques may affect the tendency of nanoparticles to aggregation. Some researchers have reported these techniques, which are ultrasonic irradiation, stabilize TiO_2 NPs in an aqueous medium, electrostatic stabilization, controlling pH level of the solution by neutralizing acidity level, and coating the surface of nanoparticles by surfactants [188]. Moreover, overcoming the van der Waals attraction of nanoparticles by utilizing steric or electrostatic stabilization is the critical factor to suppress nanoparticle aggregation or agglomeration effectively.

Ultrasonic irradiation was an effective method to disperse NPs, which depends on solvent type, concentration and suspension volume. Two ultrasonic irradiation methods, bath and probe sonications, are commonly used, although probe sonication showed a better result [187]. Even using probe sonication is not the permanent solution to suppress aggregation. Stabilizers were reported to have prolonged effects on dispersed particles [189]. As mentioned earlier, steric and electrostatic stabilization takes place when charges accumulate by the particle surfaces. More than 30 mV or less than −30 mV surface charge on the TiO_2

NPs yields no aggregation. Moreover, having higher than 1% TiO_2 NPs concentration in the AAm-based hydrogels composition resulted in sedimented particles even if a long homogenization process was used [190].

Some monomers of hydrogel compositions have a high acidity level, for instance, AAc, which can affect NPs dispersion. The hydrodynamic size of nanoparticles can be tuned by modifying the pH level of the solution. TiO_2 and SiO_2 particles have a positive surface charge when the pH level is low, and on the opposite, negative surface charge when the pH level is high [191].

TiO_2 and Silica NPs Mechanical and Tribological Properties

Chemically crosslinked co-polymeric hydrogels have been reported to have superior mechanical properties compared to the conventional chemically crosslinked homopolymeric hydrogels. This has been attributed to the formation of more uniform and compact networks in the co-polymeric hydrogels [154]. However, nanocomposite hydrogels, loaded with nano particles (NCHs), reported higher strength, improved sliding wear resistance, anisotropy and potential self-healing property compared with double-network hydrogels (DNHs), topology hydrogels (TPHs) and micromolecular microsphere hydrogels (MMHs). The swelling ratio is a crucial factor for hydrogels in biomedical applications, which supports water-stability within the hydrogel and can be achieved by utilizing titania NPs [154]. The superior mechanical strength of hydrogels is associated with the equilibrium swelling state. Seddiki et al. [133] reported that TiO_2 NPs and a high dosage of crosslinking agents (15%) are vital factors affecting swelling ratio. Furthermore, it has been reported that carboxyl groups formed complexes with TiO_2 NPs via different methods to crosslink polymer chains [192].

The concentration of TiO_2 NPs is a critical point in the reinforcement process since this substrate act as a crosslinker. The higher concentration of NPs, which is inversely proportional to the structure mesh size, would produce a higher degree of crosslinking [190]. Consequently, with smaller mesh-size, hydrogels would imbibe less fluid in the networks, which affects stress distribution over the structure. Due to this fact, the poroelasticity and viscoelasticity relaxation time would also be affected.

Silica nanoparticles (SNPs) have also been utilized to synthesize artificial cartilage and have demonstrated appreciable mechanical and biological properties [143,193]. Incorporating SNPs within polymer networks improves tissue adhesion, stiffness and shear modulus [194]. Furthermore, SNPs, interlaced with polymer chains, enhances hydrogel elasticity [195]. Zareie et al. [196] showed that by increasing SNPs amounts in the polyacrylamide networks, the number of tie points in each entanglement increased, and the compressive strength of hydrogel reached 26.2 kPa.

In addition to improving mechanical strength, SNPs have promoted the degree of crosslinking in very weak chemically crosslinked PAAm hydrogels, which have interestingly presented the ability of SNPs to function as a crosslinker [195]. Arjmandi and Ramezani [146] reported that SNPs interact with PAAm chains resulting in network crosslinks through hydrogen bonds.

Unlike other NPs, SNPs showed a significant impact on initial shear modulus and viscoelastic properties since they could immobilize the polymer chains and form NPs-polymer interphases [197]. SNPs reported increasing the number of tie points in each entanglement, which results in the improvement of the compressive strength [196]. SNPs also enhance slower chain kinetics and relaxation due to tough NPs-polymer bonds [146]. Polymer bonds relax promptly when NPs are located far from chains [198]. Viscoelasticity of the SNP loaded nanocomposite hydrogels (NCHs) was studied extensively and found to be similar to that of AC [195]. AC exhibits a time-dependent response associated with viscoelasticity, poroelasticity or the combination of both phenomena [43,199].

Tribologically, SNPs showed the dominance of adhesion mechanisms rather than other wear mechanisms, although fatigue wear took place with surface pitting at higher applied loads [200]. Utilizing 1–4% SNPs into the PAAm-alginate network resulted in low Cof values in the range 0.0035–0.0055, which is comparable to the CoF of AC (0.0001) [146]. It is attributed to the strong interfacial NPs-polymer bonding in the hydrogel matrix. The contact pressure and pore pressurization within interconnected channels are the key factors that control hydration levels in tribological assessments [168]. SNPs also affect mesh patterns, and therefore, are strongly correlated with the lubrication regimes [200].

11. Conclusions

In this paper, a comprehensive review of the literature for the AC is presented. First, the architecture of the AC, its compositions and the role of each component on mechanical and tribological properties were discussed extensively. It was explained that damaged cartilage cannot recover itself due to its avascular nature. Then, osteoarthritis roots and treatment methods were presented with conventional TKR/THR solutions as the ultimate treatment being highly invasive and with significant disadvantages especially for younger patients, and the need for revision surgery due to the limited service life of TKR/THR implants were discussed. To address the gap in treatment of younger patients with OA, developments of artificial cartilage by different synthesizing processes, materials and their pros and cons were described. The required standard and necessary tests for artificial cartilage to assess its mechanical and tribological properties based on the International Cartilage Repair Society (ICRS), Food and Drug Administration (FDA) and American Society for Testing and Materials (ASTM) were briefly reviewed. Viscoelastic properties were found as the critical point in the design of engineered soft tissues and the techniques to tune viscoelasticity to perform optimum responses under different loading scenarios were reviewed. Advanced bilayer hydrogels were discussed as a promising candidate for artificial cartilage. Both the load-bearing and lubricious layer were investigated recently; however, the weak point of the proposed lubricious layer was found to be its limited strength and service life under cyclic sliding tests.

Polymeric hydrogels have indeed provided a practical alternative to AC when OA treatment is considered. This is largely attributed to the progress attained in finding the appropriate combinations of materials as well as techniques for the synthesis of hydrogels with mechanical and biochemical properties of natural cartilage. Polymeric hydrogels stand to emerge as an attractive technology for AC replacement applications. Even though highly promising, the application of hydrogels in AC replacement are not free from challenges of biocompatibility. It is, therefore, imperative that attention be diverted to understanding the degradability of synthetic polymeric networks and the interaction of the hydrogels with cells in physiological conditions. A further area of innovation would be addressing the fabrication challenges of hydrogels which will make them safer and ready for clinical use. The mechanical properties of hydrogels are an important consideration for AC replacement application; however, mechanical characterization of hydrogels have been limited to mainly cell free scaffolds. Cells' encapsulation can potentially dictate profound changes in mechanical properties of hydrogels. Hence, mechanical characterization of cell seeded hydrogels should be a consideration for the future.

Author Contributions: Conceptualization, M.M.; writing—original draft preparation, M.M.; writing—review and editing, A.N. and M.R.; supervision, A.N. and M.R. All authors have read and agreed to the published version of the manuscript.

Funding: This research received no external funding.

Institutional Review Board Statement: Not applicable.

Informed Consent Statement: Not applicable.

Data Availability Statement: The data presented in this study are available on request from the corresponding author.

Conflicts of Interest: The authors declare no conflict of interest.

References

1. Baldino, L.; Cardea, S.; Maffulli, N. Regeneration technique for bone to tendon and muscle to tendon interfaces reconstruction. *Br. Med Bull.* **2016**, *117*, 25–37. [CrossRef] [PubMed]
2. Knecht, S.; Vanwanseele, B.; Stüssi, E. A review on the mechanical quality of articular cartilage—Implications for the diagnosis of osteoarthritis. *Clin. Biomech.* **2006**, *21*, 999–1012. [CrossRef]
3. Hunziker, E.B. Articular cartilage repair: Basic science and clinical progress. A review of the current status and prospects. *Osteoarthr. Cartil.* **2002**, *10*, 432–463. [CrossRef]
4. Maroudas, A.; Wachtel, E.; Grushko, G.; Katz, E.P.; Weinberg, P. The effect of osmotic and mechanical pressures on water partitioning in articular cartilage. *Biochim. Biophys. Acta (BBA) Gen. Subj.* **1991**, *1073*, 285–294. [CrossRef]
5. Ateshian, G.A. The role of interstitial fluid pressurization in articular cartilage lubrication. *J. Biomech.* **2009**, *42*, 1163–1176. [CrossRef] [PubMed]
6. Sardinha, V.M.; Lima, L.L.; Belangero, W.D.; Zavaglia, C.A.; Bavaresco, V.P.; Gomes, J.R. Tribological characterization of polyvinyl alcohol hydrogel as substitute of articular cartilage. *Wear* **2013**, *301*, 218–225. [CrossRef]
7. Mow, V.C.; Ratcliffe, A.; Poole, A.R. Cartilage and diarthrodial joints as paradigms for hierarchical materials and structures. *Biomaterials* **1992**, *13*, 67–97. [CrossRef]
8. Travis, J.K.; Jos, M.; Robert, L.S.; and Dietmar, W.H. Tissue Engineering of Articular Cartilage with Biomimetic Zones. *Tissue Eng. Part B Rev.* **2009**, *15*, 143–157.
9. Soltz, M.; Ateshian, G.A. A Conewise Linear Elasticity Mixture Model for the Analysis of Tension-Compression Nonlinearity in Articular Cartilage. *J. Biomech. Eng.* **2000**, *122*, 576–586. [CrossRef]
10. Daniela, A.S.-T.; Lucía, T.-J.; Luís, M.R.-L. Hydrogels for Cartilage Regeneration, from Polysaccharides to Hybrids. *Polymers* **2017**, *9*, 671.
11. Buckwalter, J.A.; Mow, V.C.; Mankin, H.J. *Articular Cartilage: Structure, Function, Metabolism, Injury and Pathogenesis of Osteoarthritis*; Lippincott Williams & Wilkins: Philadelphia, PA, USA, 2003.
12. Poole, C.A.; Flint, H.; Beaumont, W. Morphological and functional interrelationships of articular cartilage matrices. *J. Anat.* **1984**, *138*, 113–138.
13. Askew, M.J.; Mow, V.C. The Biomechanical Function of the Collagen Fibril Ultrastructure of Articular Cartilage. *J. Biomech. Eng.* **1978**, *100*, 105–115. [CrossRef]
14. Lipshitz, H.; Etheredge, R.; Glimcher, M.J. Changes in the hexosamine content and swelling ratio of articular cartilage as functions of depth from the surface. *J. Bone Jt. Surg. Am. Vol.* **1976**, *58*, 1149–1153. [CrossRef]
15. Kumar, P.; Oka, M.; Toguchida, J.; Kobayashi, M.; Uchida, E.; Nakamura, T.; Tanaka, K. Role of uppermost superficial surface layer of articular cartilage in the lubrication mechanism of joints. *J. Anat.* **2001**, *199*, 241–250. [CrossRef]
16. Mow, V.C.; Guo, X.E. Mechano-Electrochemical Properties of Articular Cartilage: Their Inhomogeneities and Anisotropies. *Annu. Rev. Biomed. Eng.* **2002**, *4*, 175–209. [CrossRef] [PubMed]
17. Graindorge, S.; Ferrandez, W.; Ingham, E.; Jin, Z.; Twigg, P.; Fisher, J. The role of the surface amorphous layer of articular cartilage in joint lubrication. *Proc. Inst. Mech. Eng. H* **2006**, *220*, 597–607. [CrossRef]
18. Stockwell, R.A. The interrelationship of cell density and cartilage thickness in mammalian articular cartilage. *J. Anat.* **1971**, *109*, 411–421.
19. Vega, S.L.; Kwon, M.Y.; Burdick, J.A. Recent advances in hydrogels for cartilage tissue engineering. *Eur. Cells Mater.* **2017**, *33*, 59–75. [CrossRef]
20. Fergusson, C.M. The aetiology of osteoarthritis. *Postgrad. Med. J.* **1987**, *63*, 439–445. [CrossRef]
21. Mostakhdemin, M.; Sadegh, A.I.; Syahrom, A. *Multi-axial Fatigue of trabecular Bone with Respect to Normal Walking*; Springer: Singapore, 2016.
22. Kiviranta, I.; Tammi, M.; Jurvelin, J.; Arokoski, J.; Säämänen, A.M.; Helminen, H.J. Articular cartilage thickness and glycosaminoglycan distribution in the canine knee joint after strenuous running exercise. *Clin. Orthop. Relat. Res.* **1992**, *283*, 302–308. [CrossRef]
23. Vanwanseele, B.; Lucchinetti, E.; Stüssi, E. The effects of immobilization on the characteristics of articular cartilage: Current concepts and future directions. *Osteoarthr. Cartil.* **2002**, *10*, 408–419. [CrossRef] [PubMed]
24. Buckwalter, J.A.; Martin, J.A. Osteoarthritis. *Adv. Drug Deliv. Rev.* **2006**, *58*, 150–167. [CrossRef]
25. Brown, C.R., Jr. *The Adult Knee*; Callaghan, J.J., Rubash, H.E., Simonian, P.T., Wickiewicz, T.L., Eds.; Lippincott Williams & Wilkins: Philadelphia, PA, USA, 2003.
26. Arjmandi, M.; Ramezani, M.; Nand, A.; Neitzert, T. Experimental study on friction and wear properties of interpenetrating polymer network alginate-polyacrylamide hydrogels for use in minimally-invasive joint implants. *Wear* **2018**, 194–204. [CrossRef]
27. Clouet, J.; Vinatier, C.; Merceron, C.; Pot-vaucel, M.; Maugars, Y.; Weiss, P.; Grimandi, G.; Guicheux, J. From osteoarthritis treatments to future regenerative therapies for cartilage. *Drug Discov. Today* **2009**, *14*, 913–925. [CrossRef]
28. Han, H.S.; Kang, S.B.; Yoon, K.S. High incidence of loosening of the femoral component in legacy posterior stabilised-flex total knee replacement. The Journal of Bone and Joint Surgery. *Br. Vol.* **2007**, *89*, 1457–1461.
29. Kreuz, P.C.; Steinwachs, M.R.; Erggelet, C.; Krause, S.J.; Konrad, G.; Uhl, M.; Südkamp, N. Results after microfracture of full-thickness chondral defects in different compartments in the knee. *Osteoarthr. Cartil.* **2006**, *14*, 1119–1125. [CrossRef]

30. Benthien, J.P.; Behrens, P. Autologous Matrix-Induced Chondrogenesis (AMIC): Combining Microfracturing and a Collagen I/III Matrix for Articular Cartilage Resurfacing. *Cartilage* **2010**, *1*, 65–68. [CrossRef] [PubMed]
31. Harris, J.D.; Siston, R.A.; Pan, X.; Flanigan, D.C. Autologous Chondrocyte Implantation: A Systematic Review. *JBJS* **2010**, *92*, 2220–2233. [CrossRef] [PubMed]
32. Solheim, E.; Hegna, J.; Inderhaug, E.; Øyen, J.; Harlem, T.; Strand, T. Results at 10–14 years after microfracture treatment of articular cartilage defects in the knee. *Knee Surg. Sports Traumatol. Arthrosc.* **2016**, *24*, 1587–1593. [CrossRef] [PubMed]
33. Hosseini, S.A.; Mohammadi, R.; Noruzi, S.; Ganji, R.; Oroojalian, F.; Sahebkar, A. Evolution of hydrogels for cartilage tissue engineering of the knee: A systematic review and meta—Analysis of clinical studies. *Jt. Bone Spine* **2021**, *88*, 105096. [CrossRef]
34. Sutter, L.; Sindermann, A.; Wyse, J.T.; Bartell, L.; Bonassar, L.; Cohen, I.; Das, M. Mechanical Structure Function Properties and Fracture Toughness of Articular Cartilage Modeled as a Biopolymer Double Network. In Proceedings of the APS March Meeting, Boston, MA, USA, 4–8 March 2019.
35. Setton, L.A.; Zhu, W.; Mow, V.C. The biphasic poroviscoelastic behavior of articular cartilage: Role of the surface zone in governing the compressive behavior. *J. Biomech.* **1993**, *26*, 581–592. [CrossRef]
36. Deva, D.C.; Luyao, C.; Kent, D.B.; Stephen, B.T.; Eric, A.N.; Corey, P.N. In vivo articular cartilage deformation: Noninvasive quantification of intratissue strain during joint contact in the human knee. *Sci. Rep.* **2016**, *6*, 19220.
37. Woo, S.L.Y.; Simon, B.R.; Kuei, S.C.; Akeson, W.H. Quasi-Linear Viscoelastic Properties of Normal Articular Cartilage. *J. Biomech. Eng.* **1980**, *102*, 85–90. [CrossRef]
38. Henak, C.R.; Anderson, A.E.; Weiss, J.A. Subject—Specific analysis of joint contact mechanics: Application to the study osteoarithritis and surgical planning. *J. Biomech. Eng.* **2013**, *135*, 021003. [CrossRef] [PubMed]
39. Hui, J.; Jack, L.L. Determination of Poisson's ratio of articular cartilage in indentation test using different sized indenters. In Proceedings of the Bioengineering Conference, Key Biscayne, FL, USA, 25–29 June 2003; pp. 565–566.
40. Zevenbergen, L.; Gsell, W.; Cai, L.; Chan, D.D.; Famaey, N.; Vander Sloten, J.; Himmelreich, U.; Neu, C.P.; and Jonkers, I. Cartilage-on-cartilage contact: Effect of compressive loading on tissue deformations and structural integrity of bovine articular cartilage. *Osteoarthr. Cartil.* **2018**, *26*, 1699–1709. [CrossRef] [PubMed]
41. Oloyede, A.; Flachsmann, R.; Broom, N.D. The Dramatic Influence of Loading Velocity on the Compressive Response of Articular Cartilage. *Connect. Tissue Res.* **1992**, *27*, 211–224. [CrossRef]
42. Radin, E.L.; Paul, I.L.; Lowy, M. A comparison of the dynamic force transmitting properties of subchondral bone and articular cartilage. *J. Bone Jt. Surg.* **1970**, *52*, 444–456. [CrossRef]
43. Wahlquist, J.A.; DelRio, F.W.; Randolph, M.A.; Aziz, A.H.; Heveran, C.M.; Bryant, S.J.; Neu, C.P.; Ferguson, V.L. Indentation mapping revealed poroelastic, but not viscoelastic, properties spanning native zonal articular cartilage. *Acta Biomater.* **2017**, *64*, 41–49. [CrossRef]
44. Katz, E.P.; Wachtel, E.J.; Maroudas, A. Extrafibrillar proteoglycans osmotically regulate the molecular packing of collagen in cartilage. *Biochim. Biophys. Acta (BBA) Gen. Subj.* **1986**, *882*, 136–139. [CrossRef]
45. Fung, Y.C.; Tong, P. *Classical and Computational Solid Mechanics*; World Scientific Publishing Co, Inc.: Singapore, 2001.
46. Nam, S.; Hu, K.H.; Butte, M.J.; Chaudhuri, O. Strain-enhanced stress relaxation impacts nonlinear elasticity in collagen gels. *Proc. Natl. Acad. Sci. USA* **2016**, *113*, 5492–5497. [CrossRef]
47. Li, L.P.; Buschmann, M.D.; Shirazi-Adl, A. A fibril reinforced nonhomogeneous poroelastic model for articular cartilage: Inhomogeneous response in unconfined compression. *J. Biomech.* **2000**, *33*, 1533–1541. [CrossRef]
48. Han, G.; Hess, C.; Eriten, M.; Henak, C.R. Uncoupled poroelastic and intrinsic viscoelastic dissipation in cartilage. *J. Mech. Behav. Biomed. Mater.* **2018**, *84*, 28–34. [CrossRef] [PubMed]
49. Wilson, W.; Huyghe, J.M.; Van Donkelaar, C.C. Depth-dependent compressive equilibrium properties of articular cartilage explained by its composition. *Biomech. Model. Mechanobiol.* **2007**, *6*, 43–53. [CrossRef] [PubMed]
50. Kurkijärvi, J.E.; Nissi, M.J.; Kiviranta, I.; Jurvelin, J.S.; Nieminen, M.T. Delayed gadolinium-enhanced MRI of cartilage (dGEMRIC) and T2 characteristics of human knee articular cartilage: Topographical variation and relationships to mechanical properties. *Magn. Reson. Med.* **2004**, *52*, 41–46. [CrossRef] [PubMed]
51. Amin, K.; Ziad, A.; Salvatore, F.; Walter, H. Effect of strain rate on transient local strain variations in articular cartilage. *J. Mech. Behav. Biomed. Mater.* **2019**, *95*, 60–66.
52. Arabshahi, Z.; Afara, I.O.; Moody, H.R.; Schrobback, K.; Kashani, J.; Fischer, N.; Oloyede, A.; Jacob, K.T. A new mechanical indentation framework for functional assessment of articular cartilage. *J. Mech. Behav. Biomed. Mater.* **2018**, *81*, 83–94. [CrossRef]
53. Deng, Y.; Sun, J.; Ni, X.; Yu, B. Tribological properties of hierarchical structure artificial joints with poly acrylic acid (AA)—Poly acrylamide (AAm) hydrogel and Ti6Al4V substrate. *J. Polym. Res.* **2020**, *27*, 157. [CrossRef]
54. Lohmander, L.S.; Englund, P.M.; Dahl, L.L.; Roos, E.M. The Long-term Consequence of Anterior Cruciate Ligament and Meniscus Injuries:Osteoarthritis. *Am. J. Sports Med.* **2007**, *35*, 1756–1769. [CrossRef]
55. Bendele, A.M. Animal models of osteoarthritis. *J. Musculoskel. Neuron. Interact.* **2001**, *1*, 363–376.
56. Katta, J.; Jin, Z.; Ingham, E.; Fisher, J. Biotribology of articular cartilage—A review of the recent advances. *Med. Eng. Phys.* **2008**, *30*, 1349–1363. [CrossRef]
57. Link, J.M.; Salinas, E.Y.; Hu, J.C.; Athanasiou, K.A. The tribology of cartilage: Mechanisms, experimental techniques, and relevance to translational tissue engineering. *Clin. Biomech.* **2019**, *79*, 104880. [CrossRef]

58. Moore, A.C.; Burris, D.L. Tribological and material properties for cartilage of and throughout the bovine stifle: Support for the altered joint kinematics hypothesis of osteoarthritis. *Osteoarthr. Cartil.* **2017**, *23*, 161–169. [CrossRef] [PubMed]
59. Oungoulian, S.R.; Chang, S.; Bortz, O.; Hehir, K.E.; Zhu, K.; Willis, C.E.; Hung, C.T.; Ateshian, G.A. Articular cartilage wear characterization with a particle sizing and counting analyzer. *J. Biomech. Eng.* **2013**, *135*, 024501. [CrossRef] [PubMed]
60. Mankin, H.J. Workshop on etiopathogenesis of osteoarthritis. *Proc. Recomm. J. Rheumatol.* **1986**, 1130–1160.
61. Jae, H.J. Knee osteoarthritis and menopausal hormone therapy in postmenopausal women: A nationwide cross-sectional study. *Menopause* **2019**, *26*, 598–602.
62. Mow, V.C.; Soslowsky, L.J. Friction, lubrication and wear of diarthrodial joints. *Basic Orthop. Biomech.* **1991**, 245–292.
63. Wu, P.-J.; Masouleh, M.I.; Dini, D.; Paterson, C.; Török, P.; Overby, D.R.; Kabakova, I.V. Detection of proteoglycan loss from articular cartilage using Brillouin microscopy, with applications to osteoarthritis. *Biomed. Opt. Express* **2019**, *10*, 2457–2466. [CrossRef]
64. Burris, D.L.; Ramsey, L.; Graham, B.T.; Price, C.; Moore, A.C. How Sliding and Hydrodynamics Contribute to Articular Cartilage Fluid and Lubrication Recovery. *Tribol. Lett.* **2019**, *67*, 46. [CrossRef]
65. Graindorge, S.L.; Stachowiak, G.W. Changes occurring in the surface morphology of articular cartilage during wear. *Wear* **2000**, *241*, 143–150. [CrossRef]
66. Gabriela, E.; Gaston, O.; Jerry, C.H.; Kyriacos, A.A. Cartilage assessment requires a surface characterization protocol: Roughness, friction, and function. *Tissue Eng. Part C Methods* **2021**, *27*, 276–286.
67. Lipshitz, H.; Etheredge, R.; Glimcher, M.J. In vitro wear of articular cartilage. *J. Bone Jt. Surg. Am. Vol.* **1975**, *57*, 527–534. [CrossRef]
68. Parkes, M.; Tallia, F.; Young, G.R.; Cann, P.; Jones, J.R.; Jeffers, J.R.T. Tribological evaluation of a novel hybrid for repair of articular cartilage defects. *Mater. Sci. Eng. C.* **2021**, *119*, 111495. [CrossRef]
69. Hossain, M.J.; Noori-Dokht, H.; Karnik, S.; Alyafei, N.; Joukar, A.; Trippel, S.B.; Wagner, D.R. Anisotropic properties of articular cartilage in an accelerated in vitro wear test. *J. Mech. Behav. Biomed. Mater.* **2020**, *109*, 103834. [CrossRef]
70. Jay, G.D.; Torres, J.R.; Rhee, D.K.; Helminen, H.J.; Hytinnen, M.M.; Cha, C.-J.; Elsaid, K.; Kim, K.-S.; Cui, Y.; Warman, M.L. Association between friction and wear in diarthrodial joints lacking lubricin. *Arthritis Rheum.* **2007**, *56*, 3662–3669. [CrossRef] [PubMed]
71. Jurvelin, J.S.; Müller, D.J.; Wong, M.; Studer, D.; Engel, A.; Hunziker, E.B. Surface and Subsurface Morphology of Bovine Humeral Articular Cartilage as Assessed by Atomic Force and Transmission Electron Microscopy. *J. Struct. Biol.* **1996**, *117*, 45–54. [CrossRef]
72. McCutchen, C.W. Mechanism of Animal Joints: Sponge-hydrostatic and Weeping Bearings. *Nature* **1959**, *184*, 1284–1285. [CrossRef]
73. Mow, V.C.; Kuei, S.C.; Lai, W.M.; Armstrong, C.G. Biphasic Creep and Stress Relaxation of Articular Cartilage in Compression: Theory and Experiments. *J. Biomech. Eng.* **1980**, *102*, 73–84. [CrossRef] [PubMed]
74. Lai, W.M.; Hou, J.S.; Mow, V.C. A Triphasic Theory for the Swelling and Deformation Behaviors of Articular Cartilage. *J. Biomech. Eng.* **1991**, *113*. [CrossRef] [PubMed]
75. Caligaris, M.; Ateshian, G.A. Effects of sustained interstitial fluid pressurization under migrating contact area, and boundary lubrication by synovial fluid, on cartilage friction. *Osteoarthr. Cartil.* **2008**, *16*, 1220–1227. [CrossRef] [PubMed]
76. Covert, R.J.; Ott, R.D.; Ku, D.N. Friction characteristics of a potential articular cartilage biomaterial. *Wear* **2003**, *255*, 1064–1068. [CrossRef]
77. Forster, H.; Fisher, J. The Influence of Loading Time and Lubricant on the Friction of Articular Cartilage. *Proc. Inst. Mech. Eng. Part H J. Eng. Med.* **1996**, *210*, 109–119. [CrossRef]
78. Katta, J.; Pawaskar, S.S.; Jin, Z.M.; Ingham, E.; Fisher, J. Effect of load variation on the friction properties of articular cartilage. *Proc. Inst. Mech. Eng. Part J J. Eng. Tribol.* **2007**, *221*, 175–181. [CrossRef]
79. Krishnan, R.; Mariner, E.N.; Ateshian, G.A. Effect of dynamic loading on the frictional response of bovine articular cartilage. *J. Biomech.* **2005**, *38*, 1665–1673. [CrossRef]
80. Northwood, E.; John, F. A multi-directional in vitro investigation into friction, damage and wear of innovative chondroplasty materials against articular cartilage. *Clin. Biomech.* **2007**, *22*, 834–842. [CrossRef]
81. Gleghorn, J.P.; Jones Aled, R.C.; Flannery, C.R.; Bonassar, L.J. Boundary mode lubrication of articular cartilage by recombinant human lubricin. *J. Orthop. Res.* **2009**, *27*, 771–777. [CrossRef] [PubMed]
82. Farnham, M.S.; Larson, R.E.; Burris, D.L.; Price, C. Effects of mechanical injury on the tribological rehydration and lubrication of articular cartilage. *J. Mech. Behav. Biomed. Mater.* **2020**, *101*, 103422. [CrossRef]
83. Santarella, F.; Simpson, C.R.; Lemoine, M.; McGrath, S.; Cavanagh, B.; Smith, A.; Murphy, C.M.; Garlick, J.A.; O'Brien, F.J.; Kearney, C.J. The lubricating effect of iPS-reprogrammed fibroblasts on collagen-GAG scaffolds for cartilage repair applications. *J. Mech. Behav. Biomed. Mater.* **2021**, *114*, 104174. [CrossRef] [PubMed]
84. Naka, M.H.; Morita, Y.; Ikeuchi, K. Influence of proteoglycan contents and of tissue hydration on the frictional characteristics of articular cartilage. *Proc. Inst. Mech. Eng. Part H: J. Eng. Med.* **2005**, *219*, 175–182. [CrossRef] [PubMed]
85. Thompson, R.C.; Oegema, T.R. Metabolic activity of articular cartilage in osteoarthritis. An in vitro study. *J. Bone Jt. Surg. Am. Vol.* **1979**, *61*, 407–416. [CrossRef]
86. Basalo, I.M.; Raj, D.; Krishnan, R.; Chen, F.H.; Hung, C.T.; Ateshian, G.A. Effects of enzymatic degradation on the frictional response of articular cartilage in stress relaxation. *J. Biomech.* **2005**, *38*, 1343–1349. [CrossRef] [PubMed]
87. Katta, J.; Jin, Z.; Ingham, E.; Fisher, J. Chondroitin sulphate: An effective joint lubricant? *Osteoarthr. Cartil.* **2009**, *17*, 1001–1008. [CrossRef]

88. Bell, C.J.; Ingham, E.; Fisher, J. Influence of hyaluronic acid on the time-dependent friction response of articular cartilage under different conditions. *Proc. Inst. Mech. Eng. Part H J. Eng. Med.* **2006**, *220*, 23–31. [CrossRef]
89. Naka, M.H.; Hattori, K.; Ohashi, T.; Ikeuchi, K. Evaluation of the effect of collagen network degradation on the frictional characteristics of articular cartilage using a simultaneous analysis of the contact condition. *Clin. Biomech.* **2005**, *20*, 1111–1118. [CrossRef]
90. Sun, Z.; Feeney, E.; Guan, Y.; Cook, S.G.; Gourdon, D.; Bonassar, L.J.; Putnam, D. Boundary mode lubrication of articular cartilage with a biomimetic diblock copolymer. *Proc. Natl. Acad. Sci. USA* **2019**, *116*, 12437–12441. [CrossRef] [PubMed]
91. Schmidt, T.A.; Gastelum, N.S.; Nguyen, Q.T.; Schumacher, B.L.; Sah, R.L. Boundary lubrication of articular cartilage: Role of synovial fluid constituents. *Arthritis Rheum.* **2007**, *56*, 882–891. [CrossRef]
92. Schmidt, T.A.; Sah, R.L. Effect of synovial fluid on boundary lubrication of articular cartilage. *Osteoarthr. Cartil.* **2007**, *15*, 35–47. [CrossRef] [PubMed]
93. Radin, E.L.; Swann, D.A.; Weisser, P.A. Separation of a Hyaluronate-free Lubricating Fraction from Synovial Fluid. *Nature* **1970**, *228*, 377–378. [CrossRef] [PubMed]
94. Obara, T.; Mabuchi, K.; Iso, T.; Yamaguchi, T. Increased friction of animal joints by experimental degeneration and recovery by addition of hyaluronic acid. *Clin. Biomech.* **1997**, *12*, 246–252. [CrossRef]
95. Forsey, R.W.; Fisher, J.; Thompson, J.; Stone, M.H.; Bell, C.; Ingham, E. The effect of hyaluronic acid and phospholipid based lubricants on friction within a human cartilage damage model. *Biomaterials* **2006**, *27*, 4581–4590. [CrossRef] [PubMed]
96. Chen, Y.; Crawford, R.W.; Adekunle, O. Unsaturated phosphatidylcholines lining on the surface of cartilage and its possible physiological roles. *J. Orthop. Surg. Res.* **2007**, *2*, 14. [CrossRef]
97. Hills, B.A.; Crawford, R.W. Normal and prosthetic synovial joints are lubricated by surface-active phospholipid: A hypothesis. *J. Arthroplast.* **2003**, *18*, 499–505. [CrossRef]
98. Pickard, J.; Ingham, E.; Egan, J.; Fisher, J. Investigation into the effect of proteoglycan molecules on the tribological properties of cartilage joint tissues. *Proc. Inst. Mech. Eng. Part H J. Eng. Med.* **1998**, *212*, 177–182. [CrossRef] [PubMed]
99. Caló, E.; Khutoryanskiy, V.V. Biomedical applications of hydrogels: A review of patents and commercial products. *Eur. Polym. J.* **2015**, *65*, 252–267. [CrossRef]
100. Ahmed, E.M. Hydrogel: Preparation, characterization, and applications: A review. *J. Adv. Res.* **2015**, *6*, 105–121. [CrossRef] [PubMed]
101. Li, L.; Yu, F.; Zheng, L.; Wang, R.; Yan, W.; Wang, Z.; Xu, J.; Wu, J.; Shi, D.; Zhu, L.; et al. Natural hydrogels for cartilage regeneration: Modification, preparation and application. *J. Orthop. Transl.* **2019**, *17*, 26–41. [CrossRef] [PubMed]
102. Pretzel, D.; Linss, S.; Ahrem, H.; Endres, M.; Kaps, C.; Klemm, D.; Kinne, R.W. A novel in vitro bovine cartilage punch model for assessing the regeneration of focal cartilage defects with biocompatible bacterial nanocellulose. *Arthritis Res. Ther.* **2013**, *15*, R59. [CrossRef]
103. Shimon, A.U.; Matthew, G.; Janice, H.L.; Joshua, C.; Thanissara, C.; Elaine, C.Y.; Jennifer, H.E. Hyaluronic Acid-Binding Scaffold for Articular Cartilage Repair. *Tissue Eng. Part A* **2012**, *18*, 2497–2506.
104. Sartori, M.; Pagani, S.; Ferrari, A.; Costa, V.; Carina, V.; Figallo, E.; Maltarello, M.C.; Martini, L.; Fini, M.; Giavaresi, G. A new bi-layered scaffold for osteochondral tissue regeneration: In vitro and in vivo preclinical investigations. *Mater. Sci. Eng. C* **2017**, *70*, 101–111. [CrossRef]
105. Kon, E.; Filardo, G.; Shani, J.; Altschuler, N.; Levy, A.; Zaslav, K.; Eisman, J.E.; Robinson, D. Osteochondral regeneration with a novel aragonite-hyaluronate biphasic scaffold: Up to 12-month follow-up study in a goat model. *J. Orthop. Surg. Res.* **2015**, *10*, 81. [CrossRef]
106. Higa, K.; Kitamura, N.; Goto, K.; Kurokawa, T.; Gong, J.P.; Kanaya, F.; Yasuda, K. Effects of osteochondral defect size on cartilage regeneration using a double-network hydrogel. *BMC Musculoskelet. Disord.* **2017**, *18*, 210. [CrossRef]
107. Erggelet, C.; Endres, M.; Neumann, K.; Morawietz, L.; Ringe, J.; Haberstroh, K.; Sittinger, M.; Kaps, C. Formation of cartilage repair tissue in articular cartilage defects pretreated with microfracture and covered with cell-free polymer-based implants. *J. Orthop. Res.* **2009**, *27*, 1353–1360. [CrossRef]
108. Schagemann, J.C.; Rudert, N.; Taylor, M.E.; Sim, S.; Quenneville, E.; Garon, M.; Klinger, M.; Buschmann, M.D.; Mittelstaed, H. Bilayer Implants: Electromechanical Assessment of Regenerated Articular Cartilage in a Sheep Model. *CARTILAGE* **2016**, *7*, 346–360. [CrossRef]
109. He, Z.; Wnag, B.; Hu, C.; Zhao, J. An overview of hydrogel based intra-articular drug delivery for the treatment of osteoarthritis. *Colloids Surf. B Biointerfaces* **2017**, *154*, 33–39. [CrossRef] [PubMed]
110. Peppas, N.A.; Merrill, E.W. Development of semicrystalline poly(vinyl alcohol) hydrogels for biomedical applications. *J. Biomed. Mater. Res.* **1977**, *11*, 423–434. [CrossRef] [PubMed]
111. Okay, O. Semicrystalline physical hydrogels with shape-memory and self-healing properties. *J. Mater. Chem. B* **2019**, *7*, 1581–1596. [CrossRef] [PubMed]
112. Yuan, J.-J.; Jin, R.-H. Fibrous Crystalline Hydrogels Formed from Polymers Possessing A Linear Poly(ethyleneimine) Backbone. *Langmuir* **2005**, *21*, 3136–3145. [CrossRef]
113. Zhang, H.; Zhang, F.; Wu, J. Physically crosslinked hydrogels from polysaccharides prepared by freeze–thaw technique. *React. Funct. Polym.* **2013**, *73*, 923–928. [CrossRef]
114. Peppas, N.A.; Huang, Y.; Torres-Lugo, M.; Ward, J.H.; Zhang, J. Physicochemical Foundations and Structural Design of Hydrogels in Medicine and Biology. *Annu. Rev. Biomed. Eng.* **2000**, *2*, 9–29. [CrossRef]

115. Hou, W.; Sheng, N.; Zhang, X.; Luan, Z.; Qi, P.; Lin, M.; Tan, Y.; Xia, Y.; Li, Y.; Sui, K. Design of injectable agar/NaCl/polyacrylamide ionic hydrogels for high performance strain sensors. *Carbohydr. Polym.* **2019**, *211*, 322–328. [CrossRef]
116. Zhang, T.; Silverstein, M.S. Highly porous, emulsion-templated, zwitterionic hydrogels: Amplified and accelerated uptakes with enhanced environmental sensitivity. *Polym. Chem.* **2018**, *9*, 3479–3487. [CrossRef]
117. Yasuda, K.; Ping, G.J.; Katsuyama, Y.; Nakayama, A.; Tanabe, Y.; Kondo, E.; Ueno, M.; Osada, Y. Biomechanical properties of high-toughness double network hydrogels. *Biomaterials* **2005**, *26*, 4468–4475. [CrossRef]
118. Cozens, E.J.; Roohpour, N.; Gautrot, J.E. Comaprative adhesion of chemically and physically crosslinked poly(acrylic acid) based hydrogels to soft tissues. *Eur. Polym. J.* **2021**, *146*, 110250. [CrossRef]
119. Zhang, R.; Lin, P.; Yang, W.; Cai, M.; Yu, B.; Zhou, F. Simultaneous superior lubrication and high load bearing by the dynamic weak interaction of a lubricant with mechanically strong bilayer porous hydrogels. *Polym. Chem.* **2017**, *8*, 7102–7107. [CrossRef]
120. Burdick, J.A.; Prestwich, G.D. Hyaluronic Acid Hydrogels for Biomedical Applications. *Adv. Mater.* **2011**, *23*, H41–H56. [CrossRef]
121. Czaja, W.K.; Young, D.J.; Kawecki, M.; Brown, R.M. The Future Prospects of Microbial Cellulose in Biomedical Applications. *Biomacromolecules* **2007**, *8*, 1–12. [CrossRef]
122. Wang, Z.; Zhu, X.; Zhang, R. Characterization and Analysis of Collective Cellular Behaviors in 3D Dextran Hydrogels with Homogenous and Clustered RGD Compositions. *Materials* **2019**, *12*, 3391. [CrossRef] [PubMed]
123. Pawar, S.N.; Edgar, K.J. Alginate derivatization: A review of chemistry, properties and applications. *Biomaterials* **2012**, *33*, 3279–3305. [CrossRef] [PubMed]
124. Luca, G.; João, F.M.; Rui, L.R. Natural polymers for the microencapsulation of cells. *NCBI* **2014**, *6*, 100.
125. Toh, W.S.; Loh, X.J. Advances in hydrogel delivery systems for tissue regeneration. *Mater. Sci. Eng. C* **2014**, *45*, 690–697. [CrossRef]
126. Zhang, D.; Duan, J.; Wang, D.; Ge, S. Effect of Preparation Methods on Mechanical Properties of PVA/HA Composite Hydrogel. *J. Bionic Eng.* **2010**, *7*, 235–243. [CrossRef]
127. Chuang, E.Y.; Chiang, C.W.; Wong, P.C.; Chen, C.H. Hydrogels for the Application of Articular Cartilage Tissue Engineering: A Review of Hydrogels. *Adv. Mater. Sci. Eng.* **2018**, *2018*, 4368910. [CrossRef]
128. Hennink, W.E.; van Nostrum, C.F. Novel crosslinking methods to design hydrogels. *Adv. Drug Deliv. Rev.* **2012**, *64*, 223–236. [CrossRef]
129. van Dijk-Wolthuis, W.N.E.; Franssen, O.; Talsma, H.; van Steenbergen, M.J.; Kettenes-van den Bosch, J.J.; Hennink, W.E. Synthesis, Characterization, and Polymerization of Glycidyl Methacrylate Derivatized Dextran. *Macromolecules* **1995**, *28*, 6317–6322. [CrossRef]
130. Stenekes, R.J.H.; De Smedt, S.C.; Demeester, J.; Sun, G.; Zhang, Z.; Hennink, W.E. Pore Sizes in Hydrated Dextran Microspheres. *Biomacromolecules* **2000**, *1*, 696–703. [CrossRef] [PubMed]
131. Sperinde, J.J.; Griffith, L.G. Synthesis and Characterization of Enzymatically-Cross-Linked Poly(ethylene glycol) Hydrogels. *Macromolecules* **1997**, *30*, 5255–5264. [CrossRef]
132. Lin, P.; Ma, S.; Wang, X.; Zhou, F. Molecularly engineered dual-crosslinked hydrogel with ultrahigh mechanical strength, toughness, and good self-recovery. *Adv. Mater.* **2015**, *27*, 2054–2059. [CrossRef]
133. Seddiki, N.; Djamel, A. Synthesis, characterization and rheological behavior of pH sensitive poly(acrylamide-co-acrylic acid) hydrogels. *Arab. J. Chem.* **2017**, *10*, 539–547.
134. Yoshikawa, M.; Wano, T.; Kitao, T. Specialty polymeric membranes 2. Pervaporation separation of aqueous lower alcohol solutions throuh modified polybutadiene membranes. *J. Membr. Sci.* **1994**, *89*, 23–36. [CrossRef]
135. Ghasemiyeh, P.; Mohammandi-Samani, S. Hydrogels as drug delivery systems; pros and cons. *Trends Pharm. Sci.* **2019**, *5*, 7–24.
136. Sennakesavan, G.; Mostakhdemin, M.; Dkhar, L.K.; Seyfoddin, A.; Fatihhi, S.J. Acrylic acid/acrylamide based hydrogels and its properties—A review. *Polym. Degrad. Stab.* **2020**, *180*, 109308. [CrossRef]
137. Hawker, C.J.; Piotti, M.E.; and Saldívar-Guerra, E. Nitroxide-Mediated Free Radical Polymerization. In *Reference Module in Materials Science and Materials Engineering*; Elsevier: Amsterdam, The Netherlands, 2016.
138. Hong, K.; Zhang, H.; Mays, J.W.; Visser, A.E.; Brazel, C.S.; Holbrey, J.D.; Reichert, M.; Rogers, R.D. Conventional free radical polymerization in room temperature ionic liquids: A green approach to commodity polymers with practical advantages. *R. Soc. Chem.* **2002**, 1368–1369. [CrossRef]
139. Rizzardo, E.; Chiefari, J.; Chong, B.Y.K.; Ercole, F.; Krstina, J.; Jeffery, J.; Le Tam, P.T.; Mayadunne, R.T.A.; Meijs, G.F.; Moad, C.L.; et al. Tailored polymers by free radical processes. *Macromol. Symp.* **1999**, *143*, 291–307. [CrossRef]
140. Nesvaba, P. Radical polymerization in industry. *Encycl. Radic. Chem. Biol. Mater.* **2012**. [CrossRef]
141. Gong, J.P.; Kurokawa, T.; Narita, T.; Kagata, G.; Osada, Y.; Nishimura, G.; Kinjo, M. Synthesis of Hydrogels with Extremely Low Surface Friction. *J. Am. Chem. Soc.* **2001**, *123*, 5582–5583. [CrossRef] [PubMed]
142. Yang, B.-Z.; Zhang, S.-Y.; Wang, P.-H.; Liu, C.-H.; Zhu, Y.-Y. Robust and rapid responsive organic—Inorganic hybrid bilayer hydrogel actuators with silicon nanoparticles as the crosslinker. *Polymer* **2021**, *228*, 123863. [CrossRef]
143. Mostakhdemin, M.; Nand, A.; Ramezani, M. A novel assessment of microstructural and mechanical behaviour of bilayer silica-reinforced nanocomposite hydrogels as a candidate for artificial cartilage. *J. Mech. Behav. Biomed. Mater.* **2021**, *116*, 104333. [CrossRef]
144. Sophia, F.A. The Basic Science of Articular Cartilage: Structure, Composition, and Function. *Sports Health A Multidiscip. Approach* **2009**, *1*, 461–468. [CrossRef]

145. Nie, X.; Chuah, Y.J.; Zhu, W.; He, P.; Peck, Y.; Wang, D.-A. Decellularized tissue engineered hyaline cartilage graft for articular cartilage repair. *Biomaterials* **2020**, *235*, 119821. [CrossRef]
146. Arjmandi, M.; Ramezani, M. Mechanical and tribological assessment of silica nanoparticle-alginate-polyacrylamide nanocomposite hydrogels as a cartilage replacement. *J. Mech. Behav. Biomed. Mater.* **2019**, *95*, 196–204. [CrossRef]
147. Carter, T.E.; Taylor, K.A.; Spritzer, C.E.; Utturkar, G.M.; Taylor, D.C.; Moorman, C.T.; Garrett, W.E.; Guilak, F.; McNulty, A.L.; DeFrate, L.E. In vivo cartilage strain increases following medial meniscal tear and correlates with synovial fluid matrix metalloproteinase activity. *J. Biomech.* **2015**, *48*, 1461–1468. [CrossRef]
148. Desireé, A.G.; Lorena, D.C.; José, O.C.S., Jr.; Roseane, M.R.-C. A review of the designs and prominent biomedical advances of natural and synthetic hydrogel formulations. *Eur. Polym. J.* **2017**, *88*, 373–392.
149. Guidance for Industry: Preparation of IDEs and INDs for Products Intended to Repair or Replace Knee Cartilage. 2001. Available online: https://www.fda.gov/media/82562/download (accessed on 4 January 2021).
150. Hurtig, M.B.; Buschmann, M.D.; Fortier, L.A.; Hoemann, C.D.; Hunziker, E.B.; Jurvelin, J.S.; Mainil-Varlet, P.; McIlwraith, C.W.; Sah, R.L.; Whiteside, R.A. Preclinical studies for cartilage repair: Recommendations from the International Cartilage Repair Society. *Cartilage* **2011**, *2*, 137–152. [CrossRef] [PubMed]
151. International ASTM, Standard Guide for In Vivo Assessment of Implantable Devices Intended to Repair or Regenerate Articular Cartilage, in ASTM F2451-05. 2010. Available online: https://www.astm.org/Standards/F2451.htm (accessed on 5 January 2021).
152. Jay, M.P.; Brian, C.W.; Edward, D.B.; Robert, L.M. A Systematic Review and Guide to Mechanical Testing for Articular Cartilage Tissue Engineering. *Tissue Eng. Part C Methods* **2019**, *25*, 593–608.
153. Lin, P.; Zhang, R.; Wang, X.; Cai, M.; Yang, J.; Yu, B.; Zhou, F. Articular Cartilage Inspired Bilayer Tough Hydrogel Prepared by Interfacial Modulated Polymerization Showing Excellent Combination of High Load-Bearing and Low Friction Performance. *ACS Macro Lett.* **2016**, *5*, 1191–1195. [CrossRef]
154. Li, Z.; Lin, Z. Recent advances in polysaccharide based hydrogels for synthesis and applications. *Aggregate* **2021**, *2*, e21. [CrossRef]
155. Kheirabadi, M.; Bagheri, R.; Kabiri, K. Structure, swelling and mechanical behavior of a cationic full-IPN hydrogel reinforced with modified nanoclay. *Iran. Polym. J.* **2015**, *24*, 379–388. [CrossRef]
156. Gong, J.P. Why are double network hydrogels so tough? *R. Soc. Chem.* **2010**, *6*, 2583–2590. [CrossRef]
157. Xu, B.; Li, H.; Wang, Y.; Zhang, G.; and Zhang, Q. Nanocomposite hydrogels with high strength cross-linked by titania. *RSC Adv.* **2013**, *3*, 7233–7236. [CrossRef]
158. Faturechi, R.; Karimi, A.; Hashemi, A.; Yousefi, H.; Navidbakhsh, M. Influence of poly(acrylic acid) on the mechanical properties of composite hydrogels. *Adv. Poly. Technol.* **2015**, *34*, 21487. [CrossRef]
159. Yang, C.H.; Wang, M.X.; Haider, H.; Yang, J.H.; Sun, J.-Y.; Chen, Y.M.; Zhou, J.; Suo, Z. Strengthening Alginate/Polyacrylamide Hydrogels Using Various Multivalent Cations. *ACS Appl. Mater. Interfaces* **2013**, *5*, 10418–10422. [CrossRef]
160. Amanda, N.B.; Junmin, Z.; Roger, M.; Jennifer, L.W.; Jung, U.Y.; Brian, J. Design and Characterization of Poly(Ethylene Glycol) Photopolymerizable Semi-Interpenetrating Networks for Chondrogenesis of Human Mesenchymal Stem Cells. *Tissue Eng.* **2007**, *13*, 2549–2560.
161. Liao, I.C.; Moutos, F.T.; Estes, B.T.; Zhao, X.; Guilak, F. Composite three-dimensional woven scaffolds with interpenetrating network hydrogels to create functional synthetic articular cartilage. *Adv. Funct. Mater.* **2013**, *23*, 5833–5839. [CrossRef]
162. Hadi, D.; Azadehsadat, H.M.; Kibret, M. Blends and Nanocomposite Biomaterials for Articular Cartilage Tissue Engineering. *Materials* **2014**, *7*, 5327–5355.
163. Danyang, H.; Yong, H.; Yun, X.; Hai, L.; Ganjun, F.; Xiangdong, Z.; Xingdong, Z. Viscoelasticity in natural tissues and engineered scaffolds for tissue reconstruction. *Acta Biomater.* **2019**, *97*, 74–92.
164. Mao, Y.; Lin, S.; Zhao, X.; Anand, L. A large deformation viscoelastic model for double-network hydrogels. *J. Mech. Phys. Solids* **2017**, *100*, 103–130. [CrossRef]
165. Zhao, X.; Huebsch, N.; Mooney, D.J.; Suo, Z. Stress-relaxation behavior in gels with ionic and covalent crosslinks. *J. Appl. Phys.* **2010**, *107*, 063509. [CrossRef]
166. Ovijit, C.; Luo, G.; Max, D.; Darinka, K.; Sidi, A.B.; James, C.W.; Nathaniel, H.; David, J.M. Substrate stress relaxation regulates cell spreading. *Nat. Commun.* **2015**, *6*, 6365.
167. Wei, H.; Xuanhe, Z.; Jinxiong, Z.; Zhigang, S. A theory of coupled diffusion and large deformation in polymeric gels. *J. Mech. Phys. Solids* **2008**, *56*, 1779–1793.
168. Emad, M.; Léo, V.; Marco, F.; Andrew, R.H.; Dale, A.M.; Adrian, J.T.; Eleanor, S.; Mahadevan, L.; Guillaume, T.C. The cytoplasm of living cells behaves as a poroelastic material. *Nat. Mater.* **2013**, *12*, 253–261.
169. Qi-Ming, W.; Anirudh, C.M.; Michelle, L.O.; Xuan-He, Z. Separating viscoelasticity and poroelasticity of gels with different length and time scales. *Acta Mech. Sin.* **2014**, *30*, 20–27.
170. Archard, J.F.; Hirst, W. The wear of metals under unlubricated conditions. *Proc. R. Soc. Lond. Ser. A Math. Phys. Sci.* **1956**, *236*, 397–410.
171. Czichos, H.; Habig, K.-H. *Tribologie-Handbuch. GWV Fachverlage GmbH, Wiesbaden: Tribologie-Handbuch: Tribometrie, Tribomaterialien, Tribotechnik*; Springer: Berlin, Germany, 2010.
172. Stachowiak, G.; Batchelor, A.W. *Engineering Tribology*; Butterworth-Heinemann: Oxford, UK, 2013.
173. Urueña, J.M.; Pitenis, A.A.; Nixon, R.M.; Schulze, K.D.; Angelini, T.E.; Gregory, S.W. Mesh Size Control of Polymer Fluctuation Lubrication in Gemini Hydrogels. *Biotribology* **2015**, 24–29. [CrossRef]

174. Thoniyot, P.; Tan, M.J.; Abdul, K.A.; Young, D.J.; Jun, L.X. Nanoparticle–Hydrogel Composites: Concept, Design, and Applications of These Promising, Multi-Functional Materials. *Adv. Sci.* **2015**, *2*, 1400010. [CrossRef]
175. Brand, R.A. Joint contact stress: A reasonable surrogate for biological processes? *Iowa Orthop. J.* **2005**, *25*, 82–94.
176. Katta, J.; Jin, Z.; Ingham, E.; Fisher, J. Friction and wear of native and GAG deficient articular cartilage. *World Biomater. Congr.* **2008**, *4*, 2306.
177. Dunn, A.C.; Sawyer, W.G.; Angelini, T.E. Gemini Interfaces in Aqueous Lubrication with Hydrogels. *Tribol. Lett.* **2014**, *54*, 59–66. [CrossRef]
178. Penskiy, I.; Gerratt, A.P.; Bergbreiter, S. Friction, adhesion and wear properties of PDMS films on silicon sidewalls. *J. Micromechanics Microengineering* **2011**, *21*, 105013. [CrossRef]
179. Bonyadi, S.Z.; Dunn, A.C. Brittle or Ductile? Abrasive Wear of Polyacrylamide Hydrogels Reveals Load-Dependent Wear Mechanisms. *Tribol. Lett.* **2020**, *68*, 16. [CrossRef]
180. Schey, J.A. Systems view of optimizing metal on metal bearings. *Clin. Orthop. Relat. Res.* **1996**, *329*, S115–S127. [CrossRef] [PubMed]
181. Lin, H.-R.; Ling, M.-H.; Lin, Y.-J. High Strength and Low Friction of a PAA-Alginate-Silica Hydrogel as Potential Material for Artificial Soft Tissues. *J. Biomater. Sci. Polym. Ed.* **2009**, *20*, 637–652. [CrossRef] [PubMed]
182. Arakaki, K.; Kitamura, N.; Fujiki, H.; Kurokawa, T.; Iwamoto, M.; Ueno, M.; Kanaya, F.; Osada, Y.; Gong, J.P.; Yasuda, K. Artificial cartilage made from a novel double-network hydrogel: In vivo effects on the normal cartilage and ex vivo evaluation of the friction property. *J. Biomed. Mater. Res. Part A* **2010**, *93*, 1160–1168.
183. Feng, L.; Anmin, W.; Chengtao, W. Analysis of friction between articular cartilage and polyvinyl alcohol hydrogel artificial cartilage. *J. Mater. Sci. Mater. Med.* **2016**, *27*, 87.
184. Li, H.; Choi, Y.S.; Rutland, M.W.; Atkin, R. Nanotribology of hydrogels with similar stiffness but different polymer and crosslinker concentrations. *J. Colloid Interface Sci.* **2020**, *563*, 347–353. [CrossRef]
185. Maliheh, H.N.; Mostafa, R.-T.; Ali, R.N.; Hamed, M.; Reza, N.; Hadi, H.; Majid, J.; Mahdi, S. Stabilizing and dispersing methods of TiO2 nanoparticles in biological studies. *J. Paramed. Sci. (JPS)* **2015**, *6*, 96–105.
186. Tso, C.-P.; Zhung, C.-M.; Shih, Y.-H.; Tseng, Y.-M.; Wu, S.-C.; Doong, R.-A. Stability of metal oxide nanoparticles in aqueous solutions. *Water Sci. Technol.* **2010**, *61*, 127–133. [CrossRef]
187. Jiang, J.; Oberdörster, G.; Biswas, P. Characterization of size, surface charge, and agglomeration state of nanoparticle dispersions for toxicological studies. *J. Nanoparticle Res.* **2009**, *11*, 77–89. [CrossRef]
188. Mandzy, N.; Grulke, E.; Druffel, T. Breakage of TiO2 agglomerates in electrostatically stabilized aqueous dispersions. *Powder Technol.* **2005**, *160*, 121–126. [CrossRef]
189. Deiss, J.L.; Anizan, P.; El Hadigui, S.; Wecker, C. Steric stability of TiO2 nanoparticles in aqueous dispersions. *Colloids Surf. A Physicochem. Eng. Asp.* **1996**, *106*, 59–62. [CrossRef]
190. Toledo, L.; Racine, L.; Pérez, V.; Henríquez, J.P.; Auzely-Velty, R.; Urbano, B.F. Physical nanocomposite hydrogels filled with low concentrations of TiO2 nanoparticles: Swelling, networks parameters and cell retention studies. *Mater. Sci. Eng. C* **2018**, *92*, 769–778. [CrossRef]
191. Azeez, F.; Al-Hetlani, E.; Arata, M.; Abdelmonem, Y.; Nazeer, A.A.; Amin, M.O.; Madkour, M. The effect of surface charge on photocatalytic degradation of methylene blue dye using chargeable titania nanoparticles. *Sci. Rep.* **2018**, *8*, 7104. [CrossRef] [PubMed]
192. Mostakhdemin, M.; Nand, A.; Arjmandi, M.; Ramezani, M. Mechanical and microscopical characterisation of bilayer hydrogels strengthened by TiO2 nanoparticles as a cartilage replacement candidate. *Mater. Today Commun.* **2020**, *25*, 101279. [CrossRef]
193. Memic, A.; Alhadrami, H.A.; Hussain, M.A.; Aldhahri, M.; Al Nowaiser, F.; Al-Hazmi, F.; Oklu, R.; Khademhosseini, A. Hydrogels 2.0: Improved properties with nanomaterial composites for biomedical applications. *Biomed. Mater.* **2015**, *11*, 014104. [CrossRef] [PubMed]
194. Shin, H.; Jo, S.; Mikos, A.G. Modulation of marrow stromal osteoblast adhesion on biomimetic oligo[poly(ethylene glycol) fumarate] hydrogels modified with Arg-Gly-Asp peptides and a poly(ethylene glycol) spacer. *J. Biomed. Mater. Res.* **2002**, *61*, 169–179. [CrossRef] [PubMed]
195. Adibnia, V.; Hill, R.J. Viscoelasticity of near-critical silica-polyacrylamide hydrogel nanocomposites. *Polymer* **2017**, *112*, 457–465. [CrossRef]
196. Zareie, C.; Bahramian, A.R.; Sefti, M.V.; Salehi, M.B. Network-gel strength relationship and performance improvement of polyacrylamide hydrogel using nano-silica; with regards to application in oil wells conditions. *J. Mol. Liq.* **2019**, *278*, 512–520. [CrossRef]
197. Janet, D.; Pearl, M.D. Diagram-of-Osteoarthritis-in-Knee-Joint. Available online: https://www.completepaincare.com/patient-education/conditions-treated/elbow-pain/diagram-of-osteoarthritis-in-knee-joint (accessed on 10 January 2021).
198. Zhan, Y.; Pan, Y.; Chen, B.; Lu, J.; Zhong, Z.; Niu, X. Strain rate dependent hyperelastic stress-stretch behavior of a silica nanoparticle reinforced poly (ethylene glycol) diacrylate nanocomposite hydrogel. *J. Mech. Behav. Biomed. Mater.* **2017**, *75*, 236–243. [CrossRef]
199. Taffetani, M.; Gottardi, R.; Gastaldi, D.; Raiteri, R.; Vena, P. Poroelastic response of articular cartilage by nanoindentation creep tests at different characteristic lengths. *Med Eng. Phys.* **2014**, *36*, 850–858. [CrossRef]
200. Arjmandi, M.; Ramezani, M. Effect of Silica Nanoparticles on Wear Mechanism of Alginate-Polyacrylamide Hydrogel Matrix as a Load-Bearing Biomaterial. *Mater. Sci. Eng.* **2019**, *823*, 15–20. [CrossRef]

polymers

MDPI

Review

Jojoba Oil: An Updated Comprehensive Review on Chemistry, Pharmaceutical Uses, and Toxicity

Heba A. Gad [1], Autumn Roberts [2], Samirah H. Hamzi [3], Haidy A. Gad [4], Ilham Touiss [5], Ahmed E. Altyar [6], Osama A. Kensara [7] and Mohamed L. Ashour [3,4,*]

1 Department of Pharmaceutics and Industrial Pharmacy, Faculty of Pharmacy, Ain Shams University, Cairo 11566, Egypt; h.gad@pharma.asu.edu.eg
2 Independent Researcher, La Route de la Haule, St. Peter, Jersey JE3 7BA, UK; autumnggroberts@yahoo.co.uk
3 Department of Pharmaceutical Sciences, Pharmacy Program, Batterjee Medical College, P.O. Box 6231, Jeddah 21442, Saudi Arabia; 120073.sameerah@bmc.edu.sa
4 Department of Pharmacognosy, Faculty of Pharmacy, Ain Shams University, Cairo 11566, Egypt; haidygad@pharma.asu.edu.eg
5 Laboratory of Bioresources, Biotechnologies, Ethnopharmacology, and Health, Faculty of Sciences, University Mohamed I, Oujda 60000, Morocco; i.touiss@ump.ac.ma
6 Department of Pharmacy Practice, Faculty of Pharmacy, King Abdulaziz University, P.O. Box 80260, Jeddah 21589, Saudi Arabia; aealtyar@kau.edu.sa
7 Department of Clinical Nutrition, Faculty of Applied Medical Sciences, Umm Al-Qura University, P.O. Box 7067, Makkah 21955, Saudi Arabia; oakensara@uqu.edu.sa
* Correspondence: mohamed.ashour@bmc.edu.sa; Tel.: +966-54-9255-376

Citation: Gad, H.A.; Roberts, A.; Hamzi, S.H.; Gad, H.A.; Touiss, I.; Altyar, A.E.; Kensara, O.A.; Ashour, M.L. Jojoba Oil: An Updated Comprehensive Review on Chemistry, Pharmaceutical Uses, and Toxicity. *Polymers* **2021**, *13*, 1711. https://doi.org/10.3390/polym13111711

Academic Editor: Bramasta Nugraha

Received: 28 April 2021
Accepted: 21 May 2021
Published: 24 May 2021

Abstract: Jojoba is a widely used medicinal plant that is cultivated worldwide. Its seeds and oil have a long history of use in folklore to treat various ailments, such as skin and scalp disorders, superficial wounds, sore throat, obesity, and cancer; for improvement of liver functions, enhancement of immunity, and promotion of hair growth. Extensive studies on Jojoba oil showed a wide range of pharmacological applications, including antioxidant, anti-acne and antipsoriasis, anti-inflammatory, antifungal, antipyretic, analgesic, antimicrobial, and anti-hyperglycemia activities. In addition, Jojoba oil is widely used in the pharmaceutical industry, especially in cosmetics for topical, transdermal, and parenteral preparations. Jojoba oil also holds value in the industry as an anti-rodent, insecticides, lubricant, surfactant, and a source for the production of bioenergy. Jojoba oil is considered among the top-ranked oils due to its wax, which constitutes about 98% (mainly wax esters, few free fatty acids, alcohols, and hydrocarbons). In addition, sterols and vitamins with few triglyceride esters, flavonoids, phenolic and cyanogenic compounds are also present. The present review represents an updated literature survey about the chemical composition of jojoba oil, its physical properties, pharmacological activities, pharmaceutical and industrial applications, and toxicity.

Keywords: jojoba; *Simmondsia*; chemistry; liquid wax; biology; toxicity; pharmaceutical/industrial uses

1. Introduction

The plant kingdom continues to hold considerable importance in our daily life. In addition to supplying humanity with food, it is considered as a potential source of thousands of novel materials such as fragrances, flavoring agents, dyes, fibers, beverages, building materials, heavy metal chelators, and many useful compounds of great therapeutic value.

Early studies of plants helped humankind make use of local flora for healing ailments. These studies have continued until now to seek out new agents for the treatment of various diseases. Recent investigations regarding plants with centuries of use in folk medicine have generated a great deal of information about the biologically active chemical components responsible for many claimed medicinal effects. As a result of thorough research involving the isolation and structure characterization techniques, many lead compounds, and prototypes from natural products have assumed reputable roles in medicine. Despite the huge number of synthetic and semisynthetic drugs, the most valuable medicinal agents still in use are obtained from medicinal plants.

There is high consumption of natural resources due to the increasing population. The resultant demand for green energy amidst fossil fuel shortages has rekindled interest in Jojoba oil (*Simmondsia chinensis* (Link) Schneider). Jojoba oil is the only unsaturated liquid wax readily extractable in large quantities from plant sources ($\approx$52% of the total seed weight), which shows a high structure similarity with the sperm whale oil. This similarity has increased the interest in Jojoba oil as a replacement for sperm whale oil (spermaceti wax) since the 1970s [1].

Simmondsia chinensis (Link) Schneider is native to North and Central American deserts but cultivated worldwide in Chile, Egypt, and Argentina [2]. Jojoba was widely used by Native Americans in the Sonora desert (California) as a foodstuff in the form of cooked fruits and in oil form as a therapeutic for multiple ailments: cancer therapy, liver and kidney disorders, obesity, parturition, sore throat, superficial wound healing, warts, psoriasis, acne, sunburn, and treatment of poison ivy exposure [3–6]. Jojoba oil is widely used in the pharmaceutical industry, especially in cosmetics, to restore the ordinary health of hair and skin. The leaf extract, combined with extracts from other plants, also acts as anti-inflammatory agents to treat sensitive skin stress [7]. Jojoba cosmetic products currently on the market include the following: bath oil, body oil, cleansing creams, cleansing pads, cleansing scrubs, nourishing facial cream, facial oil, hair conditioner, hair oil, makeup remover, and shaving cream [8–11].

In addition, the oil has many industrial applications that include an extreme temperature/extreme pressure lubricant in the form of sulfurized oil, which can bear high temperature and pressure without changing its viscosity [6,12]. Other industrial uses include the extraction and separation of isotopes such as Uranium (VI), Thorium (IV), and Plutonium (IV); in the leather industry as a fat liquor with good tanning properties [5]; as a surfactant, fire retardant, lamp oil, candle wax, polishes [13], and antifoaming agents in isolation of penicillin and tetracycline [9].

An updated and in-depth review about jojoba oil chemistry, its pharmaceutical and industrial uses, and toxicity was conducted and is presented in this work to supplement the lack of comprehensive reviews covering the plant since the 1990s. The keywords jojoba, *Simmondsia*, chemistry, pharmaceutical preparations, emulgels, nanoparticles, toxicity, and biological activity were used in many combinations to search Scifinder®, PubMed®, Web of Science ® starting 1990 until 2021. English language was used as the only filter.

2. Common Names and Botanical Characteristics

The word jojoba, pronounced "ho-ho-ba", is a distortion of the native Papago Indian word "howhowi". Jojoba is known by many other names such as bucknut, coffee nut, goatnut, pignut, nutpush, goatberry, sheepnut, and lemon leaf [14]. The seeds of the jojoba plant are dark brown, akin to large coffee beans.

Plants of the order Euphorbiales are usually herbs, shrubs, or sometimes trees [15]. They are widely distributed globally, especially in temperate, subtropical, and tropical regions [16]. They have frequently unisexual (rarely bisexual) hypogynous flowers, which are generally regular with a single whorl of a green perianth. The stamens are equal in number to perianth leaves or numerous. The pistil is composed of three carpels forming a trilocular ovary, with each chamber containing one or two anatropous, pendulous ovules in the inner angle with ventral or dorsal raphe [17]. Simmondsiaceae is a small family of one genus, *Simmondsia*, which is abundant in Southern Arizona, Sonora, and Baja California. Plants that belong to "Simmondsiaceae" are mostly woody branched shrubs that reach 2–4 m in height [4–6]. A photograph of male and female trees, flowers, and seeds of *Simmondsia chinensis* are displayed in Figure 1.

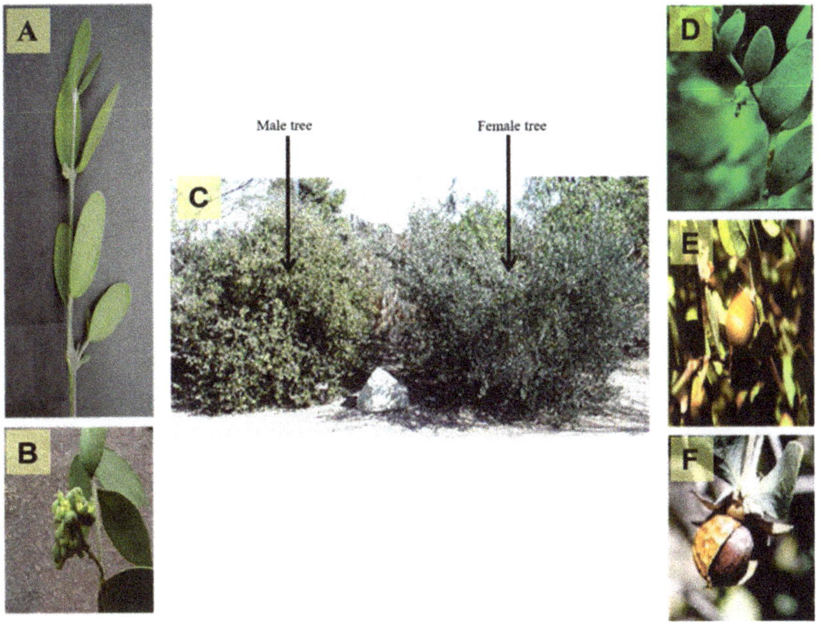

Figure 1. A photograph showing different organs of *Simmondsia chinensis*, (**A**) Branch of the plant (X 0.8), (**B**) Male flowers (X 1.0), (**C**) Old male and female trees (X 0.02), (**D**) Female flower (X 0.5), (**E**) Ripe fruit (X 0.5) and (**F**) Seed (X 0.8) (Photographer Eng. Nabil Elmougi, the jojoba farms of The Egyptian Natural Oil Company, Ismailia Desert Road, Egypt).

3. Chemical Constituents

Jojoba oil is composed of almost 98% pure waxes (mainly wax esters, few free fatty acids, alcohols, and hydrocarbons), sterols, and vitamins with few triglyceride esters, so it is widely known as liquid wax rather than oil or fat [18].

3.1. Jojoba Wax

Investigation of the different organs of the jojoba plant for the presence of the wax revealed that the seeds contain most of the wax content in the plant (almost 50–52% of the seed weight) [5]. Jojoba wax is composed mainly of esters and, to a lesser extent, free acids, free alcohols, and hydrocarbons [4]. Esters are composed by the association of long straight-chain fatty acids with long straight-chain or higher molecular weight monohydric alcohols, C20 and C22; both the acids and alcohols are cis-monounsaturated at the (ω-9) position. Small triglyceride esters are also present [19–22].

3.1.1. Wax Esters

The main components of the wax esters that have been isolated and previously identified are docosenyl eicosenoate "erucyl jojobenoate" (1), eicosenyl eicosenoate "jojobenyl jojobenoate" (2), eicosenyl docosenoate "jojobenyl erucate" (3), docosenyl docosenoate (4), eicosenyl oleate (5), and docosenyl oleate (6) (Table 1) [23]. Many other wax esters and free fatty alcohols and acids components are present in small quantities [19,24].

It was initially thought that jojoba wax esters were made up of random combinations of alcohols and acids until Miwa conducted a study on these combinations [13]. He showed a significant difference between the observed results and those calculated by a random association of acids and alcohols. For instance, it was observed that (acid/alcohol, % experimental (% random)): (C20:1/C′20:1, 28.0% (31.8%)), (C20:1/C′22:1, 10.3% (5.7%)), (C22:1/C′20:1, 41.4% (32.0%)), (C22:1/C′22:1, 1.9% (5.7%)) indicating that eicosenyl docosenoate ester is preferably biosynthesized by the association of eicosenoic acid and docosenol. These combinations demonstrate that plants favor specific associations, which correspond to their genome. From an analytical point of view, this observation constitutes a valuable tool for detecting adulterated oil and good discrimination between natural Jojoba wax and its synthetic substitutes. In the latter case, associations between fatty acids and alcohols are governed by thermodynamic rules, and random results would be observed.

Table 1. Chemical structures for the most abundant wax ester components in jojoba wax.

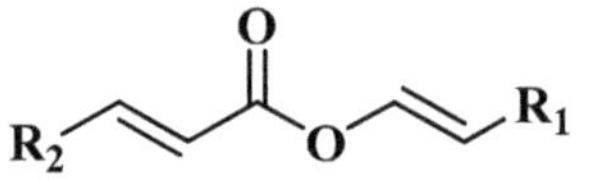

$R_1 = C_{20}H_{41}$, $R_2 = C_{17}H_{35}$	Docosenyl eicosenoate (**1**)
$R_1 = C_{18}H_{37}$, $R_2 = C_{17}H_{35}$	Eicosenyl eicosenoate (**2**)
$R_1 = C_{18}H_{37}$, $R_2 = C_{19}H_{39}$	Eicosenyl docosenoate (**3**)
$R_1 = C_{16}H_{33}$, $R_2 = C_{19}H_{39}$	Docosenyl docosenoate (**4**)
$R_1 = C_{18}H_{37}$, $R_2 = C_{17}H_{33}$ (C9)	Eicosenyl oleate (**5**)
$R_1 = C_{20}H_{41}$, $R_2 = C_{17}H_{33}$ (C9)	Docosenyl oleate (**6**)

3.1.2. Free Fatty Acids and Alcohols

It was reported that the natural oil contains small quantities of free fatty acids (0.96%) and free alcohols (1.11%), as seen in (Table 2) [13].

Table 2. The composition of free fatty alcohols and fatty acids derived from jojoba oil.

Alcohols	(%)	Acids	(%)
Tetradecanol	trace	Dodecanoic	trace
Hexadecanol	0.1	Tetradecanoic	trace
Heptadec-8-enol	trace	Pentadecanoic	trace
Octadecanol	0.2	Hexadecanoic	1.2
Octadec-9-enol	0.7	Hexadec-7-onoic	0.1
Octadec-11-enol	0.4	Hexadec-9-enoic	0.2
Eicosanol	trace	Heptadecenoic	trace
Eicos-11-enol	43.8	Octadecanoic	0.1
Hecos-12-enol	trace	Octadec-9-enoic	10.1
Docosanol	1.0	Octadec-11-enoic	1.1
Docos-12-enol	44.9	Octadecadienoic	0.1
Tetracos-15-enol	8.9	Octadecatrienoic	trace
Hexacosenol	trace	Nonadecenoic	trace
		Eicosanoic	0.1
		Eicos-l1-enoic	71.3
		Eicosadienoic	trace
		Docosanoic	0.2
		Docos-13-enoic	13.6
		Tricosenoic	trace
		Tetracosenoic	trace
		Tetracos-15-enoic	1.3

3.2. *Sterols*

There are many reports concerning the sterol content of jojoba oil [5,19]. The major content of the sterols fraction is cholesterol (7), β-Sitosterol (8), campesterol (9), stigmasterol (10), and isofucosterol (11). Most of these sterols are sketched in Figure 2, and the composition is tabulated in Table 3 [22].

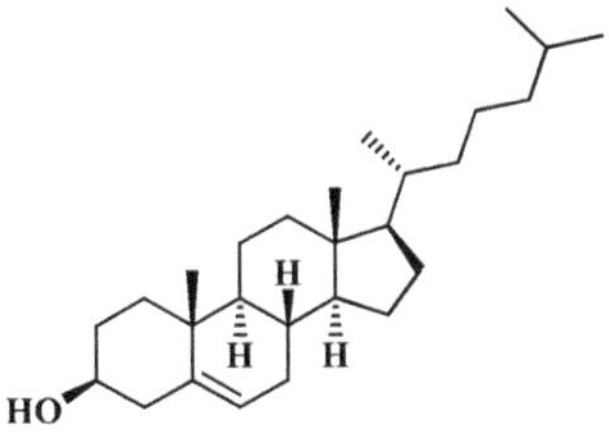

Cholesterol (7)

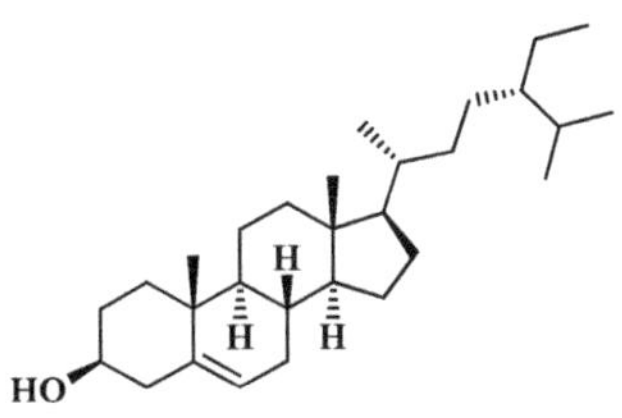

Sitosterol (8)

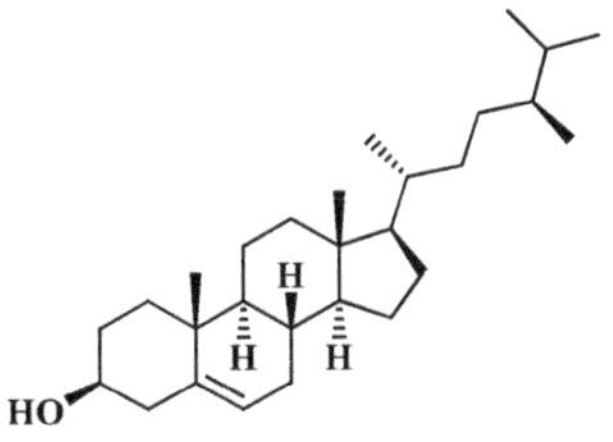

Campesterol (9)

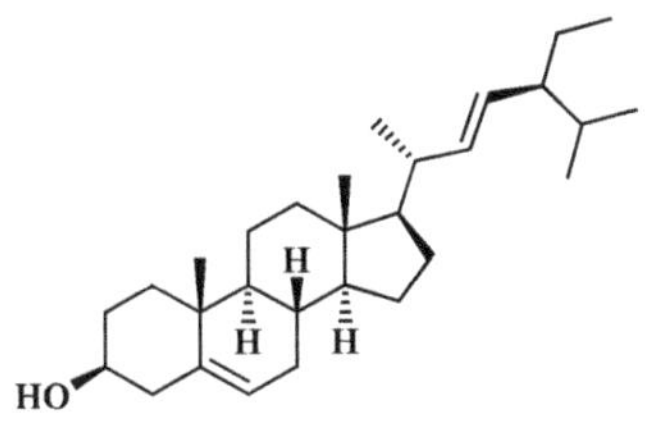

Stigmasterol (10)

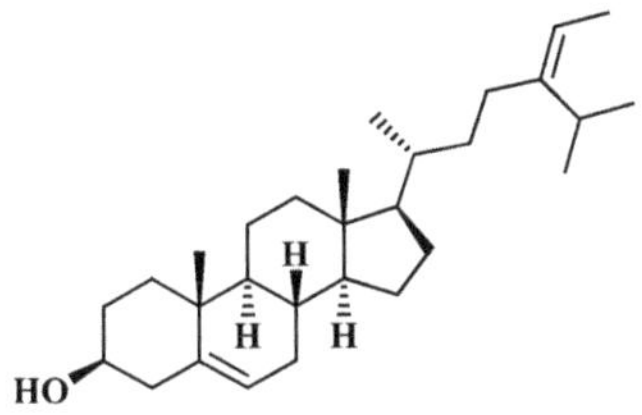

Isofucosterol (11)

Figure 2. Structures of major sterols content of jojoba oil.

Table 3. The average percentage of sterols content in jojoba oil.

Sterol	Sterol Fraction (%)	Total Wax (mg/kg Seed)
Unidentified	0.4	16
Stigmasta-5,25-dien-3β-ol	0.6	24
Fucosterol	0.6	24
Isofucosterol	4.1	163
Cholesterol	0.8	32
Stigmasterol	6.7	266
Campesterol	16.9	672
Sitosterol	69.9	2780

3.3. *Flavonoids, Phenolic, and Cyanogenic Compounds*

Although phenolic compounds are the most common secondary metabolites distributed in nature, they are only present in small quantities in jojoba, as reported in Table 4 [25]. Ten flavonoids have been identified as quercetin (12), quercetin 3′methyl ether (isorhamnetin), quercetin 3-methyl ether (14), quercetin 3,3′-dimethyl ether (15), isorhamnetin 3-*O*-glucoside (16), quercetin 3-O-glucoside (17), typhaneoside (18), isorhamnetin 3-O-rutinoside (19), quercetin 3-*O*-rutinoside (20). Some lignans are also present: (+)-lyoniresinol 4,4′-bis-*O*-β-D-glucopyranoside (21), salvadoraside (22), and eleutheroside E (23) [26]. Simmondisin (24), simmonosides A (25), simmonosides B (26), and 4, 5-dimethyl-4-*O*-alpha-D-glucopyranosylsimmondsin (27) are the main cyanogenic glycosides [20,21,27].

Table 4. Chemical structures for the most abundant flavonoids in jojoba.

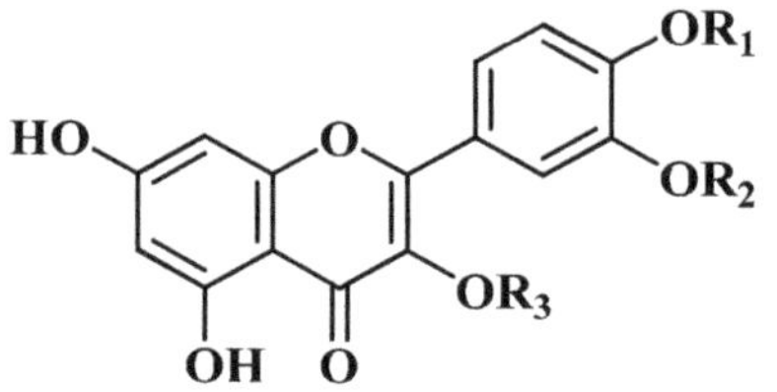

	R1	R2	R3
Quercetin (**12**)	H	H	H
Isorhamnetin (**13**)	H	Me	H
Quercetin 3-methyl ether (**14**)	H	H	Me
Quercetin 3,3′-methyl ether (**15**)	H	Me	Me
isorhamnetin 3-*O*-glucoside (**16**)	H	Me	Glc
Quercetin-3-*O*-glucoside (**17**)	H	H	Glc
Typhaneoside (**18**)	Me	H	Glc $\overset{2}{-}$ Rha, 6 | Rha
Isorhamnetin 3-*O*-rutinoside (**19**)	Me	H	Glc, 6 | Rha
Quercetin 3-*O*-rutinoside (**20**)	H	H	Glc, 6 | Rha

3.4. Fat-Soluble Vitamins

Vitamin D and its derivatives *viz.* α, γ, and δ tocopherol were isolated and quantitatively estimated in the oil where γ-tocopherol makes up approximately 79% of these compounds. Other fat-soluble vitamins such as vitamin A are also found [22].

4. Physical Characters of the Oil

Crude jojoba oil obtained directly by either cold expression or solvent extraction of the seeds, without any modifications, yields an oil with a golden or light yellow color. It has a pleasant, slightly nutty taste [6]. The thermal and oxidative stabilities of the oil are high; therefore, the oil shows high resistance toward rancidity due to the presence of natural antioxidants (α, γ, and δ tocopherol) [6]. Refined or bleached oil, obtained by passing the natural oil over activated charcoal and treating with caustic alkali substances, is nearly white with low oxidative stability due to subsequent removal of the antioxidants. The thermal stability of both natural and bleached forms is high, which is indicated by a high flash point reaching 295 °C [28]. The oil's viscosity favors using the oil and/or its derivatives as an extreme temperature/pressure lubricant [6,12]. Jojoba oil is soluble in common solvents such as benzene and chloroform. However, it is essentially immiscible in methanol. The solubility of jojoba in different organic solvents (Table 5) [29] and other physical properties (Table 6) are listed in many previous works [4–6,13,29–31].

Table 5. Solubility characteristics of jojoba oil in common organic solvents at 15 °C [a].

Solvent	mL of Solvent	Observation [b]
Water	5.0	I
	10.0	I
Acetic acid	10.0	I
	40.0	I
	50.0	S

Table 5. *Cont.*

Solvent	mL of Solvent	Observation [b]
	1.0	I
Methanol	10.0	I
	40.0	S
	1.0	I
Ethanol	5.0	I
	20.0	S
t-Amyl Alcohol	1.0	S
1-Butanol	1.0	S
	1.0	I
Acetone	3.0	I
	8.0	I
Benzene	1.0	I
Toulene	1.0	I
Carbon Tetrachloride	1.0	I
s-Tetrachlocthane	1.0	I
Diethylether	1.0	I
Tetrahydrofuran	1.0	I
Hexane	1.0	I
Cyclohexane	1.0	I
	1.0	I
Dimethylformamide	10.0	I
	30.0	S
	1.0	I
Dimethylsulfoxide	5.0	I
	20.0	S
	1.0	I
Acetonitrile	10.0	I
	30.0	S
Aniline	2.0	S
m-Cresol	2.0	S

[a] all measurement used 0.2 g [b] I = insoluble; S = soluble.

Table 6. Some physical properties of jojoba oil as reported in the literature [31].

Freezing point, °C	10.6–7.0
Melting point, °C	6.8–7.0
Boiling point at 757 mm under N2, °C	389
Heat of fusion by DSC, Cal/g	21
Refractive index at 25 °C	1.465
Dielectric constant, 27 °C	2.680
Specific conductivity, 27 °C, mho/cm	8.86.10–13
Specific gravity, 25/25 °C	0.863
MV-1 rotor in MY cup, cp	35
Plate and cone with PK-1, cp	33
Brookfield, spindle #1, 25 °C, cp	37
Cannon–Fenske, 25 °C, cp	50
Cannon–Fenske, 100 °C centistokes	27
Smoke point, °C	195
Flash point, °C	295
Fire point, °C	338
Iodine value	82
Saponification value	92
Acid value	<2
Acetyl value	2
Unsaponifiable matter, %	51
Total acids, %	52
Iodine value of alcohols	77
Iodine value of acids	<76
Average molecular weight of wax esters	606

5. Chemical Properties of the Oil

Jojoba molecules contain two double bonds at ω-9 positions in both alcohol and acid sides, which are separated by an ester bond. While in typical plant oils, double bonds are usually close to each other; in jojoba molecules, they are far apart and uneven from the center. These three active sites have been proven to be the source of many intermediates and final products with different physical and chemical characters. These derivatives are described with particular reference to the reaction that leads to the formation of a wide potential of industrial and pharmaceutical applications: the production of semisoft waxes by geometrical isomerization in the manufacture of suppository bases, production of hard waxes by hydrogenation in the manufacture of candles, production of additives by sulfurization for high-pressure/high-temperature lubricants, production of selective exectrants for the nuclear industry by phosphonation of chemically bonded jojoba oil [5,32,33].

These chemical modifications provide a wide range of polymers with diverse properties that could serve as good candidates in industrial application, especially those related to the polyhydroxyurethanes polymers that will be discussed in detail in Section 8.1.

Shani continued his basic research on the possible reaction schemes at the double bond. All-trans jojoba oil was prepared by the straight chemical route, involving the anti-addition of bromine or chlorine to the double bonds followed by displacement and elimination of the halogens with Na I. All-*trans* jojoba was obtained at a yield greater than 75% and had a melting point of 52–54 °C. Similar to those obtained from natural liquid oil, a series of products were prepared from the semisolid all-*trans* jojoba under the same conditions used for the natural liquid oil [34,35].

Thorough investigations of the all-*trans* derivatives and their physical and chemical characteristics revealed that the all-*trans* derivatives of jojoba oil had essentially the same melting points as those of the *cis* configuration. Based on these observations, Shani concluded that the polar groups played a more significant role than the geometrical configuration of the double bonds in determining the strength of the packing of the molecules in the solid phase.

5.1. *Cis/Trans Isomerization*

Unsaturated fatty materials can be converted into solid materials by geometrical isomerization of the double bonds. The *trans* isomer of jojoba is thermodynamically more stable than the *cis* form. Moreover, it has a substantially higher melting point, and its soaps have superior wetting and detergency properties. The reaction has never had any commercial significance, which is most likely because the same results can be achieved by partial hydrogenation with the additional advantages of higher oxidation stability. This phenomenon could expand the uses of this isomerized material, especially as a suppository base in the pharmaceutical industry due to its natural creamy appearance coupled with a melting point close to human body temperature [6].

Wisniak and Alfandary were the first to report on the geometrical isomerization of jojoba oil with selenium and NO_2 catalysts under a wide range of conditions. Melting points of the resultant product varied between 36 and 42 °C. Proper adjustment of the operating conditions could, if necessary, allow the preparation of a material with a melting point close to average human body temperature [36]. Later, Galun and coworkers described the thermal and photosensitized isomerization of jojoba oil. The absorption of light at wavelengths of 366 nm or more via the allowance of sensitizers enables the acquisition of the isomerized form of jojoba oil. However, this is dependent on the fact that the *cis* isomer can transform into the trans form if heated to a temperature sufficiently high and that the double bonds present in jojoba oil absorb light of wavelengths below 200 nm as a result [37,38].

5.2. Hydrogenation

Hydrogenation is a standard technique for improving the properties of vegetable and animal oils. In addition, it increases the softening and melting points of the fats and improves their color, odor, and stability. The reaction involves the chemical addition of hydrogen to the unsaturated carbon-to-carbon double bonds in fatty alcohol or the fatty acid molecule. This addition occurs by mixing the heated oil and hydrogen in the presence of nickel as a catalyst, at pressures in the order of 0–120 psi, and in hydrogenation conditions widely used in industrial purposes [5]. Total hydrogenation of the oil produces highly lustrous, pearly white crystalline laminae that are very hard. Solid wax has been suggested as a potential ingredient in polish waxes, carbon paper, waxing of fruit, and candles component [5].

In 1959, a comparison was made by Knoepfler et al. between the hydrogenation characteristics of jojoba oil obtained by extracting the oil with solvents and those obtained by the cold-hydraulic pressing of the jojoba seeds. The results revealed no significant difference between both hydrogenated forms, except in the melting point. Those prepared from cold-hydraulic pressing have a melting point of 67–68 °C, while those prepared from oil extracted by solvents have a higher melting point of 74–76 °C [32]. Wisniak and Holin have studied the hydrogenation of jojoba oil under a wide range of operating conditions and reaction kinetics in the preparation of different types of solid waxes and compared the characters of the hydrogenated jojoba oil with Beeswax and Carnauba wax. It was observed that jojoba oil is substantially better than Beeswax and relatively equal with Carnauba wax regarding hydrogenation [39]. Simpson and Miwa have done an in-depth X-ray diffraction study of hydrogenated jojoba oil to determine fatty acid and alcohol chain conformation, unit cell, and angle of tilt of the chains [40].

5.3. Halogenation

Halogenated fatty materials find extensive uses in preparing quaternary compounds, anti-rotting, flame proofing, and fungicide additives. In addition, brominated vegetable oils have long been used as weighting oil in carbonated beverages [41]. In 1979, Wisniak and Alfandary conducted an extensive study of the chlorination and bromination of jojoba oil. Their main objective was to determine the kinetics of the reaction and evaluate the influence of the operating variables. The experimental results indicated that in the dark and the temperature range used (−15 to +5 °C), a direct addition to the double bond with essentially no substitution occurred. The rate of halogenation decreased with the increase in temperature [42].

5.4. Sulfurization and Sulfur Halogenation

The sulfurization of fatty material with sulfur or other reagents containing sulfur and halogen yields various products with different physical and chemical properties. In general, when sulfur content is low (<5%), the products will be liquid and be used as additives. Increasing the sulfur content will increase the viscosity until a rubber-like mass is obtained.

In 1975, Gisser et al. conducted a deep study about the mechanical properties of sulfurized jojoba oil and sulfurized sperm oil. The results obtained revealed that there is no difference between both oils [5]. Furthermore, sulfurized jojoba oil has additional advantageous properties regarding its appearance and high viscosity; the same result was obtained by Miwa et al. [13].

5.5. Phosphonation

Dialkyl alkylphosphantes are stable organic phosphorus esters possessing unique properties and offer considerable potential for commercial exploitation. Thus, they have been recommended for use in many applications. As plasticizers, they hold great potential due to their superior stability and other unique characteristics compared to organic phosphates. They have been suggested as synthetic lubricants, additives to improve the extreme pressure properties of lubricants, functional fluids, oil, or fuel additives; pour-point depressants, pesticides, synergists, or carriers for pesticides and fertilizers, intermediates for the synthesis of corrosion inhibitors, and metal extractants. In general, several dialkyl alkylphosphantes are useful as flame-retardants, softeners, textile treating agents, and heat transfer media [5]. Wisniak has reported preliminary experimental data on the phosphonation of jojoba oil with different dialkylphosphites, using tert-butyl perbenzoate as a radical generator. The average ester chain in jojoba oil contains two double bonds so that the final product may contain up to two atoms of phosphorus per chain [33,42].

5.6. Oxidation, Epioxidation, and Ozonolysis

Jojoba oil shows good thermal stability up to a relatively high temperature. Generally, the cosmetic formulations containing jojoba oil have superior stability toward oxidation than other lipids used for this purpose. A comparative study of the relative oxidation stability of jojoba oil, sperm whale oil, carnauba wax esters, Limnanthes douglassi wax esters, and behenyl arachidate revealed that jojoba oil has high oxidative stability comparing all other oils [43]. Kampf conducted an in-depth study of the accelerated oxidation of crude jojoba oil and bleached and stripped oils. He found that crude jojoba oil contains natural antioxidants that counted for the high oxidative stability of the natural oil. The removal of these antioxidants through bleaching or stripping of the oil leads to a sharp decline in the oxidative stability of the products [5]. Epoxides of unsaturated glycerides and simple fatty acid esters are currently used as plasticizers and stabilizers for polyvinyl chloride plastics [5].

Ozonolysis is an important technique for studying the structure of unsaturated compounds such as those present in jojoba oil. Ozonides in general, but particularly jojoba ozonides, are viable intermediates for many synthetic paths. Zabicky previously used ozone as a reagent to attain intermediates to synthesize different derivatives that are widely used for industrial purposes [5].

6. Biological Activity

Extensive biological and pharmacological investigations, based on the uses of jojoba oil in folk medicine, revealed that jojoba oil and its derivatives exhibit vast biological activities in different pharmaceutical forms, whether used topically or internally. These activities can be attributed to the unique chemical composition of the wax esters [4]. Most of the relevant activities were grouped in Figure 3.

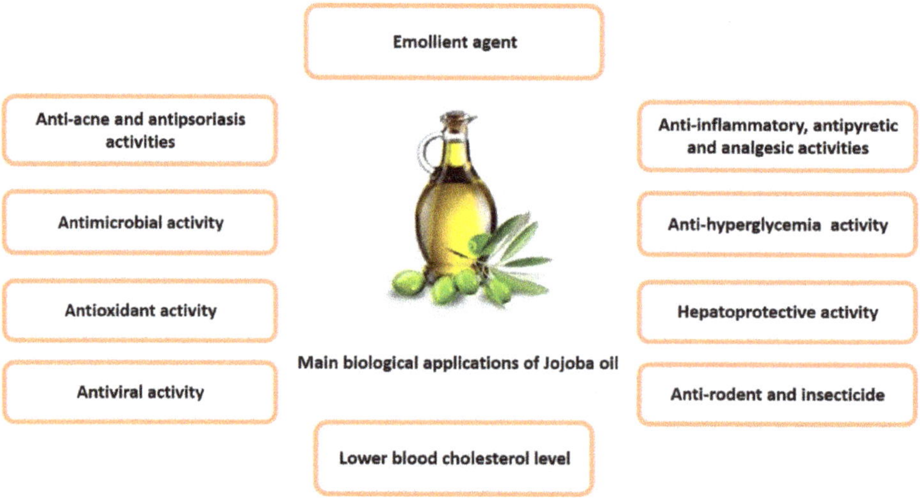

Figure 3. Summary of the main biological activities of jojoba oil.

6.1. Traditional and Folk Medicinal Uses

Jojoba has a rich ethnobotanical history due to its wide use by natives of the arid southwestern deserts of the USA and northwest of Mexico. Jesuit priests in this area recorded tribal uses of jojoba for many skin and scalp disorders. It was first reported in 1789 by the Mexican historian Francisco J. Clavijero that the Amerindians of Baja California highly prized the fruit for food and the oil as a medication [10,33]. "Two to three jojoba seeds taken in the morning are said to be good for the stomach. Seeds when ground and mixed with chocolate facilitate parturition for women. Toasted and ground seeds are found to be specific against sores that erupt on the face. The unguent oil stops chills and if eaten in certain quantity gradually eliminates them". He was also the first to describe how the Indians use the nuts to treat the wounds, where jojoba nuts were put in hot ashes until the oil starts oozing. "They were then ground on rocks, with the resultant salve-like substance applied to the wound. This salve is claimed to cure cuts, scratches and sores rapidly" [5].

Other early mentioned medical uses include curing the suppression of urine, helping in weight loss, improvement of liver functions, elevating body immunity, remedy for cancer, and promotion of growth of hair [5].

6.2. Pharmacological Uses

6.2.1. Emollient Agent

Skin surface-softening effects are represented by an increase in the extensibility or suppleness of the surface. These changes contribute to the overall softness of the skin and make it possible to accommodate stretching and movement without cracks and tears, perceived as scaliness, developing on the surface. That surface suppleness changes rapidly in response to the application of water or known emollients [6,8,10,11,44]. Jojoba oil in single-phase and emulsion systems shows an excellent lubricity without the oily, greasy feel of other lipids, especially lanolin and petrolatum [45]. It can also contribute to superior transpirational water control in the skin, thus reducing evaporation without blocking the passage of gases and water vapor. This character is due to its high molecular weight and low viscosity, and structural similarity with skin sebum, leading to a smoothing effect on dry skins and the inhibition of excess flaking of epidermal cells [5,33]. Skin indentation tests showed that the oil enhanced skin elasticity, similar to the effect of lanolin. Jojoba oil also showed a keratoplastic effect and seemed to restore the skin's natural shine [5].

Many studies have been carried out to evaluate the penetration rates, slip, and occlusive of various emollients, including jojoba oil and fully hydrogenated jojoba oil in many pharmaceutical skin care products. It was found that the derivatives of jojoba oil have excellent lubricity characteristics. It was also demonstrated that hydrogenated jojoba oil has a faster penetration rate and good occlusive properties. Thus, it is recommended to use jojoba oil alone or with other natural oils to maintain the natural appearance of the skin and the safety of that derivative as an emollient in the cosmetic formulation [7,10].

Christensen et al. in 1988 examined jojoba oil, both hydrogenated and ozonized derivatives, for their emollient activity. He found that a marked increase in skin surface suppleness appeared after 5 min which persisted for many hours, implying a potential use in dry skin products. In addition, ozonized jojoba derivatives make the skin surface water repellent and resistant to the stiffening effect encountered after washing with soap and water [6,10].

6.2.2. Anti-Acne and Antipsoriasis Activities

The historic use of jojoba oil by Mexican Indians to treat sores has recently highlighted its potential in treating acne and psoriasis. Miwa gave the scientific evidence of its use as anti-acne in 1973, who clinically examined the wax on patients suffering from acne vulgaris. The results revealed that jojoba oil could be used successfully to treat these conditions [10,13]. Its properties as a liquid wax allow the dissolution of sebum deposits within hair follicles due to an ability to penetrate the follicles and remove the comedome, thus clearing the skin.

Mosovich studied the effect of jojoba wax in the treatment of both acne vulgaris and psoriasis. He found that jojoba has high effectiveness in acne, with no secondary effects noted and no reports made of burning or itching. This efficacy indicates that jojoba oil may be used alone or in addition to other treatments. The antipsoriasis activity of jojoba oil is related to the positive keratoplastic and the slight keratolytic effect required to treat excessive scaling of the skin. Therefore, jojoba oil may be used as an additional treatment [6].

6.2.3. Anti-Inflammatory, Antipyretic, and Analgesic Activities

Possible anti-inflammatory effects of jojoba oil were investigated against both acute and chronic inflammation of the skin. The possibility that jojoba oil could be beneficial in treating pain and reducing edema resulting from thermal and sunburns was demonstrated [10]. Habashy et al. conducted a study in 2005 that demonstrated this reduction of edema and prostaglandin E2 content in rats, further supporting this potential of jojoba. The anti-inflammatory effect of jojoba oil involved the blockage of both cyclooxygenase II and lipoxygenase enzymes [7,26].

This work is confirmed by a controlled clinical trial evaluating the short-term effectiveness of jojoba liquid wax as local treatment of Napkin rash. The results were compared to standard treatment of a combination of triamcinolone acetonide, nystatin, neomycin, and gramicidin. Jojoba liquid wax was found as effective as the use of that combination in the treatment of Napkin rash. However, jojoba had the advantage of being safer due to the lack of systemic side effects that are usually present using the combination mentioned above [10].

6.2.4. Antimicrobial Activity

Jojoba oil has been shown to have an intense inhibitory action on the growth of *Tubercle bacilli*, *leprosy bacilli*, and *Brucelli* [11]. The liquid wax could help dissolve the solid wax coatings around the bacilli due to the chemical structure similarity between jojoba waxes and the fats forming the sheath of the bacilli, which prevents the penetration of the antibiotics. A combination of antibiotics and jojoba oil as penetrating oil may be effective in treating those serious diseases [6,46]. Furthermore, alcoholic extracts of the jojoba root have demonstrated antimicrobial activity against several pathogens, including *Bacillus cereus*, *Salmonella typhimurium*, and *Candida albicans*. This activity is attributed to the alkaloid, saponin, and steroid content of the root extract.

6.2.5. Other Activities

Jojoba oil has also demonstrated a beneficial effect against hyperglycemia-induced oxidative stress. Cyanogenic glycosides and other components found in the seed extract markedly decreased ROS and caspase-3 activation and improved antioxidant defense, inhibiting p22phox and increasing nuclear factors—this activity may serve as a useful tool for combating diabetes [46,47]. Manoharan et al. support this theory, having conducted a report in 2016 that discussed the potential of jojoba oil to inhibit or manage diabetes due to its antioxidant properties. Jojobenoic acid present in the alcoholic seed extract has also demonstrated protection against FB1-induced hepatotoxicity in rat liver. Similar results were confirmed in a recent study that indicated jojoba seeds induced a decrease in body weight, fat mass, insulin resistance, oxidative stress, liver steatosis and renal complications. The results demonstrated the beneficial effect of jojoba against metabolic syndrome and oxidative stress [48].

Clarke and Yermanos were the first to study the lowering effect of jojoba oil on the serum cholesterol by their studies on the blood cholesterol level in rabbits where blood cholesterol level was reduced 40% in rabbits given 2% jojoba oil and 1% cholesterol in the diet for 30 days compared to the result obtained when 1% cholesterol is given alone [49].

The concomitant administration of jojoba oil with fipronil ameliorated the toxic effects of fipronil on liver, brain, and kidney with improvement of the antioxidant status, the rate of apoptosis, and the histopathological alterations. This positive effects were evidenced by the combating effect on the oxidative stress in liver, brain, and kidney as indicated by lowering the malondialdehyde (MDA) and nitric oxide (NO) levels with elevating in glutathione (GSH) level and activities of superoxide dismutase (SOD) and catalase (CAT). In addition, there is a marked lowering of the elevated serum levels of hepatic markers alanine aminotransferase (ALT), aspartate transaminase (AST), alkaline phosphatase (ALP), and lactate dehydrogenase (LDH) and the γ-aminobutyric acid (GABA) level in the brain [50].

Biorefinery processes can be employed to produce jojobyl alcohols from jojoba oil (11-eicosenol, 13-docosenol, and 15-tetracosenol), which have been explored as antivirals. Jojoba oil also holds value in the industry as anti-rodent treatment, insecticides, and bioenergy production. Furthermore, the presence of compounds with cyclooxygenase-2 (COX-2) inhibitive properties in jojoba leaf extracts holds potential in anticancer treatments. COX-2 inhibitors lead to an increase in the rate of apoptosis and a decrease in the invasiveness of cancer cells alongside angiogenesis reduction.

7. Pharmaceutical Uses

It is preferred to formulate it into a pharmaceutical preparation to achieve a maximum benefit of any biologically active natural compound. Owing to jojoba's high skin moisturizing ability, high resistance to oxidation, its ability to penetrate the skin, and its ability to solubilize insoluble drugs, jojoba has been investigated as an excipient in different dosage forms. In an attempt to compile most of the work done on jojoba oil either as an active pharmaceutical ingredient or as an excipient, all the efforts published in PubMed have been collected, and most of the relevant information is reported in the following section. It is summarized in Table 7.

7.1. Topical Preparations

Jojoba was incorporated in topical preparations to enhance the efficacy of drugs used to treat skin diseases [1]. A previous study demonstrated the ability of jojoba oil to solubilize lycopene, which is an important antioxidant with low solubility in both water and oil. The improved solubility enables the formulation of lycopene into liquid and transparent products for pharmaceutical uses [2]. Shevachman et al. reported the successful preparation of microemulsion using jojoba wax as the oily phase using different surfactants and cosurfactants, in which the content of jojoba oil determined the transition from the water-in-oil to bicontinuous and to oil-in-water structures [3].

Diclofenac sub-micron emulsion formulated using 20% jojoba oil showed an enhanced anti-inflammatory effect compared to marketed Voltaren® Emulgel® cream, which was attributed to jojoba penetrative properties [4]. Thakur et al. reported the preparation of jojoba oil-based emulsion of benzoyl peroxide for the treatment of acne. Based on jojoba oil emollient effect, anti-inflammatory, and antibacterial properties, the study resulted in a significant reduction in skin irritation and dryness caused by benzoyl peroxide. It enhanced its therapeutic effect [5].

Methotrexate-loaded jojoba oil-based microemulsion was proved to be clinically safe and effective in treating psoriasis vulgaris due to its moisturizing and anti-inflammatory effects [6]. Another jojoba oil-based microemulsion loading the synthetic retinoid tazarotene revealed a better therapeutic effect in psoriatic patients than the marketed product with no irritation and a double increase in tazarotene skin deposition [7].

Stable valacyclovir solid lipid nanoparticles were successfully prepared using jojoba oil. The prepared nanoparticles were stable with high entrapment efficiency of valacyclovir, which can be an effective delivery system in treating viral infections in humans [8]. In addition, nanostructured lipid carriers (NLC) were developed in semisolid preparation using jojoba oil as the liquid lipid. The in vivo studies showed a great increase in skin hydration and reduction of transepidermal water loss, which may result in the improvement in the symptoms of some skin disorders such as eczema [9].

Previous studies demonstrated the successful use of jojoba oil as an excipient for different topical antifungal preparations. Shahin et al. revealed the high physical stability of clotrimazole-loaded jojoba oil-based emulgels with a superior antimycotic activity against Candida albicans compared to the commercially available formulation Candistan® and Canesten® [10,11]. In addition, fluconazole dissolved in jojoba oil in the oily phase of microemulsion gel showed superior antifungal activity against Candida albicans with the widest zone of inhibition in comparison to fluconazole solution [12]. Moreover, El-Hadidy et al. explored the use of jojoba oil to formulate the poorly water-soluble voriconazole in microemulsion (ME) for topical application. Jojoba oil-based MEs showed good physical and rheological properties upon storage for 12 months at ambient conditions, and in vitro permeation studies revealed that they were able to sustain voriconazole release up to 42 h. In addition, voriconazole-loaded MEs showed significantly better antifungal activity against *Candida albicans* than the drug solution [13].

7.2. Cosmetic Products

Jojoba oil was reported for its use as a conditioning agent due to its emollient properties. The addition of jojoba oil to thioglycolate-based straightening emulsions benefited the hair fiber, allowing a little protein loss, protection to hair thread, and improved the breakage resistance [14]. In an attempt to benefit from the jojoba oil chemical backbone, Touitou and Godin formulated skin non-penetrating sunscreens (NPSUN) as new photo protectors from UV harmful radiation. The idea depends on the conjugation of jojoba oil with UV sunscreen molecules as methoxycinnamate to form new filters. The formulated NPSUNs exhibited high skin substantivity, decreasing the need for a frequent application with no in vitro permeation of methoxycinnamate-NPSUN across the skin for 24 h [15,16].

7.3. Transdermal and Intradermal Preparations

Jojoba oil has been investigated as a penetration enhancer in the fabrication of transdermal patches to deliver olanzapine. The fabricated patch was stable with good physical properties and increased drug skin flux [17]. Intradermally administrated Bacillus Calmette–Guérin (BCG) vaccine has been successfully encapsulated in small-sized agarose microcapsules and small-diameter alginate beads prepared by the emulsification of the hydrogel within jojoba oil. The freeze-drying microcapsules were stable for 12 months of storage at room temperature [18,19].

7.4. Parenteral Preparations

Novel nanocapsules for parenteral administration were prepared using vegetable oils such mango, jojoba, pequi, oat, annatto, calendula, and chamomile as the lipid core instead of the capric/caprylic triglyceride. All the formulated nanosystems were compatible regardless of the oil type; however, nanocapsules formulated using jojoba were the most favorable due to their optimum particle size characteristics [20].

Table 7. A summary of pharmaceutical dosage forms containing jojoba oil.

Dosage Form	Drug	Ingredients	Use/effect of Jojoba Oil	Ref.
Microemulsion	Antioxidant lycopene	Jojoba oil, alcohols, nonionic surfactant (Brij 96V)	To solubilize lycopene	[51]
Microemulsion	-	Jojoba oil, alcohols, different nonionic surfactants, namely Brij 96V and Tweens, and water	To study the effect of Jojoba oil content on the type of the microemulsion	[52]
Sub-micron emulsion	Diclofenac (Diethyl ammonium)	Jojoba oil, purified egg lecithin, Cremophor EL surfactant, and water	To increase the anti-inflammatory effect of topical preparations of diclofenac	[53]
Gellified emulsion	Anti-acne agent, Benzoyl peroxide	Lipophilic surfactant (Span 60), jojoba oil, hydrophilic surfactant (Tween 20), propylene glycol, methyl paraben, propyl paraben, disodium EDTA, butylated hydroxy toluene, Carbopol 940, and water	To decrease the skin irritation and dryness caused by benzoyl peroxide	[54]
Microemulsion	Methotrexate	Jojoba oil, Tween 80, Span-85 and water	Treatment of psoriasis vulgaris.	[55]
Microemulsion	Synthetic retinoid tazarotene	Jojoba wax, labrasol/plurol isostearique and water	Treatment of psoriasis and increase in skin deposition of tazarotene	[56]
Solid lipid nanoparticles	Valacyclovir hydrochloride	Glyceryl monostearate. jojoba oil, polyethylene Glycol 400, Tween 80, and water	To benefit from jojoba oil moisturizing and stabilizing activity in the treatment of viral infections in humans	[57]
Nanostructured lipid carriers	-	Glyceryl behenate, jojoba oil, Tween 80, cetrimide, glycerine, Carbopol 934 or Carbopol 980, triethanolamine, and water	To improve symptoms of some skin disorders like eczema	[58]
Emulgels	Clotrimazole	Jojoba oil, hydroxypropyl methylcellulose (HPMC) Carbopol 934, Span 60, Brij 35, triethanolamine, propylene glycol, and water	An excipient for different topical antifungal preparations	[59]
		Hydrophobically modified co-polymers of acrylic acid, namely Pemulen TR1 and TR2, jojoba oil, and water		[60]
Cutina lipogels	Fluconazole	Cutina, Jojoba oil	An excipient for fluconazole topical drug delivery	[61]
Microemulsion gel		Jojoba oil, Brij 96, Capmul and, water		
Straightening emulsions	-	Jojoba oil, ammonium thioglycolate, self-emulsifying wax, oleth-3, mineral oil, propylene glycol, aqua, and preservative blend	As a conditioning agent added to the emulsion	[62]

Table 7. *Cont.*

Dosage Form	Drug	Ingredients	Use/effect of Jojoba Oil	Ref.
Skin non-penetrating sunscreens	-	Jojoba oil, methoxycinnamate	To link UV sunscreen molecules as methoxycinnamate to jojoba oil to form new filters	[63,64]
Transdermal patch	Olanzapine	Jojoba oil, Eudragit polymer	As a penetration enhancer in transdermal delivery	[65]
Small-sized agarose microcapsules	Bacillus Calmette–Guérin (BCG) vaccine	Agarose, jojoba oil	An excipient	[66,67]
Small-diameter alginate beads		Calcium alginate matrix, jojoba oil		
Nanocapsules		Jojoba oil, Poly(€-caprolactone) Tween 80, and Span 60	To study physical stability and the hemocompatibility of jojoba oil-based nanocapsules for parenteral administration	[68]
Solid nanoemulsion	Imiquimod, a Toll-like receptor 7 (TLR7) agonist + SIINFEKL antigen	Jojoba oil, sucrose fatty ester S-1670 and water	An excipient	[69]
O/W microemulsions	Paclitaxel	Jojoba oil, d-α-tocopherol polyethylene glycol 1000 succinate (TPGS-1000), isobutanol, and water	As an excipient to load paclitaxel for cancer treatment	[70]
Charged micelles	Small interfering RNAs (siRNAs)	Cationic lipids Bolaamphiphiles (GLH-58 and GLH-60) synthesized from jojoba oil	Starting material for the synthesis of lipids	[71]

7.5. Inhalable Preparations

The dry nanoemulsion powder prepared by jojoba oil had a good particle size distribution and an improved mass median aerodynamic diameter. The nanoemulsion showed higher anti-inflammatory effect on LPS-induced acute lung injury compared to than dexamethasone with a decrease in total protein content and downregulation of tumor necrosis factor-alpha (TNF-α), interleukins-1beta/6 (IL-1β/6), and NF-κB p65. In addition, it showed higher anti-inflammatory and anti-oxidation effect on H2O2-induced acute lung injury through the elimination of reactive oxygen species (ROS), increasing of superoxide dismutase (SOD), decreasing in of lipid peroxide malondialdehyde (MDA) and glutathione (GSH), and inhibition of caspase-3 expression [72].

7.6. Anticancer Preparations

Jojoba oil was incorporated in anticancer drug delivery systems. Solid nanoemulsion containing a combination of imiquimod, a Toll-like receptor 7 (TLR7) agonist, and model peptide antigen SIINFEKL for the topical treatment of different types of precancerous skin lesions and skin cancer, as a new perspective to avoid invasive technique and enhance dermal antigen administration [21]. Flores-Villaseñor et al. reported on the formulation of physically stable biocompatible o/w microemulsions with Jojoba oil as the oily phase for the delivery of paclitaxel. The microemulsion could load paclitaxel in a concentration of 0.3 mg/mL, which provides a new alternative nanodevice for cancer treatment [22]. In another study, authors were able to prepare positively charged micelles from bolaamphiphiles synthesized using natural jojoba oil. The prepared micelles delivered small interfering RNAs (siRNAs) to cancer cells with relatively low toxicities in vitro and in vivo and protected the nucleic acid from degradation [23].

8. Industrial Applications

8.1. Synthesis Polyurethanes Polymers

Jojoba oil has a wide range of industrial applications especially in polymers synthesis. Polymers are versatile materials that are used in a wide range of industries. Polyurethanes (Pus) are commonly used synthetic polymers involved in a wide range of applications, including furniture, automobiles, clothes, shoes, elastomers, coatings, and insulation. The usefulness of polyurethane is related to its excellent properties, including outstanding mechanical strength, strong chemical resistance, and light weight [73].

The most popular source of polyols used in the production of PUs is petrol; however, the researchers were forced to substitute petrol with clean natural resources such as vegetable oils, especially seed oils, due to the need for saving the environment. Seed oils are biodegradable, abundant, inexpensive substituents that entice many researchers to use them to produce PUs. This process converts different seed oils into reactive polyols by introducing hydroxyl groups into their structure with the consequent production of PUs with varying mechanical and thermal properties [74].

Jojoba oil has been used to produce PUs after functionalizing the oil by mercaptoethanol in a single step reaction to yield a diol with two hydroxyl functions, followed by catalyst-free reaction with different isocyanates to obtain different polyurethane prepolymers. Then, the chain extenders were added to obtain linear and cross-linked polyurethane materials characterized by exhibit good flexibility and high thermal stability [75]. The same group makes a major change through a high reactivity synthesis of cyclic carbonate monomers to generate biobased PolyHydroxyUrethane (PHU) from jojoba and castor oils. The first step involved thiol-ene coupling with thioglycolic acid to functionalize jojoba oil, followed by esterification with glycerol carbonate to yield new dicyclic carbonates. By aminolysis with different diamines, the dicyclic carbonates were used to synthesize linear PHUs. The cyclic carbonates produced are recommended due to the absence of solvents and catalysts during the manufacturing process and the production at low temperatures and thus with good reactivity [76].

More recent research has extended the development of linear PUs from synthesized diol Jojoba with different diisocyanates as a catalyst-free polycondensation reaction. PUS was versatile depending on the nature of the disocyanate used, with good thermal instability and regulated characteristics. Bio-based PUs are characterized by their improved solubility, allowing their casting with cellulose nanocrystals or cellulose nanofibrils to produce strong nanocomposites [77].

8.2. Other Industrial Uses

A rubber-like material is obtained from sulfurized jojoba oil, which is applied in linoleum manufacturing and ink printing composition, the paint and varnish industries, and the chewing gum industry [78]. One of the most extensive applications of jojoba oil includes an extreme temperature/extreme pressure lubricant in the form of sulfurized oil, which can bear high temperature and pressure without changing its viscosity [6,12,13,79]. Its stability at elevated temperatures permits the constant provision of a thin-film lubricating border, which is of remarkable necessity in decreasing frictional wear and temperature increase, which helps directly to extend the life span of the lubricating oil and indirectly to protect the automobile parts [13]. The study of the utilization of jojoba oil as a lubricant for some of the petroleum-derived products proved its improvement of certain desirable characteristics as antirust, antifoam, anti-wear, and friction reduction properties [80,81].

Nasser et al. explored the application of jojoba polymers as a lubricant and evaluated its viscosity index and pour point depressants when compared to homopolymer. The results showed that the viscosity index increases with increasing the alkyl chain length of both α- olefins and acrylate monomers. The pour point improved for additives based on alkyl acrylate. [82].

Another industrial application is its use as a surfactant due to the long alkenyl (jojobenyl, erucyl) alcohols obtained by hydrolysis, as its combination with polyethylene glycol chains customizes surfactants with desired hydrophile–lipophile balance [13].

The synthesis of methyl esters from jojoba oil allows its commercial application for the production of biodiesel. The results explored the promising future of jojoba oil as an oil feedstock for cultivation in comparatively dry areas [83,84]. The use of ultrasound technology was successfully applied to reduce the reaction time and temperature and increase biodiesel yield by reducing the cost and energy, contributing to a cleaner, safer and green technology for biodiesel production [84]. In addition, Jojoba oil is regarded as an excellent renewable feedstock to produce replacements for petroleum-derived transportation fuels and chemicals [85]. A recent study showed that the blend of jojoba oil with diesel fuel leads to a clear reduction in NOx and hydrocarbon (HC) emissions but indirectly impacts CO emission due to its high viscosity. Moreover, jojoba oil in the blends adversely influences thermal radiation to furnace walls due to the less sooting tendency of the flame when jojoba is present [86].

Moreover, jojoba oil has been used in the leather industry as a fat-liquoring agent, which verified significant improvement in the mechanical properties of leather, such as tensile strength and elongation at break [5,87].

The application of jojoba oil as an alternative collector for the selective separation of apatite and calcite minerals showed high selectivity between calcite and apatite, improving their selective flotation by using jojoba oil at a slightly acid medium, without the use of depressants [88].

Jojoba oil has been implemented with castor oil for the synthesis of PolyHydroxyUrethane polymer [76]. Other industrial uses include extraction and separation of isotopes such as Uranium (VI), Thorium (IV), and Plutonium (IV); and antifoaming agents in isolation of penicillin and tetracycline [9]. Jojoba oil replaced sperm whale oil as lamp oil, and it is used as solid wax to mix with and improve paraffin candies, microporous polyethylene film from microencapsulation of oil, and fatty acid amides as a lubricant for polyethylene film extrusion [13].

9. Toxicity of Jojoba Oil

No acute toxicity was found when crude jojoba oil was fed to mice; i.e., the LD_{50} is more than 160 g/Kg. In ocular irritation tests on rabbits, jojoba oil refined by deodorization or deodorization and discolorations caused some reversible conjunctival irritation 1 h after oil application. The reverse action was completely cleared 24 h after ocular application. In 15- and 30-day-old guinea pigs, patch tests did not cause pathological inflammation. A light swelling of the epidermis occurred 30 days after topical application, which was less pronounced than that induced by liquid paraffin and more than that induced by olive oil. However, the effects on the animal skin were reversible and may have been caused by the occlusive nature of the oil film. In addition, prolonged daily subcutaneously injections in rats did not result in any histopathological changes of blood or urine analyses. Only a mild local reversible granulomatous reaction in the injected area indicated that jojoba oil is slightly irritant. Patch tests on humans did not reveal allergic reactions except in hyperallergic people. Prick tests with people exposed earlier to jojoba oil for two years revealed no allergic reactions to either the crude or refined oil.

A mixture of jojoba oil and hydrogenated jojoba wax was not mutagenic both with and without activation in the Ames assay [8,10,44,89]. Taguchi measured the safety of Jobacohol, which was produced by sodium reduction and molecular distillation. No acute toxicity was found in mice, and eye irritation was quite low. Repeated patch tests in rabbits, where Jobacohol was compared with oleyl alcohol with both dissolved in jojoba oil, showed no difference between these materials. Irritation was quite low, and it was concluded that Jobacohol is quite safe. Jobacohol also showed no irritation in primary skin irritation tests in marmots and no sensitization in maximization-of-sensitization tests. Negative results were also obtained in mutagenicity tests with *Salmonella typhimurium* and *Escherichia coli* [6].

Tests of primary irritation on humans with either healthy skin or humans suffering from contact dermatitis were also carried out. The results revealed no skin irritation concerning Jobacohol or oleyl alcohol. Phototoxicity tests on humans also showed that Jobacohol was quite free of this effect [6].

10. Conclusions

In this review, we shed light on one of the most economically important crops, jojoba. Although limited phytochemical work has previously been conducted on the different plant extracts, the composition of the liquid wax obtained by direct expression of the seeds has been thoroughly investigated. The plant appears to be a source of golden oil, which shows high structural similarity to spermaceti wax, involved in many pharmaceutical products. Traditionally, it is used for many skin and scalp disorders. The seed cake is used safely as a food and has many applications in the food industry due to its high fat and protein content. Most of the previously conducted biological work has been directed to prove the claimed emollient effect and then further extended to evaluate the oil's anti-inflammatory, analgesic, and antipyretic properties. In addition, the plant has shown substantial activity as an antibacterial and antiviral agent. Interestingly, the plant extract shows a promising antidiabetic and antihypercholesterolemia. In conclusion, the jojoba tree represents an attractive source for the future development of new medication that could be identified and characterized using the new tools available in biochemical, physicochemical, and biological domains.

Author Contributions: H.A.G. (Heba A. Gad), H.A.G. (Haidy A. Gad) and S.H.H. collecting of data and writing original draft; A.R. revising the whole manuscript; I.T., A.E.A. and O.A.K. reviewing and editing; M.L.A. conceptualization, writing the original draft supervising and finalizing. All authors have read and agreed to the published version of the manuscript.

Funding: This research received no external funding.

Institutional Review Board Statement: Not applicable.

Informed Consent Statement: Not applicable.

Data Availability Statement: The data presented in this study are available on request from the corresponding author.

Conflicts of Interest: The authors declare no conflict of interest.

References

1. Spencer, G.F.; Plattner, R.D.; Miwa, T. Jojoba oil analysis by high pressure liquid chromatography and gas chromatography/mass spectrometry. *J. Am. Oil Chem. Soc.* **1977**, *54*, 187–189. [CrossRef]
2. Khairi, M.M.A. Genetics and Breeding of Jojoba [Simmondsia chinensis (Link) Schneider]. In *Advances in Plant Breeding Strategies: Industrial and Food Crops*; Al-Khayri, J.M., Jain, S.M., Johnson, D.V., Eds.; Springer: Cham, Switzerland, 2019; Volume 6, pp. 237–276. [CrossRef]
3. Li, T.S.C. *Medicinal Plants: Culture, Utilization, and Phytopharmacology*; Technomic Pub. Co.: Lancaster, PA, USA, 2000; 517p.
4. National Research Council (U.S.). Advisory Committee on Technology Innovation. Ad Hoc Panel. In *Jojoba: New Crop for Arid Lands, New Raw Material for Industry*; National Academy Press: Washington, DC, USA, 1985; 102p.
5. Wisniak, J. *The Chemistry and Technology of Jojoba Oil*; American Oil Chemists' Society: Champaign, IL, USA, 1987; 272p.
6. Baldwin, A.R.; American Oil Chemists' Society. *Seventh International Conference on Jojoba and Its Uses: Proceedings*; American Oil Chemists' Society: Champaign, IL, USA, 1988; 453p.
7. Habashy, R.R.; Abdel-Naim, A.B.; Khalifa, A.E.; Al-Azizi, M.M. Anti-inflammatory effects of jojoba liquid wax in experimental models. *Pharmacol. Res.* **2005**, *51*, 95–105. [CrossRef] [PubMed]
8. Matsumoto, Y.; Ma, S.; Tominaga, T.; Yokoyama, K.; Kitatani, K.; Horikawa, K.; Suzuki, K. Acute Effects of Transdermal Administration of Jojoba Oil on Lipid Metabolism in Mice. *Medicina* **2019**, *55*, 594. [CrossRef] [PubMed]
9. Al-Obaidi, J.R.; Halabi, M.F.; AlKhalifah, N.S.; Asanar, S.; Al-Soqeer, A.A.; Attia, M.F. A review on plant importance, biotechnological aspects, and cultivation challenges of jojoba plant. *Biol. Res.* **2017**, *50*, 25. [CrossRef]
10. Pazyar, N.; Yaghoobi, R.; Ghassemi, M.R.; Kazerouni, A.; Rafeie, E.; Jamshydian, N. Jojoba in dermatology: A succinct review. *G. Ital. Dermatol. Venereol.* **2013**, *148*, 687–691. [PubMed]
11. Ranzato, E.; Martinotti, S.; Burlando, B. Wound healing properties of jojoba liquid wax: An in vitro study. *J. Ethnopharmacol.* **2011**, *134*, 443–449. [CrossRef]
12. Bhatia, V.K.; Chaudhry, A.; Sivasankaran, G.A.; Bisht, R.P.S.; Kashyap, M. Modification of jojoba oil for lubricant formulations. *J. Am. Oil Chem. Soc.* **1990**, *67*, 1–7. [CrossRef]
13. Miwa, T.K. Structural determination and uses of jojoba oil. *J. Am. Oil Chem. Soc.* **1984**, *61*, 407–410. [CrossRef]
14. Quattrocchi, U. *CRC World Dictionary of Medicinal and Poisonous Plants: Common Names, Scientific Names, Eponyms, Synonyms, and Etymology*; CRC: Boca Raton, FL, USA, 2012.
15. Stuessy, T.F. *Plant Taxonomy: The Systematic Evaluation of Comparative Data*; Columbia University Press: New York, NY, USA, 1990; 514p.
16. Wunderlin, R.P. *Guide to the Vascular Plants of Central Florida*; University Presses of Florida: Gainesville, FL, USA, 1982; 472p.
17. Ashour, M.L.; Ayoub, N.A.; Singab, A.N.B.; Al Azizi, M.M. *Simmondsia chinensis* (Jojoba): A comprehensive pharmacognostic study. *J. Pharmacogn. Phytochem.* **2013**, *2*, 97–120.
18. Kramer, J.K.G.; Sauer, F.D.; Pigden, W.J. *High and Low Erucic Acid Rapeseed Oils: Production, Usage, Chemistry, and Toxicological Evaluation*; Academic Press: New York, NY, USA, 1983; 582p.
19. Van Boven, M.; Daenens, P.; Maes, K.; Cokelaere, M. Content and composition of free sterols and free fatty alcohols in jojoba oil. *J. Agric. Food Chem.* **1997**, *45*, 1180–1184. [CrossRef]
20. Van Boven, M.; Holser, R.; Cokelaere, M.; Flo, G.; Decuypere, E. Gas chromatographic analysis of simmondsins and simmondsin ferulates in jojoba meal. *J. Agric. Food Chem.* **2000**, *48*, 4083–4086. [CrossRef] [PubMed]
21. Van Boven, M.; Leyssen, T.; Busson, R.; Holser, R.; Cokelaere, M.; Flo, G.; Decuypere, E. Identification of 4,5-didemethyl-4-O-alpha-D-glucopyranosylsimmondsin and pinitol alpha-D-galactosides in jojoba seed meal (*Simmondsia chinensis*). *J. Agric. Food Chem.* **2001**, *49*, 4278–4283. [CrossRef] [PubMed]
22. Busson-Breysse, J.; Farines, M.; Soulier, J. Jojoba wax: Its esters and some of its minor components. *J. Am. Oil Chem. Soc.* **1994**, *71*, 999. [CrossRef]
23. Tank Chintankumar, J.; Borkhataria Chetan, H.; Baria Ashok, H.; Patel Rakesh, P.; Tamizharasi, S.; Sureja, D.K.; Patel, I.D.; Parmar, G.R. Formulation and evaluation of aceclofenac loaded maltodextrin based proniosome. *Int. J. ChemTech Res.* **2009**, *1*, 567–573.
24. Graille, J.; Pina, M.; Ploch, D. Routine analysis of jojoba wax fatty acids and alcohols by single column capillary GC. *J. Am. Oil Chem. Soc.* **1986**, *63*, 111–116. [CrossRef]
25. Culling, C.F.A. *Handbook of Histopathological and Histochemical Techniques: Including Museum Techniques*, 3rd ed.; Butterworth-Heinemann: Oxford, UK, 2013.
26. Abdel-Mageed, W.M.; Bayoumi, S.A.; Salama, A.A.; Salem-Bekhit, M.M.; Abd-Alrahman, S.H.; Sayed, H.M. Antioxidant lipoxygenase inhibitors from the leaf extracts of *Simmondsia chinensis*. *Asian Pac. J. Trop. Med.* **2014**, *7S1*, S521–S526. [CrossRef]
27. Abdel-Mageed, W.M.; Bayoumi, S.A.; Al-Wahaibi, L.H.; Li, L.; Sayed, H.M.; Abdelkader, M.S.; El-Gamal, A.A.; Liu, M.; Zhang, J.; Zhang, L.; et al. Noncyanogenic Cyanoglucoside Cyclooxygenase Inhibitors from *Simmondsia chinensis*. *Org. Lett.* **2016**, *18*, 1728–1731. [CrossRef] [PubMed]
28. Landis, P.S.; Craver, R.H.; Barton, D.E. Pyrolysis studies with jojoba oil. *J. Agric. Food Chem.* **1992**, *40*, 456–457. [CrossRef]

29. Landis, P.S.; Craver, R.H. Solubility of jojoba oil in organic solvents. *J. Am. Oil Chem. Soc.* **1984**, *61*, 1879–1880. [CrossRef]
30. Bower, D.I. *An Introduction to Polymer Physics*; Cambridge University Press: Cambridge, UK, 2002; 444p.
31. Wisniak, J.; Liberman, D. Some physical properties of *Simmondsia* oil. *J. Am. Oil Chem. Soc.* **1975**, *52*, 259–261. [CrossRef]
32. Knoepfler, N.B.; Vix, H.L.E. Vegetable Oils, Review of Chemistry and Research Potential of *Simmondsia Chinensis* (Jojoba) Oil. *J. Agric. Food Chem.* **1958**, *6*, 118–121. [CrossRef]
33. Wisniak, J. Potential uses of jojoba oil and meal—A review. *Ind. Crop. Prod.* **1994**, *3*, 43–68. [CrossRef]
34. Shani, A. Functionalization at the double bond region of jojoba oil: I. bromine derivatives. *J. Am. Oil Chem. Soc.* **1981**, *58*, 845–850. [CrossRef]
35. Shani, A. Functionalization at the double bond region of jojoba oil: II. Diels-alder adducts of jojobatetraene. *J. Am. Oil Chem. Soc.* **1982**, *59*, 228–230. [CrossRef]
36. Wisniak, J.; Alfandary, P. Geometrical Isomerization of Jojoba Oil. *Ind. Eng. Chem. Prod. Res. Dev.* **1975**, *14*, 177–180. [CrossRef]
37. Galun, A.B.; Grinberg, S.; Kampf, A.; Shaubi, E. Oxidation and halogenation of jojoba wax. *J. Am. Oil Chem. Soc.* **1984**, *61*, 1088–1089. [CrossRef]
38. Galun, A.B.; Shaubi, E. Thermal isomerization of jojoba wax. *J. Am. Oil Chem. Soc.* **1984**, *61*, 564–569. [CrossRef]
39. Wisniak, J.; Holin, M. Hydrogenation of Jojoba Oil. *Ind. Eng. Chem. Prod. Res. Dev.* **1975**, *14*, 226–231. [CrossRef]
40. Simpson, T.D.; Miwa, T.K. X-ray study of hydrogenated jojoba wax. *J. Am. Oil Chem. Soc.* **1977**, *54*, 54. [CrossRef]
41. Soontag, N.O.V. Halogenation. *J. Am. Oil Chem. Soc.* **1963**, *40*, 199–203. [CrossRef]
42. Wisniak, J.; Alfandary, P. Sperm Whale Oil Replacements from Halogenation of Jojoba Oil. *Ind. Eng. Chem. Prod. Res. Dev.* **1979**, *18*, 358–364. [CrossRef]
43. Hagemann, J.W.; Rothfus, J.A. Oxidative stability of wax esters by thermogravimetric analysis. *J. Am. Oil Chem. Soc.* **1979**, *56*, 629–631. [CrossRef]
44. Meier, L.; Stange, R.; Michalsen, A.; Uehleke, B. Clay jojoba oil facial mask for lesioned skin and mild acne–results of a prospective, observational pilot study. *Forsch. Komplementmedizin* **2012**, *19*, 75–79. [CrossRef]
45. Lovell, C.R. *Plants and the Skin*; Blackwell Scientific Publications: Oxford, UK, 1993; 272p.
46. Baccouch, N.; Ben Salah, H.; Belhadj, S.; Hentati, O.; Abdennabi, R.; Gharsallah, N.; Elfeki, A.; Ayedi, M.; Allouche, N. Chemical characterization and biological activities of *Simmondsia chinensis* (Link) C. K. Schneid seeds oil. *Cell. Mol. Biol.* **2018**, *64*, 11–16. [CrossRef]
47. Belhadj, S.; Hentati, O.; Hamdaoui, G.; Fakhreddine, K.; Maillard, E.; Dal, S.; Sigrist, S. Beneficial Effect of Jojoba Seed Extracts on Hyperglycemia-Induced Oxidative Stress in RINm5f Beta Cells. *Nutrients* **2018**, *10*, 384. [CrossRef]
48. Belhadj, S.; Dal, S.; Khaskhoussi, F.; Maillard-Pedracini, E.; Hentati, O.; Sigrist, S. Anorexic and metabolic effect of jojoba: Potential treatment against metabolic syndrome and hepatic complications. *Nutr. Metab.* **2020**, *17*, 24. [CrossRef] [PubMed]
49. Clarke, J.A.; Yermanos, D.M. Effects of ingestion of jojoba oil on blood cholesterol levels and lipoprotein patterns in New Zealand white rabbits. *Biochem. Biophys. Res. Commun.* **1981**, *102*, 1409–1415. [CrossRef]
50. Abou-Zeid, S.M.; Tahoun, E.A.; AbuBakr, H.O. Ameliorative effects of jojoba oil on fipronil-induced hepatorenal- and neurotoxicity: The antioxidant status and apoptotic markers expression in rats. *Environ. Sci. Pollut. Res.* **2021**. [CrossRef]
51. Garti, N.; Shevachman, M.; Shani, A. Solubilization of lycopene in jojoba oil microemulsion. *J. Am. Oil Chem. Soc.* **2004**, *81*, 873–877. [CrossRef]
52. Shevachman, M.; Shani, A.; Garti, N. Formation and investigation of microemulsions based on jojoba oil and nonionic surfactants. *J. Am. Oil Chem. Soc.* **2004**, *81*, 1143–1152. [CrossRef]
53. Schwarz, J.S.; Weisspapir, M.R.; Shani, A.; Amselem, S. Enhanced antiinflammatory activity of diclofenac in jojoba oil submicron emulsion cream. *J. Appl. Cosmetol.* **1996**, *14*, 19–24.
54. Thakur, N.K.; Bharti, P.; Mahant, S.; Rao, R. Formulation and characterization of benzoyl peroxide gellified emulsions. *Sci. Pharm.* **2012**, *80*, 1045–1060. [CrossRef] [PubMed]
55. Ramez, S.A.; Soliman, M.M.; Fadel, M.; Nour El-Deen, F.; Nasr, M.; Youness, E.R.; Aboel-Fadl, D.M. Novel methotrexate soft nanocarrier/fractional erbium YAG laser combination for clinical treatment of plaque psoriasis. *Artif. Cells Nanomed. Biotechnol.* **2018**, *46*, 996–1002. [CrossRef] [PubMed]
56. Nasr, M.; Abdel-Hamid, S.; Mofath, N.H.; Fadel, M.; Alyoussef, A.A. Jojoba Oil Soft Colloidal Nanocarrier of a Synthetic Retinoid: Preparation, Characterization and Clinical Efficacy in Psoriatic Patients. *Curr. Drug Deliv.* **2017**, *14*, 426–432. [CrossRef] [PubMed]
57. Archana, C.; Amaldoss, M.J.N. Synthesis and Characterization of Valacyclovir HCl Hybrid Solid Lipid Nanoparticles by Using Natural Oils. *Recent Pat. Drug Deliv. Formul.* **2019**, *13*, 46–61. [CrossRef]
58. Estanqueiro, M.; Conceição, J.; Amaral, M.H.; Sousa Lobo, J.M. Characterization, sensorial evaluation and moisturizing efficacy of nanolipidgel formulations. *Int. J. Cosmet. Sci.* **2014**, *36*, 159–166. [CrossRef]
59. Shahin, M.; Abdel Hady, S.; Hammad, M.; Mortada, N. Novel Jojoba Oil-Based Emulsion Gel Formulations for Clotrimazole Delivery. *AAPS PharmSciTech* **2011**, *12*, 239–247. [CrossRef] [PubMed]
60. Shahin, M.; Hady, S.A.; Hammad, M.; Mortada, N. Optimized formulation for topical administration of clotrimazole using Pemulen polymeric emulsifier. *Drug Dev. Ind. Pharm.* **2011**, *37*, 559–568. [CrossRef] [PubMed]
61. El Laithy, H.M.; El-Shaboury, K.M.F. The development of Cutina lipogels and gel microemulsion for topical administration of fluconazole. *AAPS PharmSciTech* **2002**, *3*, E35. [CrossRef] [PubMed]

62. de Dias, T.C.S.; Baby, A.R.; Kaneko, T.M.; Velasco, M.V.R. Protective effect of conditioning agents on Afro-ethnic hair chemically treated with thioglycolate-based straightening emulsion. *J. Cosmet. Dermatol.* **2008**, *7*, 120–126. [CrossRef]
63. Touitou, E.; Godin, B. Skin nonpenetrating sunscreens for cosmetic and pharmaceutical formulations. *Clin. Dermatol.* **2008**, *26*, 375–379. [CrossRef]
64. Touitou, E.; Godin, B. New approaches for UV-induced photodamage protection. *J. Appl. Cosmetol.* **2006**, *24*, 139.
65. Geeta, A.; Sanju, D.; HariKumar, S.L. Natural Oils as Skin Permeation Enhancers for Transdermal Delivery of Olanzapine: In Vitro and In Vivo Evaluation. *Curr. Drug Deliv.* **2012**, *9*, 172–181. [CrossRef]
66. Esquisabelr, A.; Hernáandez, M.; Igartuaa, M.; Gascóan, R.; Calvo, B.; Pedraz, J.L. Production of BCG alginate-PLL microcapsules by emulsification/internal gelation. *J. Microencapsul.* **1997**, *14*, 627–638. [CrossRef] [PubMed]
67. Esquisabel, A.; Hernández, R.M.; Igartua, M.; Gascón, A.R.; Calvo, B.; Pedraz, J.L. Preparation and stability of agarose microcapsules containing BCG. *J. Microencapsul.* **2002**, *19*, 237–244. [CrossRef] [PubMed]
68. Venturini, C.G.; Bruinsmann, F.A.; Oliveira, C.P.; Contri, R.V.; Pohlmann, A.R.; Guterres, S.S. Vegetable Oil-Loaded Nanocapsules: Innovative Alternative for Incorporating Drugs for Parenteral Administration. *J. Nanosci. Nanotechnol.* **2016**, *16*, 1310–1320. [CrossRef] [PubMed]
69. Gogoll, K.; Stein, P.; Lee, K.D.; Arnold, P.; Peters, T.; Schild, H.; Radsak, M.; Langguth, P. Solid nanoemulsion as antigen and immunopotentiator carrier for transcutaneous immunization. *Cell. Immunol.* **2016**, *308*, 35–43. [CrossRef] [PubMed]
70. Flores-Villaseñor, S.E.; Peralta-Rodríguez, R.D.; Padilla-Vaca, F.; Meléndez-Ortiz, H.I.; Ramirez-Contreras, J.C.; Franco, B. Preparation of Peppermint Oil-Based Nanodevices Loaded with Paclitaxel: Cytotoxic and Apoptosis Studies in HeLa Cells. *AAPS PharmSciTech* **2019**, *20*, 198. [CrossRef] [PubMed]
71. Gupta, K.; Afonin, K.A.; Viard, M.; Herrero, V.; Kasprzak, W.; Kagiampakis, I.; Kim, T.; Koyfman, A.Y.; Puri, A.; Stepler, M.; et al. Bolaamphiphiles as carriers for siRNA delivery: From chemical syntheses to practical applications. *J. Control. Release* **2015**, *213*, 142–151. [CrossRef]
72. Zhang, G.; Xie, F.; Sun, Y.; Yu, X.; Xiao, Z.; Fang, R.; Li, J.; Li, Q.; Du, L.; Jin, Y. Inhalable Jojoba Oil Dry Nanoemulsion Powders for the Treatment of Lipopolysaccharide- or H2O2-Induced Acute Lung Injury. *Pharmaceutics* **2021**, *13*, 486. [CrossRef]
73. Raquez, J.M.; Deléglise, M.; Lacrampe, M.F.; Krawczak, P. Thermosetting (bio)materials derived from renewable resources: A critical review. *Prog. Polym. Sci.* **2010**, *35*, 487–509. [CrossRef]
74. Ghasemlou, M.; Daver, F.; Ivanova, E.P.; Adhikari, B. Polyurethanes from seed oil-based polyols: A review of synthesis, mechanical and thermal properties. *Ind. Crop. Prod.* **2019**, *142*, 111841. [CrossRef]
75. Mokhtari, C.; Malek, F.; Caillol, S.; Negrell, C. Synthesis of Bio-Based Polyurethanes from Jojoba Oil. *Eur. J. Lipid Sci. Technol.* **2018**, *120*, 1700414. [CrossRef]
76. Mokhtari, C.; Malek, F.; Manseri, A.; Caillol, S.; Negrell, C. Reactive jojoba and castor oils-based cyclic carbonates for biobased polyhydroxyurethanes. *Eur. Polym. J.* **2019**, *113*, 18–28. [CrossRef]
77. Mokhtari, C.; Malek, F.; Halila, S.; Belgacem, M.-N.; Khiari, R. New Biobased Polyurethane Materials from Modified Vegetable Oil. *J. Renew. Mater.* **2021**, *9*, 1213–1223. [CrossRef]
78. Daugherty, P.M.; Sineath, H.H.; Wastler, T.A. Industrial raw materials of plant origin. IV. A survey of *Simmondsia chinensis* (Jojoba). *Econ. Bot.* **1958**, *12*, 296–304. [CrossRef]
79. Wisniak, J. Chemistry and Technology of Jojoba Oil: State of the Art. In *Sixth International Conference on Jojoba and Its Uses: Proceedings Beer-Shiva, Israel, 21–26 October 1984*; American Oil Chemists' Society: Beer-Shiva, Israel, 1984.
80. Bisht, R.P.S.; Sivasankaran, G.A.; Bhatia, V.K. Additive properties of jojoba oil for lubricating oil formulations. *Wear* **1993**, *161*, 193–197. [CrossRef]
81. Anand, O.; Chhibber, V. Vegetable oil derivatives: Environment-friendly lubricants and fuels. *J. Synth. Lubr.* **2006**, *23*, 91–107. [CrossRef]
82. Nasser, R.; Nassar, A.; Ahmed, N. Jojoba Polymers As Lubricating Oil Additives. *Pet. Coal* **2015**, *57*, 120–129.
83. Abdelmoez, W.; Tayeb, A.M.; Mustafa, A.; Abdelhamid, M. Green Approach for Biodiesel Production from Jojoba Oil Supported by Process Modeling and Simulation. *Int. J. Chem. React. Eng.* **2016**, *14*, 185–193. [CrossRef]
84. Sarojini, G.; Kannan, P.; Pravin, G. Production of biodiesel from jojoba oil using ultra sonicator. *J. Environ. Biol.* **2019**, *40*, 802–806. [CrossRef]
85. Kozliak, E.; Mota, R.; Rodriguez, D.; Overby, P.; Kubátová, A.; Stahl, D.; Niri, V.; Ogden, G.; Seames, W. Non-catalytic cracking of jojoba oil to produce fuel and chemical by-products. *Ind. Crop. Prod.* **2013**, *43*, 386–392. [CrossRef]
86. Al Omari, S.A.B.; Hamdan, M.O.; Selim, M.Y.E.; Elnajjar, E. Combustion of jojoba-oil/diesel blends in a small scale furnace. *Renew. Energy* **2019**, *131*, 678–688. [CrossRef]
87. Nashy, E.-S.H.A.; Megahed, M.G.; Abd El-Ghaffar, M.A. Preparation of Fat-Liquor Based on Jojoba Oil Under Phase Transfer Catalysis. *J. Am. Oil Chem. Soc.* **2011**, *88*, 1239–1246. [CrossRef]
88. Santos, E.P.; Dutra, A.J.B.; Oliveira, J.F. The effect of jojoba oil on the surface properties of calcite and apatite aiming at their selective flotation. *Int. J. Miner. Process.* **2015**, *143*, 34–38. [CrossRef]
89. Di Berardino, L.; Di Berardino, F.; Castelli, A.; Della Torre, F. A case of contact dermatitis from jojoba. *Contact Dermat.* **2006**, *55*, 57–58. [CrossRef] [PubMed]

polymers

MDPI

Article

Effects of Gamma Radiation on the Sterility Assurance, Antibacterial Ability, and Biocompatibility of Impregnated Hydrogel Macrosphere Protein and Drug Release

Po-Sung Fu [1,2], Jen-Chyan Wang [1,3,4], Pei-Ling Lai [3], Shih-Ming Liu [5], Ya-Shun Chen [5], Wen-Chen Chen [4,5,*] and Chun-Cheng Hung [1,3,4,*]

1 School of Dentistry, College of Dental Medicine, Kaohsiung Medical University, Kaohsiung 807378, Taiwan; posung.elegant@msa.hinet.net (P.-S.F.); jechwz@kmu.edu.tw (J.-C.W.)
2 Department of Dentistry, Kaohsiung Municipal Ta-Tung Hospital, Kaohsiung 80145, Taiwan
3 Division of Prosthodontics, Department of Dentistry, Kaohsiung Medical University Hospital, Kaohsiung 807378, Taiwan; casting0118@gmail.com
4 Dental Medical Devices and Materials Research Center, College of Dental Medicine, Kaohsiung Medical University, Kaohsiung 807378, Taiwan
5 Advanced Medical Devices and Composites Laboratory, Department of Fiber and Composite Materials, Feng Chia University, Taichung 40724, Taiwan; 0203home@gmail.com (S.-M.L.); yaschen@fcu.edu.tw (Y.-S.C.)
* Correspondence: wencchen@mail.fcu.edu.tw (W.-C.C.); chuchh@kmu.edu.tw (C.-C.H.)

Abstract: Devices and medicines used in the medical field must be sterile. Gamma (γ)-irradiation is commonly used for sterilization because its high rate of penetration ensures uniform sterilization. To confirm that hydrogel macrosphere carriers inherit excellent liquid absorption with no cytotoxicity after γ-irradiation sterilization, investigating whether the physiochemical properties of hydrogel macrospheres differ before and after sterilization is essential. The present study evaluated the influence of the recommended 25-kGy γ-irradiation dose on the physicochemical characteristics and in vitro release of bovine serum albumin and vancomycin (an antibiotic medication) from alginate/gelatin with a w/w ratio of 1/4 crosslinking gel macrospheres. Gel macrosphere properties before and after sterilization were compared according to optical and scanning electron microscopy, infrared spectroscopy analysis, the amino residual crosslinking index, water absorption, degradation, sterility assurance, in vitro drug release, antibacterial ability, and cytotoxicity. The crosslinking index was almost unchanged; however, the γ-irradiation caused in situ hydrogel debonding and recrosslinking, which led to a decrease in the water absorption and increase in the degradation rate of the macrospheres after immersion. The release of gel macrospheres carrying vancomycin did not significantly affect antibacterial ability or biocompatibility after γ-irradiation. Accordingly, we conclude that γ-irradiation is suitable for macrospherical formulation.

Keywords: hydrogels; crosslinking; degradable; gamma (γ)-irradiation; sterilization; sterility assurance; antibacterial ability

Citation: Fu, P.-S.; Wang, J.-C.; Lai, P.-L.; Liu, S.-M.; Chen, Y.-S.; Chen, W.-C.; Hung, C.-C. Effects of Gamma Radiation on the Sterility Assurance, Antibacterial Ability, and Biocompatibility of Impregnated Hydrogel Macrosphere Protein and Drug Release. *Polymers* **2021**, *13*, 938. https://doi.org/10.3390/polym13060938

Academic Editor: Bramasta Nugraha

Received: 17 February 2021
Accepted: 14 March 2021
Published: 18 March 2021

1. Introduction

Hydrogel scaffolds with three-dimensional (3D) structures are generally used to provide physical and structural support to cells because the composition of the hydrogel is similar to an extracellular matrix. Hydrogels consisting of microspheres (in micrometers) or macrospheres (in millimeters) possess highly interconnected pores, which are key to maximizing blood absorption to enhance cell growth [1–4]. Therefore, hydrogel microspheres or macrospheres can potentially alter the function or performance of an implant in terms of drug delivery, regenerative therapies in assisting native regeneration, and restorative therapy toward repairing tissue or organs. Accordingly, biodegradable or absorbable hydrogel microspheres or macrospheres are the most widely used shapes in wound dressings, tissue engineering, regenerative medicine, and drug delivery [5–7].

Hydrogel scaffolds are mainly fabricated using physical and chemical crosslinking methods [8,9]. Hydrogel scaffolds fabricated through physical crosslinking are mainly formed due to the interaction of environmental conditions with hydrogen bonds and proteins. The physical crosslinking process involves freeze-thawing [10,11], stereo complex formation [12–14], ionic interaction [15–17], and hydrogen bonding [18]. The chemical crosslinking process involves Schiff base formation [19], grafting [20,21], radical polymerization [22–24], the condensation reaction [25,26], and high-energy irradiation [27,28]. A chemically crosslinked hydrogel is mainly formed through free radical polymerization, chemical reaction, energy irradiation, and catalytic enzyme crosslinking [29–31].

In biomedicine, the applied forms of hydrogel microspheres or macrospheres are solid, semisolid, and liquid hydrogels. Solid hydrogels have a network structure of ions and covalent crosslinks, and inorganic metals or microparticles or nanoparticles can be added to hydrogel to increase its antibacterial ability and enhance its mechanical properties [32–35]. Due to their excellent adhesion properties, semisolid hydrogels are advantageous for prolonging drug delivery and improving drug availability [36–38]. Liquid hydrogels easily incorporate drugs, proteins, and cells and are suitable for wound dressing. Besides, liquid hydrogels can be used to administer medication as a controlled release dose through injection [39–42].

Medical equipment, devices, and drugs are most commonly sterilized using gamma (γ)-irradiation. The main advantage of γ-irradiation is its high level of penetration and isothermal characteristics, which can appropriately manage heat-sensitive materials include inorganic metal oxides, polymer blends, or liquid crystals. In addition, γ-irradiation ensures uniform sterilization; thus, the risk of microbial contamination can be avoided after products are packaged. Historically, the United States permitted a relatively high sterility assurance level (SAL) of 10^{-3} for items such as surgical drapes and gowns. However, in recognition of certain Pharmacopeia requirements, as of 1998, the Conformitè Europëenne (CE) marking requires a SAL of at least 10^{-6}. Due to the number of microorganisms and the drug resistance of materials, the most common γ-irradiation dose is 25 kGy [43–47].

Sterilization can be achieved by a combination of heat, chemicals, irradiation, high pressure, and filtration like steam under pressure, dry heat, ultraviolet, radiation, gas vapor sterilants, chlorine dioxide gas, etc. However, for products that cannot be sterilized in the final containers, aseptic processing is necessary. Besides, natural polymers undergoing radioactive sterilization may cause energy transfer, which leads to covalent bond breakage and the generation of free radicals that can change the physicochemical properties and activities of materials, thereby producing toxic substances. Therefore, confirming whether toxic products are generated after newly developed medical products are sterilized using γ-irradiation is essential. According to our preliminary test, the basic chemical structure of hydrogels was changed greatly and showed less stability at radiation doses of 30 and 50 kGy than 25 kGy due to amide degradation by γ-irradiation.

The current study aimed to determine whether the use of 25 kGy of γ-irradiation to sterilize a relatively large amount of hydrogel macrospheres on a millimeter-scale prevents or reduces cytotoxicity or changes in physical properties in the context of hydrogel macrospheres impregnated with protein or drugs.

2. Materials and Methods

2.1. *Raw Materials*

The raw materials used in this study were gelatin (80–100 Blooms [USP-NF, BP, Ph. Eur.] pure, pharmaceutical grade, PANREAC, EU), alginic acid sodium salt from brown algae (low viscosity, Sigma-Aldrich®, St Louis, MO, USA), *N*-(3-dimethylaminopropyl)-*N*′-ethylcarbodiimide hydrochloride (EDC, molecular weight 191.70 g/mole, Sigma-Aldrich®, St Louis, MO, USA), vancomycin (GENTLE PHARMA CO., LTD, Yunlin County, Taiwan), and sucrose (KATAYAMA CHEMICAL CO., LTD, Osaka, Japan).

2.2. Preparation of Gel Macrospheres

Porous spheres were fabricated through solvent casting and particulate leaching. The preparation procedures were based on previously described methods [48,49]. A colloidal suspension was prepared after heating to 50 °C and mixing sodium alginate with gelatin in a *w*/*w* ratio of 1:4 and suspending the mixture in 10 mL of deionized distilled (DD) water. The colloidal suspension was also mixed with saccharose particles in a particle:colloid ratio of 4 g:1 mL, which formed more than 70% of the interconnected pores within the gel macrospheres after particle leaching. After the colloid was evenly mixed, an autoinjector was used to control the discharge rate and produced fixed-volume macrospheres. The fixed-volume particles containing colloidal were added dropwise into the solution with cross-linkers of 1% EDC and 0.5% anhydrous calcium chloride at 4 °C. Subsequently, the gel macrospheres were removed and reimmersed in 1% EDC solution for 24 h to complete the crosslinking reaction. The crosslinked gel macrospheres were soaked in DD water for 3 h at 25 °C and were washed three times for leaching the particles. The macrospheres were then dried in a vacuum. Air pressure was reduced to approximately 26 μbar through lyophilization for 3 d.

2.3. Bovine Serum Albumin and Vancomycin Loading as Well as Release Measures

The porous macrospheres were immersed separately in 0.1% bovine serum albumin (BSA) and 25 mg/mL vancomycin solution to conduct protein and antibiotic loading at 4 °C for 24 h. The solution was frozen at −20 °C for 3 h and dried in a vacuum through lyophilization for 24 h to fabricate gel macrospheres with BSA and vancomycin. The designated group of macrospheres with vancomycin after irradiation was HyS-Van25.

The release rates of the macrospheres with BSA and vancomycin were investigated using DD water. BSA- and vancomycin-loaded macrospheres weighing 0.01 g were suspended in Eppendorf tubes with 1 mL of immersion solution. The release rates of BSA and vancomycin were determined after 5 and 22 days, respectively, in a water bath at 37 °C. Triplicate tests were used at each time point (n = 3). The immersion solutions were withdrawn at each time point. The amount of BSA released from the porous spheres was evaluated using a bicinchoninic acid (BCA) protein assay kit (Prod#23225; Thermo Fisher Scientific, Rockford, IL, USA) by measuring the optical density (OD) at a wavelength of 570 nm in an enzyme-linked immunosorbent assay (ELISA) macroplate reader (EZ Read 400, Biochrom, Cambridge, UK). To determine the content of vancomycin released by the spherical drug carrier, the OD of the amino acid in vancomycin was measured at a wavelength of 562 nm to compare the relative quantitative regression curves.

2.4. Sterilization by γ-Irradiation

The hydrogel macrospheres were sterilized using γ-radiation. The commonly used unit of absorbed radiation dose is the gray (Gy), which is equivalent to 1 joule of energy absorbed per kilogram of material. Hydrogel macrospheres (HyS-w/o γ) with protein BSA or antibiotic vancomycin and blank macrospheres were placed in 3-mL glass vials labeled and packed. The samples were irradiated using ^{60}Co-γ as the radiation source at China Biotech Corporation, Taichung, Taiwan. According to United States Pharmacopeial Convention (USP) recommendations, a sterilized dose of 25 kGy was used. After γ-ray irradiation, the sterilized hydrogel microspheres of HyS-w/γ were subjected to a sterility assurance test and appearance confirmation before the samples could be used for further testing and analysis. The relevant tests are described subsequently.

2.5. Characterization of Gel Macrospheres after Sterilization

2.5.1. Morphological Observations

Dried and wetted porous macrospheres of HyS-w/γ and HyS-w/o γ were observed using an optical microscope (OM; Primotech, ZEISS, Oberkochen, Germany). The wetted macrospheres were first immersed in excess DD water and placed at 37 °C for 24 h. The water-containing macrospheres were then removed, rinsed with saturated sponges, and placed on a glass slide for observation. The cross-sectional morphology was then examined through scanning electron microscopy (SEM; S-3000 N, Hitachi, Tokyo, Japan) and compared with the OM images to investigate the pore changes and morphological characteristics of the macrospheres before and after sterilization.

2.5.2. Changes in the Crosslinking Index after Radiation

The residual number of amino groups observed was approximately related to the crosslinking index of hydrogels. Accordingly, ninhydin (2,2-dihydroxy-1,3-indanedione) reagent (Sigma-Aldrich) was used to investigate the residual amino groups of macrospheres before and after sterilization. Ninhydin reagent can react with amines and amino acids during colorimetric assays. Residual amino measurements were conducted according to the manufacturer's instructions, and the OD was measured at a wavelength of 570 nm. The crosslinking index of the macrospheres before and after radiation was compared by measuring the content of unreacted free amine groups in the sample and subsequent calculation by using the following formula:

$$\text{Fixation index } (\%) = \frac{[(\text{amine-reactive})_{\text{fresh}} - (\text{amine-reactive})_{\text{fixed}}]}{(\text{amine-reactive})_{\text{fresh}}} \times 100\% \quad (1)$$

$(\text{amine-reactive})_{\text{fresh}}$: the free amine group content before crosslinking
$(\text{amine-reactive})_{\text{fixed}}$: the free amine group content before and after sterilization

2.5.3. Differences in Water Absorption and Degradation Rate after Sterilization

A water absorption test was performed to determine the swelling ratio or water content in the hydrogel macrospheres of HyS-w/γ and HyS-w/o γ. Each group of hydrogel macrospheres (W_0) was weighed and immersed in double-distilled (DD) water at 37 °C for 5, 10, 15, and 30 min as well as 1, 2, 4, 6, 8, and 24 h. The samples were taken out and rinsed, and the excess water was removed from the surfaces. The weights of the hydrated specimens (W_{wa}) were immediately measured and compared with the weights of the dried porous spheres (W_{wa}) (n = 3). The formula for measuring the water absorption of the hydrogel macrosphere is as follows:

$$\text{Water absorption} = (W_{wa} - W_o)/W_o \quad (2)$$

The degradation rate was measured by immersing the macrospheres in DD water for 1 day, weighing the standard hydrate saturation of the macrospheres (W_h), and again immersing the macrospheres in DD water at 37 °C for 1–13 d. After removing the test piece, the excess water was removed from the surface. The residual weight (W_r) was measured using a precision balance after water absorption. The following formula was used to calculate the degradation rate of each group of macrospheres after different periods:

$$\text{Degradation rate} = (W_h - W_r)/W_h \times 100\% \quad (3)$$

2.5.4. Sterility Assurance, Antibacterial Ability, and Cell Viability of Hydrogel Macrospheres with Drugs

Sterility Assurance

The sterility of any product is defined by the viability of a microorganism on the product after sterilization. Negative control (NC), positive control (PC), and experimental groups are essential for selecting the appropriate sterility assurance of medical devices. The NC group was sterile deionized water mixed with a liquid medium. The PC group was bacteria-containing water mixed with a liquid medium, which became turbid after 1 day of cultivation. The culture environment was heated to 35 °C, and the culture was cultivated without carbon dioxide to prevent the bacteria from growing excessively fast. The experimental group was sterilized gel macrospheres soaked in a hydrogel: culture solution with a ratio of 0.1 g:2.5 mL. Finally, the supernatant and agar culture were examined to observe whether agar colonies were formed after 1 day of cultivation.

In Vitro Cytotoxicity Following ISO 10993-5:2009

For the biological evaluation of the macrospheres, cytotoxicity tests were conducted following ISO 10993-5:2009. The newborn mouse fibroblast cell line of L929 was used in the aforementioned tests. The used cells were cultured with an alpha-modified Eagle's medium (α-MEM, Gibco®, Life technologies Co., NY, USA) containing house serum (Biolegend Co., South Logan, UT, USA) in an incubator containing 5% CO_2 at 37 °C. The medium was replaced once every 2 days. When the cell cultures grew to 80% capacity, they were subcultured. The PC was 15% dimethyl sulfoxide (DMSO), with each 1 mL of cell culture medium containing 150 µL of DMSO filtered through a 0.22-µm filter membrane. The NC was high-density polyethylene (HDPE) with a weight-to-medium volume ratio (g/mL) of 1:10. The medium was placed in a water bath at 37 °C for 24 h, and the extract of HDPE was set as the NC. The control group used the normal cell culture medium to cultivate the L929 cell line.

For each group, six replicate tests were measured ($n = 6$). The extraction solution was prepared by placing the irradiated macrospheres in the cell culture medium with a weight-to-medium volume ratio (g/mL) of 1:10 and heating it to 37 °C. After 24 h of incubation, the resultant supernatant liquid was the extract of the experimental group. The cell concentration of 1×10^4 cells/well was transferred into a 96-well microliter plate and cultured overnight in an incubator; the original medium was aspirated, and the sample extract (100 µL/well) was added to cultivate the cells. After culturing for 24 h, the aspirated cell culture medium was used for the experimental group. A general cell culture medium (100 µL/well) was then added and mixed with a cell proliferation assay kit (XTT; 50 µL/well). The mixture was then placed in a 5% CO_2 incubator at 37 °C for 4 h. Subsequently, the OD_{490} was measured using an ELISA reader (the XTT assay OD is proportional to the cell activity), and the cell morphology was observed.

Bacterial Endotoxin Testing

First, the test sample extract was prepared by adding 1 mL of pyrogen-free water to each 0.04-g batch of macrospheres and conducting ultrasonic-assisted shaking for 1 min. The extract was then placed at room temperature for 1 h before shaking again for 1 min. Then, a serial amount of pyrogen-free water was used for dilution. The NC group was prepared with 100 µL of pyrogen-free water, and the PC group was prepared using 50 µL of the 4λ endotoxin standard and 50 µL of pyrogen-free water. The positive product control group comprised 50 µL of undiluted test sample extract and 50 µL of the 4λ endotoxin standard.

Second, the sample group was prepared by diluting 50 µL of undiluted extract into 2×, 4×, 8×, and 16× dilutions by using pyrogen-free water. A volume of 100 µL of limulus amoebocyte lysate endotoxin reagent was prepared for cleaning the validation and sample groups with a reagent concentration of 0.25 endotoxin units (EU)/mL. The cleaning was conducted at 37 °C for 1 h. The standard tube agglutination test was performed; however, no agglutination was observed in the NC group.

Antibacterial Activity

An agar diffusion test was performed to measure the degree of antibacterial activity. The medium was tryptic soy agar, and the strains were Staphylococcus aureus (*S. aureus*) and Escherichia coli (*E. coli*). The antibiotic-loaded sterilized macrospheres were attached to the agar culture plate coated with bacteria, and the inhibition zone sizes were observed after incubating at 37 °C for 24 h. The quantitative inhibition sample was tested with the broth dilution method. The sample was immersed in 1 mL of bacterial suspension with a cell density at an OD_{595} value of 0.2 and incubated at 37 °C for 1, 4, 8, and 24 h. The control sterilized control, and experimental groups were measured after removing the bacterial liquid at each time point and measuring the OD_{595} value with an ELISA reader.

2.6. Statistical Analysis

IBM SPSS was used to determine characteristics such as average pore diameter, deviation rate, and degree of crosslinking and overlap. The experimental data were statistically analyzed, and the experimental data of the two groups were compared using the t-test. Moreover, Tukey's test was used to analyze the comparison of the groups.

3. Results and Discussion

3.1. Changes in the Physiochemical Properties of Hydrogel Macrospheres after Sterilization

The external optical and internal microstructure images of the hydrogel macrospheres are displayed in Figure **??**. The size of the prepared particle macrospheres was approximately 2 mm, and no noticeable effects on the appearance and size of the macrospheres were observed after sterilization with γ-ray irradiation (Figure **??**a). Observations of the internal pores of the macrospheres before and after water absorption (Figure **??**b) indicated that obvious pores appeared regardless of whether the spheres had been sterilized.

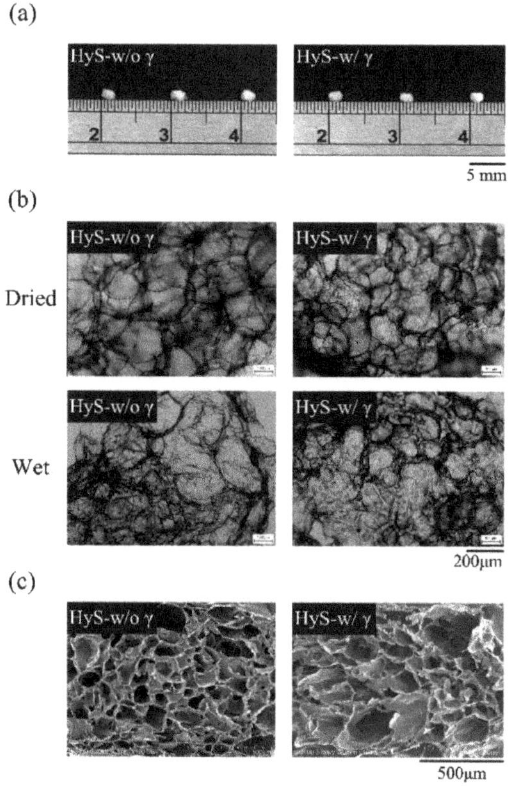

Figure 1. Freeze-dried hydrogel macrospheres after (HyS-w/γ) and before (HyS-w/o γ) sterilization of internal macrosphere microstructures of (**a**) photographs, (**b**) OM images, and (**c**) SEM images.

This observation confirms that after sterilization, the hydrogel macrospheres retained their original pore structures (Figure **??**b,c). Notably, the largest measured frequency of the internal pore diameter distribution in the hydrogel macrospheres shifted to the right, which indicated that the pores increased in size after sterilization (Figure 2a,b), and the significant difference was observed after statistical analysis ($p < 0.05$). The porosity changes in the macrospheres before and after sterilization were further analyzed using the SPSS software, which indicated that although the porosity of the macrospheres decreased marginally after sterilization (Figure 2c), no significant difference was observed after further statistical analysis ($p > 0.05$). The preliminary conclusion is that the hydrogel macrospheres maintained a uniform pore structure before and after sterilization with γ-ray irradiation.

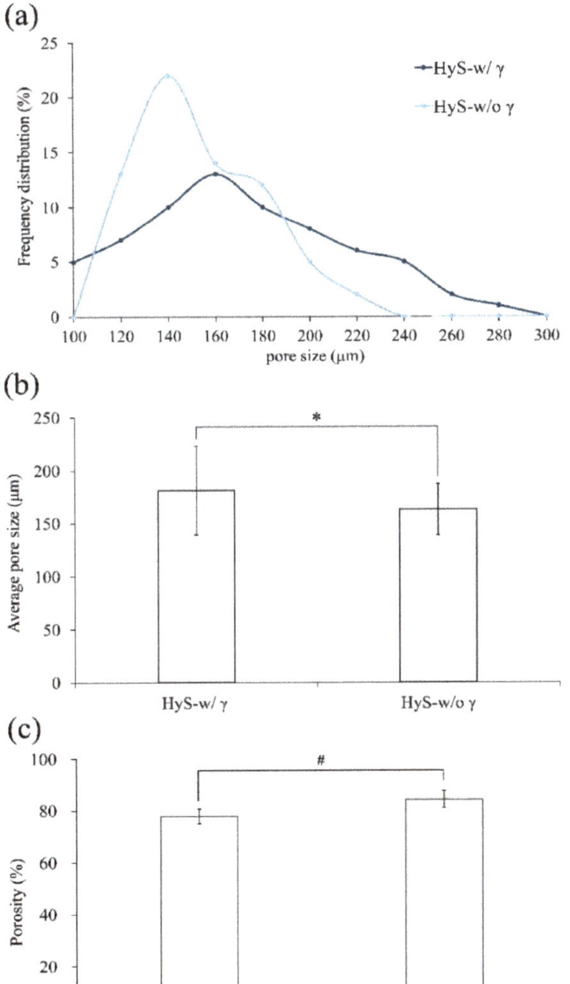

Figure 2. Comparisons of the (**a**) pore size distribution, (**b**) average pore size ($n = 60$; *: $p < 0.05$), and (**c**) porosity of hydrogel macrospheres before (HyS-w/o γ) and after (HyS-w/γ) sterilization ($n = 60$; #: $p > 0.05$).

The Fourier-transform infrared (FTIR) spectroscopy analysis results of the hydrogel macrospheres before and after sterilization are presented in Figure 3a. The characteristic peaks are as follows: the bands at 1080 and 1030 cm^{-1} for the COC group correspond to sodium alginate [50]; the vibrations at 1259 and 1240 cm^{-1} indicate amide III; the band regions at 1370–1440 and 1510–1580 cm^{-1} indicate amide II [51]; and the bands at 1655, 1629, and 1600 cm^{-1} indicate amide I of gelatin [52]. Notably, a new functional imine group (HC=N) was discovered in the band of 1610–1621 cm^{-1} for the sterilized HyS-w/γ macrospheres. [53,54] A study indicated that the amide group may decompose and transform into a new imine or nitrile group after irradiation [55]. Accordingly, the possible mechanisms of amide decomposition into more active imine or nitrile groups are displayed in Figure 3b. The amides between hydrogels decomposed immediately after irradiation and these active sites provided new sites for intermolecular recrosslinking to form a 3D interlocking structure. This process may have induced the internal pore size fluctuation and the following analysis results.

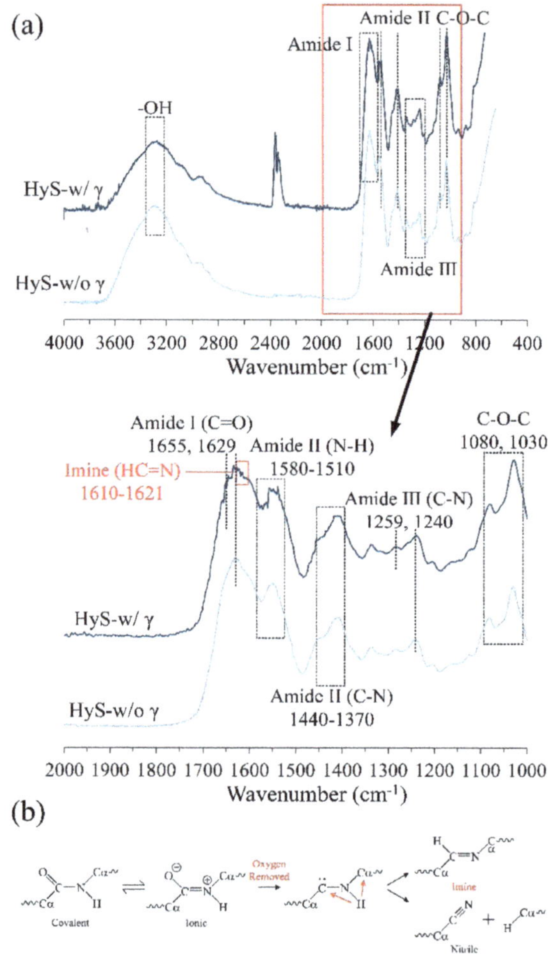

Figure 3. (**a**) Full and specific absorption bands obtained through the FTIR spectrum analysis of macrospheres before (HyS-w/o γ) and after (HyS-w/γ) sterilization. (**b**) Schematic of the mechanisms of amide bond decomposition into active imine or nitrile groups after irradiation, which can generate new intermolecular crosslinking sites in hydrogels.

The fixation index of the internal crosslinking degree of the hydrogel was directly proportional to the amount of residual free amine (Figure 4a). When the hydrogel reacted with EDC, the free amine of gelatin and carbonyl in hyaluronic acid reacted when EDC was added to produce a stable amide bond. The fixed index of crosslinking hydrogels was evaluated according to the opposite quantity of the residual amine group. Accordingly, the irradiation did not significantly affect the crosslinking degree between the hydrogels; however, γ-ray irradiation caused amide bond breakage, which exposed certain active amino groups. However, in situ crosslinking occurred again immediately; thus, the measured differences in the crosslinking degree between the groups before and after irradiation (HyS-w/o γ and HyS-w/γ) were limited.

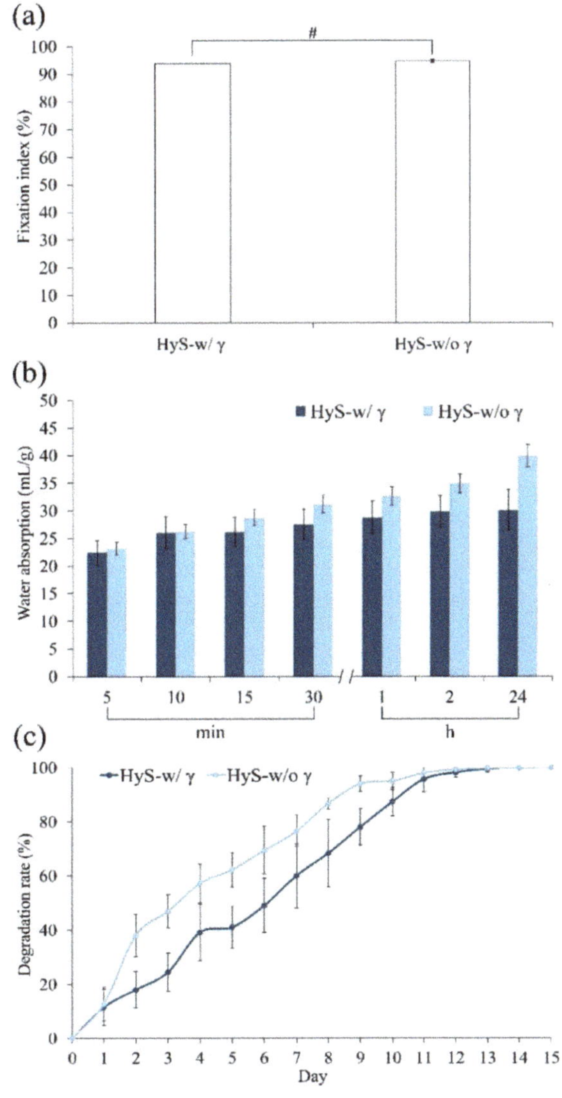

Figure 4. Physiochemical analysis of hydrogel macrospheres before (HyS-w/o γ) and after (HyS-w/γ) sterilization corresponds to amine fixation index (n = 6, #: $p > 0.05$) (**a**), water absorption ratio (n = 10) (**b**), and degradation rate (n = 10) (**c**).

The water absorption test results were noticeably different (Figure 4b). The degree of water absorption observed in the HyS-w/γ group plateaued from 10 min to 2 h. Subsequently, the degree of water adsorption marginally increased, and finally, macrospheres appeared after 24 h of immersion. The absorption rate reached approximately 30 mL/g.

However, the degree of water absorption in the HyS-w/o γ group continued to increase until 24 h elapsed, ultimately reaching approximately 40 mL/g. The water absorption rate of the macrospheres between the HyS-w/o γ and HyS-w/γ groups significantly differed after 15 min of immersion. We speculate that the difference observed between the HyS-w/o γ and HyS-w/γ groups might have occurred because certain hydrophilic bonds crosslinked with the active imine, which resulted in the strengthening of the intermolecular force and the significant reduction of the water absorption rate of HyS-w/γ after irradiation.

The in vitro degradations of hydrogels indicate that the HyS-w/o γ group degraded faster than the sterilized HyS-w/γ group within 10 days of immersion (Figure 4c); however, both groups of immersed macrospheres were completely disintegrated after 13 days. This phenomenon confirms the hypothesis that most of the internally active groups exposed on the pore surfaces bonded with one other at an accelerated rate due to irradiation, which exacerbated the reduction in water absorption and contributed to the delay in hydrogel degradation.

Sterilization can be achieved by a combination of heat, chemicals, irradiation, high pressure, and filtration like steam under pressure, dry heat, ultraviolet, radiation, gas vapor sterilants, chlorine dioxide gas, etc. [43–47]. In this study, hydrogels with high viscosity were used in the design and manufacturing of the final product on the scale of macrosphere. The sterilization method of filtration is suitable for thermolabile solutions that can pass through sterile bacteria-retaining filters. However, hydrogels with high viscosity cannot pass through sterile bacteria-retaining filters. The sterilization method of heat, e.g., steam under pressure and dry heat destroys the amino, amide, or hydroxy groups in hydrogel macrospheres, and are not considerably thermal stable for our study. Therefore, the sterilization method of heat is still unsuitable [47].

The sterilization method of chemical or gas sterilization is done with ethylene oxide or other highly volatile substances. Due to the porous macrospheres created by hydrogels that have high water or gas adsorption efficiency and stability, there is the possible issue of toxic residues remaining intact within the hydrogels in the macrospheres. Hence, gas sterilization is also not suitable here. The reviewed literature suggest that for the sterilization of hydrogels (excluding irradiation sterilization), gas sterilization or aseptic process are suitable and more credible compared to other methods [47]. Aseptic processing is conducted only for products that cannot be sterilized in final containers. Accordingly, raw materials and products of aseptic processing that have been sterilized by one of the above sterilization processes are transferred to pre-sterilized containers and sealed; both operations need to be carried out under controlled aseptic conditions. However, the whole process will cost more and the risk is higher than with irradiation sterilization. Therefore, the aseptic material filling process is suggested only if the final commercial products cannot be sterilized in the final containers. The sterilization method of irradiation, especially γ-irradiation, has a high level of penetration, is isothermal, and offers good assurance of product sterility, no chemical residue, and immediate availability of the product after sterilization. Thus, it is suitable for hydrogel macrospheres. The effect of γ-ray doses (25, 30, 50 kGy) on hydrogels is the reason why this research focused on 25 kGy (provided in Appendix A (Figure A1)).

3.2. *Sterility Assurance as Well as Protein and Antibiotic-Releasing Abilities*

The endotoxin test was based on a simple gel-clot method for detecting and semi-quantifying endotoxins according to lysate clotting. If the sample endotoxin contained more than 0.25 EU/mL, the reagent gel clotted. According to the ANSI/AAMI ST72 standard, the endotoxin content of each medical device package should be less than 20 EU/mL, so that it meets the requirements of pyrogen-free labware and the reagent preparation environment. The endotoxin test consisted of three control groups and five experimental groups of undiluted and diluted extracts under different magnifications to determine whether they would gel-clot. The EU concentration per mL was then reversed and converted for the hydrogels. The test results revealed that the undiluted, 2-,

4-, and 8-fold diluted reagent groups gel-clotted; however, the 16-fold diluted reagents did not gel-clot (Figure 5), which indicated that the endotoxin content of the macrospheres was between 2 and 4 EU/mL after adjusting on the standard curve; thus, this sample was endotoxin/pyrogen-free. For sterility validation, the quantitative measurement results of L929 cell viability displayed in Figure A2a reveal that the cell survival rate of HyS-w/γ was 83%, indicating that the hydrogel macrospheres were not cytotoxic after sterilization according to EN ISO 10993-5 Clause 4.1. The additional qualitative results of the L929 cells displayed in Figure A2b further validate that the HyS-w/γ process did not affect cell phenotype and growth after 24 h of cell culture.

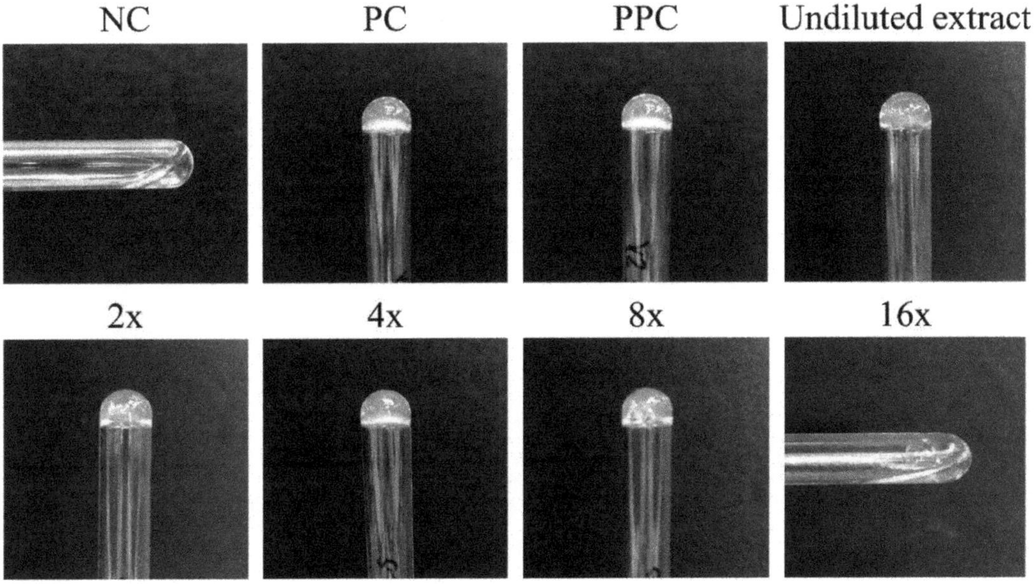

Figure 5. Bacterial endotoxin results of sterilized hydrogel macrospheres (NC: negative control; PC: positive control; PPC: positive product control; 2×, 4×, 8×, and 16× indicate extracts diluted with pyrogen-free water).

To confirm whether the irradiation would stimulate a reaction between the hydrogels and the carrying additives, we measured the release ability of the hydrogel macrospheres impregnated with protein and antibiotics before and after sterilization. The curves in Figure 6a indicate the BSA releases of HyS-w/γ and HyS-w/o γ at different time points after immersion. Both groups demonstrated no considerable variations in BSA releases after 1-h tests. The release rate of HyS-w/γ marginally increased after 1 h, and the average BSA release in the microspheres was approximately 2.14 g/L. The BSA releases tended to plateau after 4 h of macrosphere immersion, and the BSA release amount was 2.47 g/L after 5 d, which indicated that the HyS-w/γ macrospheres maintained its release capability after γ-ray irradiation.

We also examined the hydrogels impregnated with vancomycin and the accumulated release amounts of immersed macrospheres after sterilization (HyS-Van25) in DD water after 22 days of immersion (Figure 6b). The cumulative releases reached 19% within 24 h following HyS-Van25 immersion, which continuously released for up to 20 days. Different release slopes represent different release mechanisms. The release curve can be divided into two slope values at 11 days, which correspond to the complete degradation depicted in Figure 4c. The small slope value indicates that the vancomycin release in the first stage of HyS-Van25 immersion was dominated by diffusion, and the large slope value represents the vancomycin transport process in the second stage. Diffusion and structure erosion accompanied these mechanisms, thus causing another wave of rapid release.

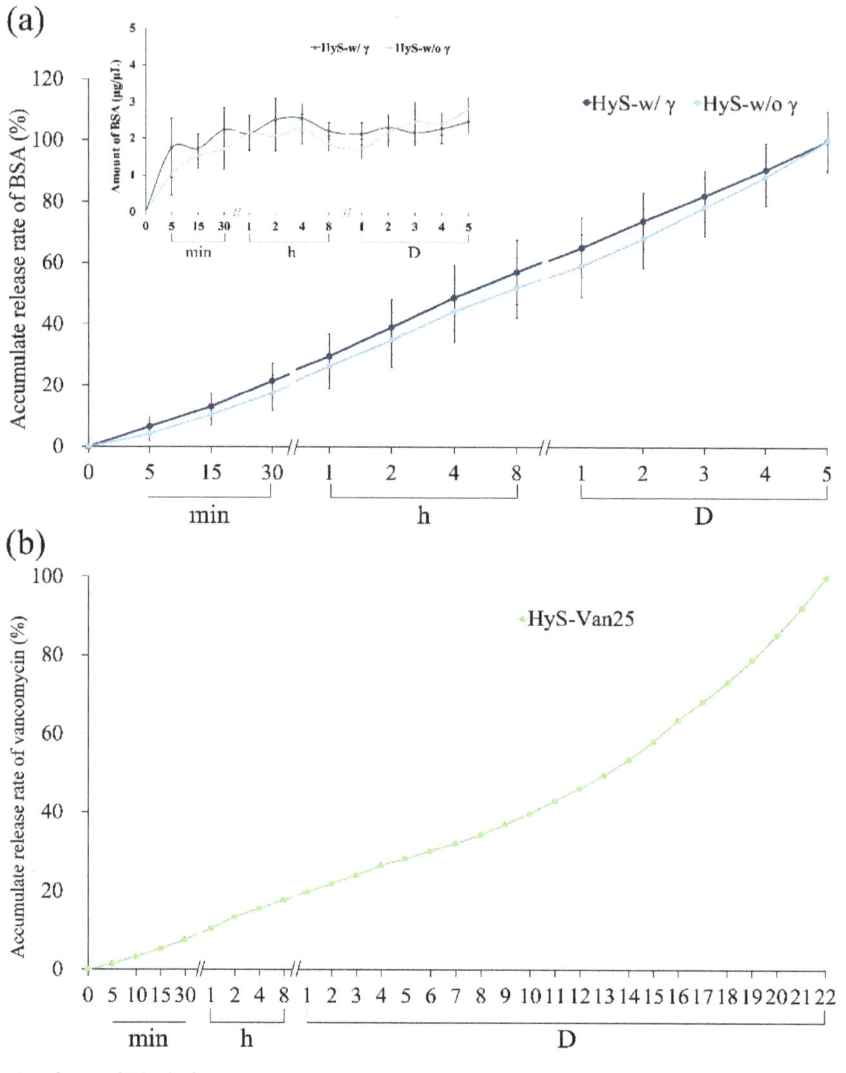

Figure 6. Protein release of BSA before (HyS-w/o γ) and after (HyS-w/γ) sterilization of hydrogel macrospheres in vitro (n = 10) (**a**) and cumulative antibiotic release of hydrogel macrospheres impregnated with vancomycin after sterilization (HyS-Van25, n = 10) (**b**).

3.3. Antibacterial and Biocompatible Abilities of HyS-Van25 after Irradiation

Figure 7a illustrates that after hydrogel sterility testing, compared with the contaminated PC group, the HyS-w/γ culture plate and the NC group were both completely sterile, which validated the hydrogel macrosphere sterilization procedures. The results of the qualitative and quantitative antibacterial testing of HyS-Van25 on *E. coli* and *S. aureus* are presented in Figure 7b,c, respectively. The qualitative results reveal evident antibacterial properties against both *E. coli* and *S. aureus*. According to the manufacturer's instructions, vancomycin has excellent antibacterial ability against gram-positive bacteria, which results in better responses of HyS-Van25 against gram-positive *E. coli* than against gram-negative *S. aureus* (Figure 7c). The quantitative results of the antibacterial effects of HyS-Van25 against *E. coli* and *S. aureus* indicate that HyS-Van25 samples cultured with *S. aureus* for 4 h exhibit superior antibacterial efficiency to the same samples cultured with *E. coli* for 8 h. After 24 h of bacterial culture, the OD of HyS-Van25 was higher than that of the control group, which may have occurred because hydrogel degradation (Figure 4c) caused the solution to become turbid. Therefore, the instrument obtained a false reading. The results of the quantitative and qualitative cytotoxicity evaluations of HyS-Van25 extract cultured with the L929 cell line after 24 h are presented in Figure 8. The results revealed that even after 25-kGy γ-ray sterilization (HyS-Van25), hydrogel macrospheres were not cytotoxic (Figure 8a) and did not noticeably affect the phenotype and growth of cells (Figure 8b).

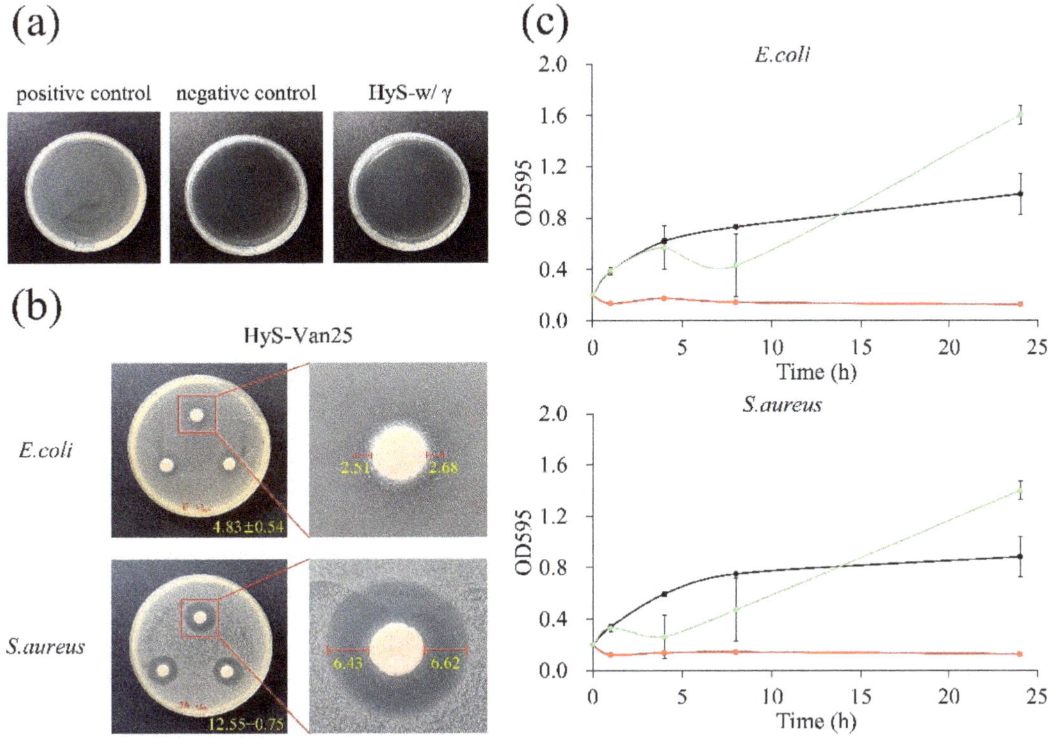

Figure 7. (**a**) Qualitative analysis of the sterility assurance of hydrogel macrospheres after sterilization (HyS-w/γ). (**b**) Qualitative results of the disk diffusion antibacterial effect of hydrogel macrospheres impregnated with vancomycin (HyS-Van25, $n = 3$) against *E. coli* and *S. aureus* after 24 h of interaction. Right figures indicate the inhibitory zones formed by the presence of macrospheres with a diameter of 6 mm. (**c**) Quantitative antibacterial results of hydrogel macrospheres impregnated with vancomycin after irradiation (HyS-Van25, $n = 3$) against *E. coli* and *S. aureus* after 24 h of interaction under broth dilution.

As for the ATR spectrum, when the samples are not sterilized by γ-ray and sterilized by 25-kGy irradiation, there is not much difference in the spectra (Appendix A, Figure A1). It only changes at 1610 cm^{-1}, which significantly affects the water absorption ratio of hydrogel macrospheres (Figure 4b). However, after 30- and 50-kGy irradiation sterilization, a certain functional group displayed an absorption band near 1259 cm^{-1}, which may affect its physical and chemical properties. Even on irradiation sterilization, each hydrogel system with and without protein or antibiotic releasing ability requires case-by-case testing to select the most suitable doses and an effective method to allow for the main properties to remain unaltered. The impact of irradiation sterilization on the physicochemical properties of the alginate/gelatin with a *w*/*w* ratio of 1/4 crosslinking gel macrospheres was understudied, and therefore further research of varying hydrogel system is needed.

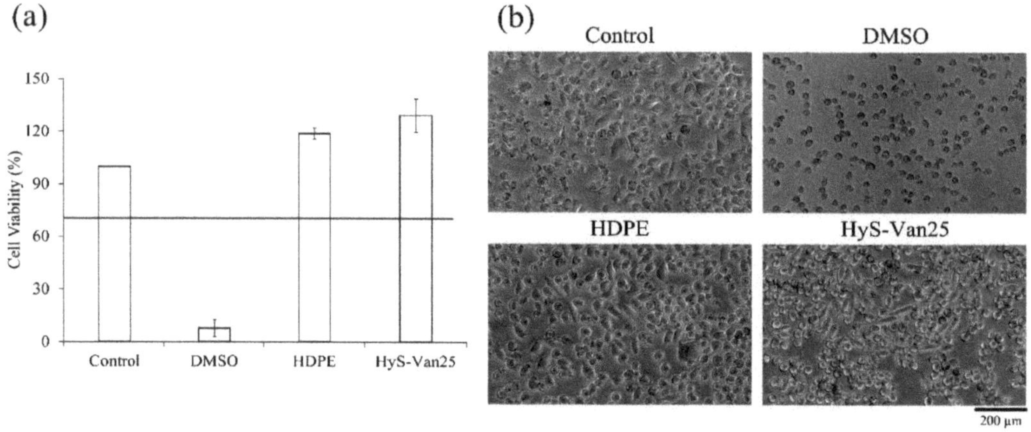

Figure 8. (**a**) Quantitative cell viability (n = 6) and (**b**) qualitative cell morphologies of L929 cells cultured for 24 h in a solution of hydrogel macrospheres impregnated with vancomycin after sterilization (HyS-Van25).

4. Conclusions

The produced hydrogel macrospheres possessed an interconnected pore structure, and after γ-ray sterilization, the degree of crosslinking of the hydrogel macrospheres marginally reduced due to the partially decrosslinked amide in the hydrogels. This amide caused the water absorption of HyS-w/γ to decrease marginally and led to an initial degradation rate higher than that of HyS-w/o γ. However, both macrosphere groups completely degraded after 13 days of immersion. After sterilization, the hydrogel macrospheres' ability to release BSA and vancomycin did not significantly change, which indicated that no chemical reaction occurred after 25-kGy γ-irradiation. Moreover, after loading vancomycin, the antibiotic was successfully released without cytotoxicity. The qualitative results indicated that favorable antibacterial ability remained for *E. coli* and *S. aureus*; however, the quantitative antibacterial effect on *S. aureus* was significant only when the culturing time was less than 8 h. The sterilization of the hydrogel macrospheres did not have any obvious influence on the structure of the macrospheres. However, sterilization exhibited several minor effects. According to the FTIR analysis results, a new active imine group was generated due to the breakage of the original intermolecular covalent amide bond. The experimental results indicated that macrospheres are an excellent drug or protein carrier and that the common 25-kGy dose of γ-ray irradiation used to sterilize medical devices can be used to validate hydrogel macrospheres and extended applications that can be combined with bone grafts in the future.

Author Contributions: Conceptualization and Methodology, P.-S.F., J.-C.W., W.-C.C. and C.-C.H.; Formal Analysis and Investigation, P.-S.F., P.-L.L., S.-M.L. and Y.-S.C.; Resources, P.-S.F., J.-C.W., W.-C.C. and C.-C.H.; Data Curation, P.-S.F., P.-L.L., S.-M.L. and Y.-S.C.; Writing—Original Draft Preparation, P.-S.F., S.-M.L., Y.-S.C. and W.-C.C.; Writing—Review & Editing, P.-S.F., J.-C.W., W.-C.C. and C.-C.H.; Visualization, Validation & Supervision, W.-C.C. and C.-C.H.; Project Administration and Funding Acquisition, P.-S.F. and W.-C.C. All authors have read and agreed to the published version of the manuscript.

Funding: This research was major supported by the Southern Taiwan Science Park Bureau, Ministry of Science and Technology, Taiwan, R.O.C. under contract 107CB02, and multi-supported by Kaohsiung Municipal Ta-Tung Hospital plan [grant number kmtth-109-040] and by the Ministry of Science and Technology, Taiwan [grant number MOST 108-2745-8-035-003 -; 109-2622-E-035-014-CC2].

Institutional Review Board Statement: Not applicable.

Informed Consent Statement: Not applicable.

Data Availability Statement: Not applicable.

Acknowledgments: The authors express their thanks to the staff at Realbone Technology Co., LTD, Kaohsiung 82151, Taiwan for generously providing the raw materials and supporting the GMP processes in this research project.

Conflicts of Interest: The authors declare no conflict of interest.

Appendix A

For comparison, the γ-ray dose effect on hydrogels and preliminarily determined influence of the recommended 25-kGy γ-irradiation dose in this study, the results using varying doses of 25, 30, and 50-kGy γ-irradiation doses in a one-step gamma-ray sterilization process through ATR spectra are shown in Figure A1. An absorption spectra in the frequency range of the amide I band for α-helix (~1655 cm^{-1}), β-sheet (~1630 cm^{-1}), and random coil (~1645 cm^{-1}) structures were changed into a new functional imine group (HC=N) band (1610~1621 cm^{-1}) in all radiation dose groups. Besides, the new peaks from the nitrite group of amide III were observed at 1259 cm^{-1} due to the decomposition and transformation into a new imine or nitrile group of hydrogel after 30 and 50- kGy γ-irradiation doses.

For comparison, the L929 cell survival rate of the control group with a pure medium was set as 100%. The cell viability results in Figure A2a indicate that according to the ISO 10993-5 standard, the cell survival rate of the PC group with 15% DMSO was lower than 10%, which suggests that the L929 cells were toxic. The cell survival rate of HyS-w/γ was 83%, which indicates that the hydrogel macrospheres were not cytotoxic after sterilization according to EN ISO 10993-5 Clause 4.1. The qualitative results of the L929 cells displayed in Figure A2b indicate that the control group and HDPE group had normal cell-type morphologies; thus, the sterilization process was validated. In the PC group, the cells were spherical, which indicated a state of apoptosis in the L929 cells. The cell morphology of the HyS-w/γ group was similar to that of the control group without apoptosis, which indicates that the sample did not cause cell apoptosis or death.

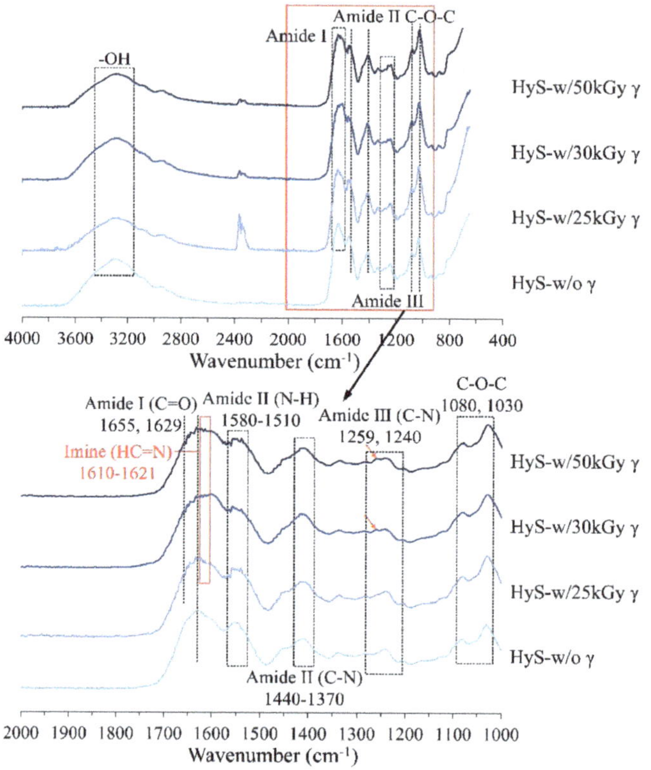

Figure A1. Full and specific absorption bands were obtained through the ATR spectrum analysis of macrospheres before (HyS-w/o γ) and different γ-radiation kGy after (HyS-w/γ) sterilization.

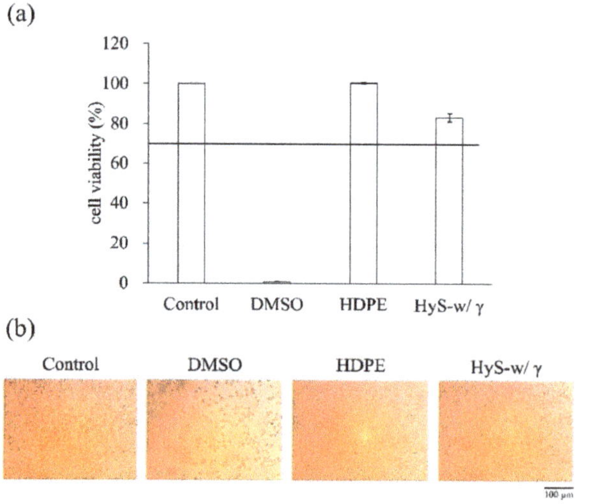

Figure A2. (**a**) Quantitative and (**b**) qualitative ($n = 6$) cytotoxicity test results of hydrogel macrosphere extract cultured with L929 cells for 24 h.

References

1. Hamidi, M.; Azadi, A.; Rafiei, P. Hydrogel nanoparticles in drug delivery. *Adv. Drug Deliv. Rev.* **2008**, *60*, 1638–1649. [CrossRef] [PubMed]
2. Vashist, A.; Ahmad, S. Hydrogels: Smart Materials for Drug Delivery. *Orient. J. Chem.* **2013**, *29*, 861–870. [CrossRef]
3. Peppas, N.A. *Biomedical Applications of Hydrogels Handbook*; Springer Science & Business Media: Berlin, Germany, 2010.
4. Tillet, G.; Boutevin, B.; Ameduri, B. Chemical reactions of polymer crosslinking and post-crosslinking at room and medium temperature. *Prog. Polym. Sci.* **2011**, *36*, 191–217. [CrossRef]
5. Laftah, W.A.; Hashim, S.; Ibrahim, A.N. Polymer Hydrogels: A Review. *Polym. Technol. Eng.* **2011**, *50*, 1475–1486. [CrossRef]
6. Raghavendra, G.M.; Varaprasad, K.; Jayaramudu, T. *Biomaterials: Design, Development and Biomedical Applications, Nanotechnology Applications for Tissue Engineering*; Elsevier: Amsterdam, The Netherlands, 2015; pp. 21–44.
7. Varaprasad, K.; Vimala, K.; Raghavendra, G.M.; Jayaramudu, T.; Sadiku, E.; Ramam, K. *Cell Encapsulation in Polymeric Self-Assembled Hydrogels, Nanotechnology Applications for Tissue Engineering*; Elsevier: Amsterdam, The Netherlands, 2015; pp. 149–171.
8. Liang, K.; Bae, K.H.; Kurisawa, M. Recent advances in the design of injectable hydrogels for stem cell-based therapy. *J. Mater. Chem. B* **2019**, *7*, 3775–3791. [CrossRef]
9. Hu, W.; Wang, Z.; Xiao, Y.; Zhang, S.; Wang, J. Advances in crosslinking strategies of biomedical hydrogels. *Biomater. Sci.* **2019**, *7*, 843–855. [CrossRef] [PubMed]
10. Hassan, C.M.; Peppas, N.A. *Structure and Applications of Poly (Vinyl Alcohol) Hydrogels Produced by Conventional Crosslinking or by Freezing/Thawing Methods, Biopolymers·PVA Hydrogels, Anionic Polymerisation Nanocomposites*; Springer: Berlin/Heidelberg, Germany, 2000; pp. 37–65.
11. Lozinsky, V.; Plieva, F. Poly (vinyl alcohol) cryogels employed as matrices for cell immobilization. 3. Overview of recent research and developments. *Enzym. Microb. Technol.* **1998**, *23*, 227–242. [CrossRef]
12. Tsuji, H.; Horii, F.; Nakagawa, M.; Ikada, Y.; Odani, H.; Kitamaru, R. Stereocomplex formation between enantiomeric poly(lactic acid)s. 7. Phase structure of the stereocomplex crystallized from a dilute acetonitrile solution as studied by high-resolution solid-state carbon-13 NMR spectroscopy. *Macromolecules* **1992**, *25*, 4114–4118. [CrossRef]
13. Tsuji, H. Poly(lactide) Stereocomplexes: Formation, Structure, Properties, Degradation, and Applications. *Macromol. Biosci.* **2005**, *5*, 569–597. [CrossRef]
14. Rastin, H.; Zhang, B.; Bi, J.; Hassan, K.; Tung, T.T.; Losic, D. 3D printing of cell-laden electroconductive bioinks for tissue engineering applications. *J. Mater. Chem. B* **2020**, *8*, 5862–5876. [CrossRef]
15. Zhao, Q.S.; Ji, Q.X.; Xing, K.; Li, X.Y.; Liu, C.S.; Chen, X.G. Preparation and characteristics of novel porous hydrogel films based on chitosan and glycerophosphate. *Carbohydr. Polym.* **2009**, *76*, 410–416. [CrossRef]
16. Ebara, M.; Kotsuchibashi, Y.; Narain, R.; Idota, N.; Kim, Y.-J.; Hoffman, J.M.; Uto, K.; Aoyagi, T. *Smart Hydrogels, Smart Biomaterials*; Springer: Berlin/Heidelberg, Germany, 2014; pp. 9–65.
17. Rastin, H.; Zhang, B.; Mazinani, A.; Hassan, K.; Bi, J.; Tung, T.T.; Losic, D. 3D bioprinting of cell-laden electroconductive MXene nanocomposite bioinks. *Nanoscale* **2020**, *12*, 16069–16080. [CrossRef] [PubMed]
18. Takigami, M.; Amada, H.; Nagasawa, N.; Yagi, T.; Kasahara, T.; Takigami, S.; Tamada, M. Preparation and Properties of CMC Gel. *Trans. Mater. Res. Soc. Jpn.* **2007**, *32*, 713–716. [CrossRef]
19. Hennink, W.; Van Nostrum, C. Novel crosslinking methods to design hydrogels. *Adv. Drug Deliv. Rev.* **2012**, *64*, 223–236. [CrossRef]
20. Athawale, V.; Lele, V. Graft copolymerization onto starch. II. Grafting of acrylic acid and preparation of it's hydrogels. *Carbohydr. Polym.* **1998**, *35*, 21–27. [CrossRef]
21. Said, H.M.; Alla, S.G.A.; El-Naggar, A.W.M. Synthesis and characterization of novel gels based on carboxymethyl cellulose/acrylic acid prepared by electron beam irradiation. *React. Funct. Polym.* **2004**, *61*, 397–404. [CrossRef]
22. Schulze, J.; Hendrikx, S.; Schulz-Siegmund, M.; Aigner, A. Microparticulate poly(vinyl alcohol) hydrogel formulations for embedding and controlled release of polyethylenimine (PEI)-based nanoparticles. *Acta Biomater.* **2016**, *45*, 210–222. [CrossRef]
23. Liu, Y.; Vrana, N.E.; Cahill, P.A.; McGuinness, G.B. Physically crosslinked composite hydrogels of PVA with natural macromolecules: Structure, mechanical properties, and endothelial cell compatibility. *J. Biomed. Mater. Res. Part B Appl. Biomater.* **2009**, *90*, 492–502. [CrossRef]
24. Hennink, W.; de Jong, S.; Bos, G.; Veldhuis, T.; van Nostrum, C. Biodegradable dextran hydrogels crosslinked by stereocomplex formation for the controlled release of pharmaceutical proteins. *Int. J. Pharm.* **2004**, *277*, 99–104. [CrossRef]
25. Varaprasad, K.; Mohan, Y.M.; Ravindra, S.; Reddy, N.N.; Vimala, K.; Monika, K.; Sreedhar, B.; Raju, K.M. Hydrogel–silver nanoparticle composites: A new generation of antimicrobials. *J. Appl. Polym. Sci.* **2010**, *115*, 1199–1207. [CrossRef]
26. Jayaramudu, T.; Raghavendra, G.M.; Varaprasad, K.; Raju, K.M.; Sadiku, E.R.; Kim, J. 5-Fluorouracil encapsulated magnetic nanohydrogels for drug-delivery applications. *J. Appl. Polym. Sci.* **2016**, *133*. [CrossRef]
27. Sperinde, J.J.; Griffith, L.G. Synthesis and Characterization of Enzymatically-Cross-Linked Poly(ethylene glycol) Hydrogels. *Macromolecules* **1997**, *30*, 5255–5264. [CrossRef]
28. Zhao, L.; Mitomo, H.; Zhai, M.; Yoshii, F.; Nagasawa, N.; Kume, T. Synthesis of antibacterial PVA/CM-chitosan blend hydrogels with electron beam irradiation. *Carbohydr. Polym.* **2003**, *53*, 439–446. [CrossRef]
29. Khademhosseini, A.; Langer, R. Microengineered hydrogels for tissue engineering. *Biomaterials* **2007**, *28*, 5087–5092. [CrossRef] [PubMed]
30. Rad, E.R.; Vahabi, H.; Formela, K.; Saeb, M.R.; Thomas, S. Injectable poloxamer/graphene oxide hydrogels with well-controlled mechanical and rheological properties. *Polym. Adv. Technol.* **2019**, *30*, 2250–2260.

31. Rastin, H.; Ormsby, R.T.; Atkins, G.J.; Losic, D. 3D Bioprinting of Methylcellulose/Gelatin-Methacryloyl (MC/GelMA) Bioink with High Shape Integrity. *ACS Appl. Bio Mater.* **2020**, *3*, 1815–1826. [CrossRef]
32. Dong, R.; Pang, Y.; Su, Y.; Zhu, X. Supramolecular hydrogels: Synthesis, properties and their biomedical applications. *Biomater. Sci.* **2015**, *3*, 937–954. [CrossRef]
33. Fisher, O.Z.; Khademhosseini, A.; Langer, R.; Peppas, N.A. Bioinspired Materials for Controlling Stem Cell Fate. *Accounts Chem. Res.* **2009**, *43*, 419–428. [CrossRef] [PubMed]
34. Lowman, A.; Peppas, N. *Encyclopedia of Controlled Drug Delivery*; John Wiley & Sons: New York, NY, USA, 1999; p. 397.
35. Varaprasad, K.; Vimala, K.; Ravindra, S.; Reddy, N.N.; Raju, K.M. Development of sodium carboxymethyl cellulose-based poly (acrylamide-co-2acrylamido-2-methyl-1-propane sulfonic acid) hydrogels for in vitro drug release studies of ranitidine hydrochloride an anti-ulcer drug. *Polym. Plast. Technol. Eng.* **2011**, *50*, 1199–1207. [CrossRef]
36. Yuan, N.; Xu, L.; Zhang, L.; Ye, H.; Zhao, J.; Liu, Z.; Rong, J. Superior hybrid hydrogels of polyacrylamide enhanced by bacterial cellulose nanofiber clusters. *Mater. Sci. Eng. C* **2016**, *67*, 221–230. [CrossRef]
37. Liow, S.S.; Dou, Q.; Kai, D.; Karim, A.A.; Zhang, K.; Xu, F.; Loh, X.J. Thermogels: In Situ Gelling Biomaterial. *ACS Biomater. Sci. Eng.* **2016**, *2*, 295–316. [CrossRef]
38. Loh, X.J.; Goh, S.H.; Li, J. New Biodegradable Thermogelling Copolymers Having Very Low Gelation Concentrations. *Biomacromolecules* **2007**, *8*, 585–593. [CrossRef] [PubMed]
39. Dou, Q.Q.; Liow, S.S.; Ye, E.; Lakshminarayanan, R.; Loh, X.J. Biodegradable Thermogelling Polymers: Working Towards Clinical Applications. *Adv. Heal. Mater.* **2014**, *3*, 977–988. [CrossRef] [PubMed]
40. Loh, X.J.; Goh, S.H.; Li, J. Hydrolytic degradation and protein release studies of thermogelling polyurethane copolymers consisting of poly [(R)-3-hydroxybutyrate], poly (ethylene glycol), and poly (propylene glycol). *Biomaterials* **2007**, *28*, 4113–4123. [CrossRef] [PubMed]
41. Xu, G.; Wang, X.; Deng, C.; Teng, X.; Suuronen, E.J.; Shen, Z.; Zhong, Z. Injectable biodegradable hybrid hydrogels based on thiolated collagen and oligo(acryloyl carbonate)–poly(ethylene glycol)–oligo(acryloyl carbonate) copolymer for functional cardiac regeneration. *Acta Biomater.* **2015**, *15*, 55–64. [CrossRef] [PubMed]
42. Jaikumar, D.; Sajesh, K.; Soumya, S.; Nimal, T.; Chennazhi, K.; Nair, S.V.; Jayakumar, R. Injectable alginate-O-carboxymethyl chitosan/nano fibrin composite hydrogels for adipose tissue engineering. *Int. J. Biol. Macromol.* **2015**, *74*, 318–326. [CrossRef]
43. Kowalski, J.; Tallentire, A. Substantiation of 25 kGy as a sterilization dose: A rational approach to establishing verification dose. *Radiat. Phys. Chem.* **1999**, *54*, 55–64. [CrossRef]
44. Kowalski, J.B.; Aoshuang, Y.; Tallentire, A. Radiation sterilization—Evaluation of a new approach for substantiation of 25 kGy. *Radiat. Phys. Chem.* **2000**, *58*, 77–86. [CrossRef]
45. Kowalski, J.B.; Herring, C.; Baryschpolec, L.; Reger, J.; Patel, J.; Feeney, M.; Tallentire, A. Field evaluations of the VDmax approach for substantiation of a 25kGy sterilization dose and its application to other preselected doses. *Radiat. Phys. Chem.* **2002**, *64*, 411–416. [CrossRef]
46. World Health Organization. *The International Pharmacopoeia*; World Health Organization: Geneva, Switzerland, 1979.
47. Galante, R.; Pinto, T.J.; Colaço, R.; Serro, A.P. Sterilization of hydrogels for biomedical applications: A review. *J. Biomed. Mater. Res. Part B Appl. Biomater.* **2018**, *106*, 2472–2492. [CrossRef]
48. Ko, C.-L.; Tien, Y.-C.; Wang, J.-C.; Chen, W.-C. Characterization of controlled highly porous hyaluronan/gelatin cross-linking sponges for tissue engineering. *J. Mech. Behav. Biomed. Mater.* **2012**, *14*, 227–238. [CrossRef]
49. Ko, C.-L.; Wu, H.-Y.; Lin, Y.-S.; Yang, C.-H.; Chen, J.-C.; Chen, W.-C. Modulating the release of proteins from a loaded carrier of alginate/gelatin porous spheres immersed in different solutions. *Biomed Mater. Eng.* **2017**, *28*, 515–529. [CrossRef] [PubMed]
50. Tallawi, M.; Germann, N. Self-crosslinked hydrogel with delivery carrier obtained by incorporation of oxidized alginate microspheres into gelatin matrix. *Mater. Lett.* **2020**, *263*, 127211. [CrossRef]
51. Rajalekshmi, R.; Shaji, A.K.; Joseph, R.; Bhatt, A. Scaffold for liver tissue engineering: Exploring the potential of fibrin incorporated alginate dialdehyde–gelatin hydrogel. *Int. J. Biol. Macromol.* **2021**, *166*, 999–1008. [CrossRef] [PubMed]
52. Chawla, D.; Kaur, T.; Joshi, A.; Singh, N. 3D bioprinted alginate-gelatin based scaffolds for soft tissue engineering. *Int. J. Biol. Macromol.* **2020**, *144*, 560–567. [CrossRef]
53. Araki, K.; Yagi, N.; Ikemoto, Y.; Yagi, H.; Choong, C.-J.; Hayakawa, H.; Beck, G.; Sumi, H.; Fujimura, H.; Moriwaki, T.; et al. Synchrotron FTIR micro-spectroscopy for structural analysis of Lewy bodies in the brain of Parkinson's disease patients. *Sci. Rep.* **2015**, *5*, 17625. [CrossRef] [PubMed]
54. Perkasa, D.P.; Erizal, E.; Darmawan, D.; Rasyid, A. Effect of Gamma Irradiation on Mechanical and Thermal Properties of Fish Gelatin Film Isolated from Lates Calcarifer Scales. *Indones. J. Chem.* **2013**, *13*, 28–35. [CrossRef]
55. Johnson, P.S.; Cook, P.L.; Liu, X.; Yang, W.; Bai, Y.; Abbott, N.L.; Himpsel, F.J. Universal mechanism for breaking amide bonds by ionizing radiation. *J. Chem. Phys.* **2011**, *135*, 044702. [CrossRef]

MDPI
St. Alban-Anlage 66
4052 Basel
Switzerland
Tel. +41 61 683 77 34
Fax +41 61 302 89 18
www.mdpi.com

Polymers Editorial Office
E-mail: polymers@mdpi.com
www.mdpi.com/journal/polymers

www.ingramcontent.com/pod-product-compliance
Lightning Source LLC
LaVergne TN
LVHW070444100526
838202LV00014B/1663
* 9 7 8 3 0 3 6 5 3 3 3 6 0 *